W.B. SAUNDERS COMPANY

A Division of Elsevier Inc.

Elsevier Inc. • 1600 John F. Kennedy Boulevard • Suite 1800 • Philadelphia, Pennsylvania 19103-2899

http://www.chestmed.theclinics.com

CLINICS IN CHEST MEDICINE   Volume 28, Number 3
September 2007   ISSN 0272-5231
Editor: Sarah E. Barth   ISBN-13: 978-1-4160-5046-9
     ISBN-10: 1-4160-5046-9

Clinics in Chest Medicine (ISSN 0272-5231) is published quarterly by Elsevier Inc., 360 Park Avenue South, New York, NY 10010-1710. Months of issue are March, June, September, and December. Business and Editorial Offices: 1600 John F. Kennedy Blvd., Suite 1800, Philadelphia, PA 19103-2899. Customer Service Office: 6277 Sea Harbor Drive, Orlando, FL 32887-4800. Periodicals postage paid at New York, NY and additional mailing offices. Subscription prices are $211.00 per year (US individuals), $330.00 per year (US institutions), $103.00 per year (US students), $232.00 per year (Canadian individuals), $396.00 per year (Canadian institutions), $135.00 per year (Canadian students), $270.00 per year (international individuals) $396.00 per year (international institutions), and $135.00 per year (international students). International air speed delivery is included in all *Clinics* subscription prices. All prices are subject to change without notice. **POSTMASTER:** Send address changes to *Clinics in Chest Medicine*, Elsevier Periodicals Customer Service, 6277 Sea Harbor Drive, Orlando, FL 32887-4800. Customer Service: 1-800-654-2452 (US). From outside of the US, call 1-407-345-4000.

Clinics in Chest Medicine is covered in *Index Medicus, Current Contents/Clinical Medicine, EMBASE/Excerpta Medica, Science Citation Index,* and *ISI/BIOMED.*

Printed in the United States of America.

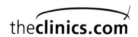

CLINICS IN CHEST MEDICINE

Chronic Obstructive Pulmonary
Disease

GUEST EDITOR
Carolyn L. Rochester, MD

September 2007 • Volume 28 • Number 3

SAUNDERS

An Imprint of Elsevier, Inc.
PHILADELPHIA   LONDON   TORONTO   MONTREAL   SYDNEY   TOKYO

GUEST EDITOR

CAROLYN L. ROCHESTER, MD, Medical Director of Pulmonary Rehabilitation; and Director of Pulmonary Clinics, VA Connecticut Healthcare System (Newington Campus), New Haven; Associate Professor of Medicine, Section of Pulmonary & Critical Care, Yale University School of Medicine, West Haven, Connecticut

CONTRIBUTORS

NICOLINO AMBROSINO, MD, Head, Pulmonary Unit, Cardio-Thoracic Department, University Hospital, Pisa, Italy

ANTONIO ANZUETO, MD, Professor, Department of Medicine, University of Texas Health Science Center; Chief, Pulmonary Diseases Section, South Texas Veterans Health Care System, Audie L. Murphy Memorial Veterans Hospital, San Antonio, Texas

SELIM M. ARCASOY, MD, FCCP, FACP, Associate Professor of Clinical Medicine, Division of Pulmonary, Allergy, and Critical Care Medicine, Columbia University College of Physicians and Surgeons, Lung Transplantation Program; New York Presbyterian Hospital of Columbia and Cornell University, New York, New York

JEAN BOURBEAU, MD, Associate Professor of Medicine, Division of Pulmonary Medicine, McGill University; and Director, COPD Clinic and Pulmonary Rehabilitation, Montréal Chest Institute, McGill University Health Center, Montréal, Québec, Canada

BARTOLOME R. CELLI, MD, Professor of Medicine, Tufts University Medical School; Division of Pulmonary and Critical Care Medicine, Caritas Saint Elizabeth's Medical Center, Boston, Massachusetts

CLAUDIA G. COTE, MD, Associate Professor of Medicine, University of South Florida, Tampa; Medical Director, Pulmonary Rehabilitation Program, Bay Pines Veterans Administration Health Care System, Bay Pines, Florida

KRISTINA CROTHERS, MD, Section of Pulmonary and Critical Care Medicine, Department of Internal Medicine, Yale University School of Medicine, New Haven, Connecticut

HARRY R. GOSKER, PhD, Department of Respiratory Medicine, Nutrition and Toxicology Research Institute, University of Maastricht, The Netherlands

NICOLA A. HANANIA, MD, MS, Associate Professor of Medicine; and Director, Asthma Clinical Research Center, Section of Pulmonary and Critical Care Medicine, Baylor College of Medicine, Houston, Texas

JOHN R. HURST, PhD, Clinical Senior Lecturer, Academic Unit of Respiratory Medicine, Royal Free and University College Medical School, Royal Free Hospital, London, United Kingdom

RAMON C. LANGEN, PhD, Department of Respiratory Medicine, Nutrition and Toxicology Research Institute, University of Maastricht, The Netherlands

DAVID J. LEDERER, MD, MS, Assistant Professor of Medicine, Division of Pulmonary, Allergy, and Critical Care Medicine, Columbia University College of Physicians and Surgeons, Lung Transplantation Program; New York Presbyterian Hospital of Columbia and Cornell University, New York, New York

WILLIAM MACNEE, MBChB, MD, FRCP, Professor of Respiratory and Environmental Medicine, ELEGI Colt Research Laboratories, MRC Centre for Inflammation Research, Queen's Medical Research Institute, University of Edinburgh, Edinburgh, Scotland, United Kingdom

DIANE NAULT, RN, MSc, Clinical Nurse Specialist, Service Régional de Soins Respiratoires à Domicile, Hôpital Maisonneuve-Rosemont, Centre Affilié à l'Université de Montréal, Montréal, Québec, Canada

LINDA NICI, MD, Clinical Associate Professor of Medicine, Brown University School of Medicine; Associate Chief, Pulmonary and Critical Care Section, Providence Veterans Administration Medical Center, Providence, Rhode Island

GERARDO PALMIERO, MD, Assistant, Pulmonary Unit, Cardio-Thoracic Department, University Hospital, Pisa, Italy

JANE Z. REARDON, MSN, RN, Acute Care Nurse Practitioner, Departments of Medicine and Nursing, Hartford Hospital, Hartford, Connecticut

ALEXANDER H. REMELS, MSc, Department of Respiratory Medicine, Nutrition and Toxicology Research Institute, University of Maastricht, The Netherlands

ANNEMIE M. SCHOLS, PhD, Professor, Department of Respiratory Medicine, Nutrition and Toxicology Research Institute, University of Maastricht, The Netherlands

AMIR SHARAFKHANEH, MD, Assistant Professor of Medicine, Section of Pulmonary and Critical Care Medicine, Baylor College of Medicine, Houston, Texas

ANDREW C. STONE, MD, MPH, Providence, Rhode Island

SOO-KYUNG STRAMBI, PT, Physiotherapist, Pulmonary Unit, Cardio-Thoracic Department, University Hospital, Pisa, Italy

JOS VAN DER VELDEN, BSc, Department of Respiratory Medicine, Nutrition and Toxicology Research Institute, University of Maastricht, The Netherlands

JADWIGA A. WEDZICHA, MD, Professor of Respiratory Medicine, Academic Unit of Respiratory Medicine, Royal Free and University College Medical School, Royal Free Hospital, London, United Kingdom

CONTRIBUTORS

CONTENTS

The pathogenesis of chronic obstructive pulmonary disease (COPD) encompasses a number of injurious processes, including an abnormal inflammatory response in the lungs to inhaled particles and gases. Other processes, such as failure to resolve inflammation, abnormal cell repair, apoptosis, abnormal cellular maintenance programs, extracellular matrix destruction (protease/antiprotease imbalance), and oxidative stress (oxidant/antioxidant imbalance) also have a role. The inflammatory responses to the inhalation of active and passive tobacco smoke and urban and rural air pollution are modified by genetic and epigenetic factors. The subsequent chronic inflammatory responses lead to mucus hypersecretion, airway remodeling, and alveolar destruction. This article provides an update on the cellular and molecular mechanisms of these processes in the pathogenesis of COPD.

Chronic obstructive pulmonary disease (COPD) has become a major and growing health problem, with a mortality rate that continues to increase. Several factors, have been identified as individual predictors of mortality in COPD. This article reviews individual predictors for mortality. It also discusses the ability of an integrated, multidimensional tool to more broadly characterize COPD severity, assess response to therapeutic interventions and exacerbations, and predict mortality.

Much of the morbidity and mortality in chronic obstructive pulmonary disease relates to symptomatic deteriorations in respiratory health termed exacerbations. Exacerbations also are associated with changes in lung function and both airway and systemic inflammation. The most common causes of exacerbation are micro-organisms: respiratory viruses such as rhinovirus, and various bacterial species. This article reviews and discusses current understanding of the biology of exacerbations, considering the definition, epidemiology, etiology, and the nature and evolution of the changes in symptoms, lung function, and inflammation that characterize these important events.

tolerance, and health status; and decrease in exacerbations and mortality are the goals of management. Inhaled short-acting bronchodilators are recommended for symptoms in mild disease, whereas inhaled long-acting bronchodilators are recommended for maintenance therapy of daily symptoms. When symptoms are not controlled using one bronchodilator, combining bronchodilators may be more effective. Combining a long-acting β-agonist with an inhaled corticosteroid is more effective than either agent alone. Several novel therapies are in different stages of development.

FORTHCOMING ISSUES

RECENT ISSUES

THE CLINICS ARE NOW AVAILABLE ONLINE!

Access your subscription at:
http://www.theclinics.com

ELSEVIER
SAUNDERS

Clin Chest Med 28 (2007) ix–x

CLINICS
IN CHEST
MEDICINE

Preface

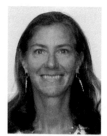

Carolyn L. Rochester, MD
Guest Editor

Chronic obstructive pulmonary disease (COPD) continues to cause disabling symptoms and impair the functional status and quality of life of millions of people worldwide. COPD is anticipated to become the third leading cause of death by the year 2020 [1]. Since the time of the last issue of *Clinics in Chest Medicine* on COPD published in December 2000, extraordinary efforts have been made by investigators and clinicians worldwide to gain an increased understanding of the pathogenesis and to refine the therapeutic management of this disabling disease. It has become recognized increasingly that heterogeneous clinical phenotypes of COPD exist, both with regard to varying degrees of emphysema and airways inflammation and remodeling in the lung, and with regard to the systemic manifestations and functional impact of the disease. It is also now well recognized that several factors in addition to lung function (including exercise tolerance and nutritional status among others) impact patient mortality risk. In recent years, investigations began to focus on unraveling differences in pathogenesis and genetic propensity to develop the varying COPD phenotypes. Increased emphasis has also been placed on assessing patient centered outcomes (such as exercise tolerance, symptoms,

and health status) and measuring changes in lung function in response to various therapeutic interventions. The ability of treatment interventions to impact the systemic manifestations of COPD and to alter mortality also has become a subject of great interest.

I hope that this issue of *Clinics in Chest Medicine* will provide the reader with current state-of-the-art knowledge of these many aspects of COPD. The introductory article by Dr. MacNee discusses the many facets of the pathogenesis of COPD. The discussion relates many cellular and molecular events to the structural and functional changes found in the lungs of COPD patients. The article by Drs. Cote and Celli reviews current knowledge regarding predictors of mortality and discusses multi-dimensional tools used to assess disease severity and predict outcomes in COPD patients. The article by Drs. Hurst and Wedzicha discusses COPD exacerbations, which are recognized increasingly to play an important role in the decline in lung function and development of disability over time. The article by Drs. Remels, Schols, and colleagues provides a state-of-the-art discussion of the mechanisms of skeletal muscle dysfunction and systemic inflammation in COPD, and the article by Drs. Stone and Nici highlights other systemic manifestations of the disease, including the impact of COPD on the cardiovascular system. Ms. Reardon's comprehensive article on the adverse health effects of environmental tobacco smoke and Dr. Crothers' article on COPD among HIV-infected patients are also unique and very important novel contributions to this issue of *Clinics in Chest Medicine*.

It is now appreciated that effective management of COPD requires a multidisciplinary, long-term, integrated approach to care. From the therapeutic standpoint, Drs. Hanania and Shar-afkhaneh provide a thorough update on pharmacologic treatment of COPD, and Dr. Anzueto discusses existing strategies to modify the disease. Increasingly, health care providers are recognizing that optimal comprehensive care of patients who have COPD also requires investment by and participation of the patient in his or her own care and effective partnership between patients and their health care providers. The article by Dr. Bourbeau and Ms. Nault provides a review of self-management strategies and effective means of patient—health care provider partnering in the management of COPD. The discussion by Drs. Ambrosino, Palmiero and Strambi considers existing and novel strategies to optimize the benefits of pulmonary rehabilitation. Finally, in the last several years, much knowledge has accrued regarding the benefits and risks of surgical therapies for COPD, and Drs. Lederer and Arcasoy review this topic in detail.

I thank each of the authors for their participation in this project, for their wonderful, scholarly contributions, and for their incredible hard work! I also extend my sincere gratitude to Sarah Barth and her colleagues at W.B. Saunders for their patience and efforts to bring this project to fruition. It has, indeed, been my great pleasure to have the opportunity to serve once again as a Guest Editor for *Clinics in Chest Medicine* and to work with such a superbly skilled and dedicated group of colleagues!

Carolyn L. Rochester, MD
Medical Director of Pulmonary Rehabilitation and
Director of Pulmonary Clinics
VA Connecticut Healthcare System
Newington Campus
333 Cedar Street, Building LCI-105
New Haven, CT 06520, USA

Associate Professor of Medicine
Section of Pulmonary & Critical Care
Yale University School of Medicine
West Haven, CT, USA

E-mail address: carolyn.rochester@yale.edu

Reference

[1] Global strategy for diagnosis, management and prevention of COPD. Available at: http://www.Goldcopd.com. Accessed June 2007.

ELSEVIER
SAUNDERS

Clin Chest Med 28 (2007) 479–513

CLINICS
IN CHEST
MEDICINE

Pathogenesis of Chronic Obstructive Pulmonary Disease

William MacNee, MBChB, MD, FRCP

ELEGI Colt Research Laboratories, MRC Centre for Inflammation Research,
Queen's Medical Research Institute, University of Edinburgh, 47 Little France Avenue,
Edinburgh EH16 4TJ, Scotland, UK

Chronic obstructive pulmonary disease (COPD) is a slowly progressive condition characterized by airflow limitation, which is largely irreversible [1]. Cigarette smoking is the main etiologic factor in this condition, far outweighing any other risk factors. The pathogenesis of COPD is therefore strongly linked to the effects of cigarette smoke on the lungs. The extent of smoking history and the severity of airflow limitation are generally related, but with huge individual variation. Fletcher and colleagues [2], in an 8-year prospective study of working men in west London, showed that the average decline in forced expiratory volume in 1 second (FEV_1) in smokers is faster (60 mL/year) than in nonsmokers (30 mL/year). Smokers who develop COPD have an average decline in FEV_1 of greater than 60 mL per year, but only a proportion of smokers develop clinically significant COPD.

It is from these studies that the concept of the susceptible smoker developed. It has been suggested that central to the pathogenesis of this condition is an abnormal inflammatory response in the lungs to the inhalation of toxic particles and gases, derived from tobacco smoke, air pollution, or occupational exposures. Tobacco smoking elicits an inflammatory response in the lungs of all smokers, but in those who develop COPD it is enhanced and fails to resolve after quitting smoking, which suggests that smokers who develop COPD have an abnormal regulation of the inflammatory response in the lungs.

The factors that lead to a susceptibility to COPD are still poorly understood and may

involve several factors, including genetic and epigenetic factors, infections, altered immune regulation, or impaired resolution of inflammation and abnormal repair mechanisms. However, the relationship between the inflammatory responses in the lung and the accelerated decline in FEV_1, which characterizes this condition, is far from clear. COPD is a heterogeneous disease in which the involvement of large and small airways (bronchitis/bronchiolitis) and lung parenchyma (emphysema) varies greatly among patients. The mechanisms resulting in these pathogenic changes are likely to be different also.

Pathologic changes in chronic obstructive pulmonary disease

Chronic bronchitis

Chronic bronchitis is defined as cough and sputum production for most days over 3 months for 2 consecutive years. This clinical definition does not include the presence of airflow limitation. It is thought to result from the innate immune response to inhaled toxic particles and gases, particularly in tobacco smoke. The epithelium of the central airways and the mucus-producing glands are inflamed in chronic bronchitis [3,4]. This airway inflammation is associated with increased mucus production, reduced mucociliary clearance, and increased permeability of the airspace epithelial barrier.

The contribution of mucus hypersecretion to the airflow limitation in COPD is still uncertain. In the early stages of COPD, its contribution is small because mucus production in smokers with normal lung function does not appear to predict later development of COPD [5]. However, in the later stages of the disease, chronic mucus

Research for this article was supported by National Institutes of Health # 1 ROI HL72282–01.

E-mail address: w.macnee@ed.ac.uk

hypersecretion may contribute to the acceleration of the loss of FEV_1 due to an increased risk of exacerbations [6]. Chronic mucus hypersecretion may result from the inflammatory response in the submucosal glands (Fig. 1) [4]. Inflammatory cells release serine proteases that are potent secretagogues for mucus [7]. Oxidants derived from cigarette smoke and released from inflammatory leukocytes may also be involved in overproduction of mucin by induction of the mucin MUC5AC gene [8].

Emphysema

Emphysema is defined as enlargement of the airspaces, distal to the terminal bronchioles, due to destruction of the alveolar walls (Fig. 2) [9]. Distal airspace enlargement with alveolar destruction reduces maximal expiratory airflow by decreasing the lung elastic recoil force that drives air out of the lungs. The centrilobular, or centriacinar, form of emphysema results from dilatation or destruction of the respiratory bronchioles and is the type of emphysema most closely associated with tobacco smoking. The panlobular, or panacinar, form of emphysema, which is usually associated with α_1-antitrypsin (α_1-AT) deficiency, results in more even dilatation and destruction of the entire acinus. It has been suggested that one or the other of these types predominates in severe disease and that the centriacinar type is more associated with severe small-airway obstruction [10]. The distribution of these types of emphysema is different, with an upper lobe predominance common in centrilobular emphysema and lower lobe predominance in panacinar emphysema. The reason is not clear, and whether different pathogenic mechanisms are involved in the different types of emphysema is also unknown.

The degree of emphysema and the pack-years of smoking are related, but this

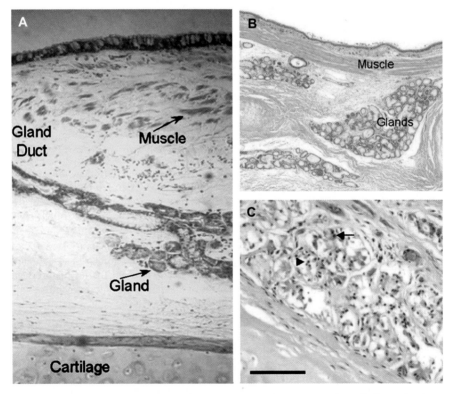

Fig. 1. Pathologic changes of the central airways in COPD. A central bronchus (*A*) from the lung of a cigarette smoker with normal pulmonary function. Only small amounts of bronchial smooth muscle are present and the epithelial glands are small. In contrast, a subject (*B*) with chronic bronchitis has bronchial smooth muscle that appears as a thick bundle and enlarged bronchial glands. (*C*) The enlarged bronchial glands at a higher magnification. Evidence also indicates a chronic inflammatory process involving polymorphonuclear leukocytes (*arrowhead*) and mononuclear cells, including plasma cells (*arrow*). (*Courtesy of* James C. Hogg, Vancouver, Canada.)

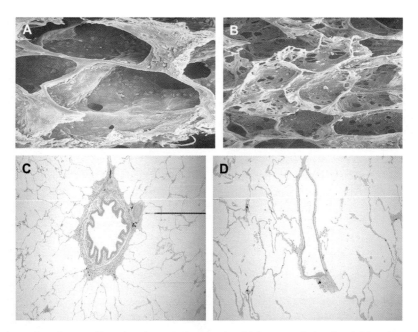

Fig. 2. Pathology of emphysema. Scanning electron micrographs of (*A*) a normal alveoli and (*B*) early emphysema with holes in alveolar walls. (*C*) Histologic section of a normal airway with surrounding alveolar attachments. (*D*) Enlargement of distal airspaces and reduced alveolar attachments in collapsed airway in emphysema.

relationship is not strong. Only around 40% of heavy smokers develop substantial lung destruction from emphysema, and emphysema can be found in some individuals who have normal lung function [3].

Small-airway disease

A major site of airway obstruction in COPD is the smaller conducting airways (<2 mm in diameter) [11]. Niewoehner and coworkers [12] were the first to demonstrate that inflammation involving clusters of monocytes and macrophages occurred in the bronchioles of asymptomatic smokers who died of nonsmoking-related causes out of hospital. Recent studies have confirmed that the small airways of smokers with and without COPD have structural abnormalities (Fig. 3) [13]. A relationship exists between the severity of COPD and the extent of occlusion of the airway lumen by inflammatory mucous exudates. Inflammation and peribronchial fibrosis contribute to the fixed airway obstruction in the small airways in COPD, and progression of the inflammation, resulting in the destruction of the alveolar attachments on the outer walls of the small airways, may also contribute.

Inflammation in the lungs of smokers without chronic obstructive pulmonary disease

Inflammation occurs in the peripheral airways of all smokers, even before COPD is established, and is made up of inflammatory cell infiltrate in the airway wall consisting of mononuclear cells and clusters of macrophages in the respiratory bronchioles. These lesions occur initially in the absence of any significant tissue destruction or fibrosis, and may be reversible. A similar inflammatory process with T lymphocytes and macrophages has been described in the large airways of smokers [14]. Evidence indicates that acute cigarette smoke exposure can result in tissue damage, with degradation of products of external matrix proteins and lipid peroxidation products [15]. In contrast to the inflammatory effects of chronic cigarette smoking, acute cigarette smoking in general has a suppressive effect on cells and inflammatory cytokines [15].

These early inflammatory changes in the airways are likely to represent a nonspecific innate immune response to airway injury from tobacco smoke. It is unclear why, in addition, some smokers develop structural abnormalities that eventually lead to clinically detectable COPD, whereas others continue to show an inflammatory

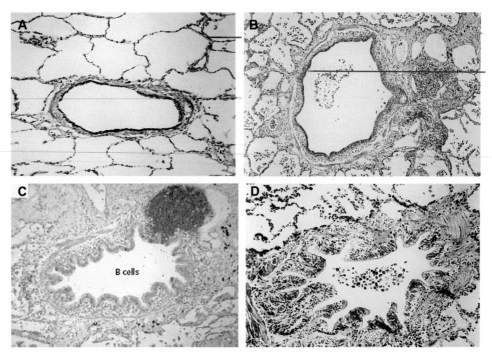

Fig. 3. Pathologic changes in the peripheral airways in COPD. Histologic sections of peripheral airways from cigarette smoker (*A*) with a nearly normal small airway. (*B*) Bronchiolitis with the presence of inflammatory exudates in the wall and lumen of the airway. (*C*) A small airway infiltrated with B cells and a lymphoid follicle (LF). (*D*) Small airway remodeling with reduced lumen, structural reorganization of the airway wall, increased smooth muscle, and deposition of peribronchial connective tissue. (*Courtesy of* James C. Hogg, Vancouver, Canada.)

infiltrate but maintain otherwise normal airways and lung parenchyma and only mild functional changes that do not become clinically relevant [16].

Smoking cessation alters the inflammatory response in the lungs of asymptomatic smokers and in patients who have COPD [17]. Cross-sectional studies are available on the effects of smoking cessation on lung inflammation in smokers and in ex-smokers without chronic symptoms [18,19]. Ex-smokers show less goblet cell hyperplasia, and less squamous metaplasia in the small, but not the large, airways. Smooth muscle mass in the peripheral and central airways, fibrotic tissue deposition in the airway wall, and the degree of alveolar destruction is not different in asymptomatic ex-smokers and current smokers, nor is the inflammatory response different [14,15]. Recent longitudinal studies of the effects of smoking cessation have shown that signs of inflammation in the airways suggesting chronic bronchitis (edema, erythema, and mucus) decreased by 3 months and disappeared after 6 months of smoking cessation. Inflammation, as assessed in sputum obtained

from bronchial biopsies, decreased 1 year after smoking cessation in asymptomatic smokers [20].

Longitudinal studies of the effects of cigarette smoking on pathology and inflammatory response in the lungs are limited.

Inflammation in the lungs of persons with chronic obstructive pulmonary disease

Studies of lung or bronchial biopsies and induced sputum have shown evidence of lung inflammation in all cigarette smokers [12,18,19]. However, it appears that an enhanced or abnormal inflammatory response to inhaling particles or gases, which goes beyond the normal protective inflammatory response in the lungs, is a characteristic feature of COPD and has the potential to produce lung injury [21]. The innate and adaptive inflammatory and immune responses are involved in the lung inflammation in smokers and in COPD patients. Recent studies have begun to characterize the inflammation in the lung in COPD in terms of its type, site, degree, and the relationship to severity of disease [13].

The cellular component of the inflammatory response in chronic obstructive pulmonary disease

Bronchial biopsies from smokers with symptoms of chronic bronchitis who have not developed airflow limitation demonstrate that the airway epithelium remains intact; however, there is squamous metaplasia of the epithelium and an increase in the numbers of goblet cells [4]. In contrast to asthma, the airway epithelial reticular basement membrane is not thickened [22]. Patients who have mild to moderate COPD have an increase in inflammatory cell infiltration in the central airways, compared with nonsmokers or smokers who have not developed the disease [23].

T Lymphocytes

In the bronchial epithelium [24] and submucosa [25] in COPD patients, monocytes are the major cells, with scanty neutrophils. Of the monocyte component, T lymphocytes (mainly CD8+, cytotoxic T lymphocytes) and macrophages (CD68+ cells) predominate (Table 1) [26–28], in contrast to asthma, where CD4+ T-helper (T helper 2) lymphocytes predominate. Thus, the CD8+/CD4+ ratio increases in COPD [29]. Morphometric analyses of bronchial biopsies show that the CD8+/CD4+ ratios of T cells were 1.3, 11.8, and 4.3 (mean/mm^3) in healthy smokers, in those with stable chronic bronchitis, and in those with exacerbated chronic bronchitis, respectively [30]. CD8+ T cells are also observed in the sputum [31,32], bronchial glands [33], bronchial smooth muscle [34,35], and around lymphoid follicles [13]. It has been suggested also that the presence of increased CD8+ T lymphocytes differentiates between smokers who do and do not develop COPD, and that T-cell numbers, smoking history, the amount of alveolar destruction, and the severity of the airflow limitation are correlated [25,29]. However, smokers with normal lung function also show, to a lesser extent, an increased number of airway CD8+ cells, compared with control nonsmokers [23]. Indeed, T lymphocyte infiltration is decreased in bronchial biopsy specimens from subjects with severe COPD [28].

The mechanisms by which CD8+ T lymphocytes accumulate in the airways in COPD are not fully understood. The T cells in the peripheral airways in COPD patients have an increased expression of CXCR3. CXCR3 is a receptor activated by interferon-inducible protein (IP)-10, and the expression of IP-10 itself is increased in bronchiolar epithelial cells. This increase could contribute to the accumulation of CD8+ cells, which preferentially express CXCR3. Circulating CD8+ cells are also increased in number in COPD patients who do not smoke [36], and CD4+ cells are increased in COPD patients, particularly as the disease progresses [37,38], which suggests chronic immune stimulation. CD8+ cells have a well-recognized role in respiratory viral infections, contributing to viral clearance, through contact-dependent effector functions, mediated by perforin, CD95 l/Fas ligand, and, in addition, by interferon gamma (INF-γ) and tumor necrosis factor alpha (TNF-α). The latter two cytokines are mediators of T-cell–mediated lung injury [39]. It may be that chronic colonization or recurrent infection during exacerbations of the lower respiratory tract of COPD patients by bacterial and viral pathogens is responsible for this enhanced inflammatory response [13]. It is also possible that cigarette smoke itself damages airway cells, creating new autoantigens that drive the immunoinflammatory response (see later discussion) [40].

The role of T cells in the pathogenesis of COPD is not fully understood. CD8+ cells have the potential to release TNF-α, perforins, and granzymes. CD8+ T lymphocytes isolated from the sputum of smokers are activated and release perforin, an enzyme that produces cell necrosis and apoptosis [41]. In addition, CD8+ cells activate the Fas/Fas ligand apoptotic pathway. An association has been shown between CD8+ cells and apoptosis of alveolar epithelial cells in subjects with emphysema [42]. The role of Fas ligand in COPD is uncertain; one study reported that soluble Fas ligand levels were elevated in the plasma in severe COPD [43], whereas another group found the levels to be unchanged in COPD, compared with control subjects [44].

Neutrophils

Neutrophils are another component of the inflammatory response in COPD. Increased numbers of activated neutrophils are found in bronchoalveolar lavage fluid (BALF) and sputum from patients who have COPD [45]. The lack of significant increased neutrophil numbers in the lung parenchyma may be because these cells make a rapid transit through the airways and the lung parenchyma. The mechanisms of neutrophil passage

Table 1
Variation of inflammatory cells and markers of inflammation in the bronchial submucosa

Cell type	CD45	CD3	Neutrophils	Eosinophils	Mast	CD68	CD8	CD4
Severe COPD	—	↓ [28]	↑ [56]	→ [56]	→ [56]	↑ [56]	↓ [28]	→ [28]
Mild/moderate COPD	↑ [14,22]	↑ [14,22,26,27] → [28]	→ [14,22] ↑ [56]	→ [14,22,56]	→ [14,22,56]	↑ [14,22] → [56]	↑ [22,27] → [14,28]	→ [14,22,27,28]
Control smokers	→ [22]	→ [22,28] ↑ [27]	→ [22,56]	→ [22,56]	→ [22,56]	→ [22,56]	↑ [27] → [22,28]	→ [22,27,28]
Control nonsmokers	→ [14,22]	→ [14,22,26,27]	→ [14,22]	→ [14,22]	→ [14,22]	→ [14,22]	→ [14,22,27]	→ [14,22,27]

Numbers close to the arrows indicate references.
↑ significantly increased values in comparison with that indicated by →.
→ basal values or values nonsignificantly changed.
↓ significantly decreased values in comparison with that indicated by →.
Data from Di Stefano A, Caramori G, Ricciardolo FL, et al. Cellular and molecular mechanisms in chronic obstructive pulmonary disease: an overview. Clin Exp Allergy 2004;34(8):1156–67.

into the airway lumen in COPD are not entirely clear. Cigarette smoking is known to increase circulating neutrophil counts and to cause sequestration of neutrophils in the lung capillaries [46] by decreasing their deformability. Cigarette smoke also has a direct stimulating effect on granulocyte production in the bone marrow, possibly mediated by granulocyte macrophage colinase stimulating factor (G-CSF) release from macrophages [47]. It is possible that neutrophils are activated within the pulmonary microcirculation to release reactive oxidant species and proteases that may have a direct injurious effect. Once sequestered in the pulmonary microcirculation, it is possible that an imbalance between pro- and anti-inflammatory cytokines may result in neutrophil migration into the airspaces. Expression of anti-inflammatory mediators, such as secretory component and Clara cell protein, and also of IL-10, is decreased in the airway lumen of smokers with COPD [48,49], whereas cytokines, such as IL-8 and monocyte chemoattractant protein (MCP-1), which promote the chemotaxis of neutrophils and monocytes, respectively, and TNF-α, which activates adhesion molecules, are increased [45,50]. Up-regulation of E-selectin and intercellular adhesion molecule (ICAM)-1 on submucosal vessels and on the bronchial epithelium of subjects with COPD [51] suggests that these adhesion molecules may be involved in the recruitment of neutrophils from the circulation and in their migration from bronchial subepithelial mucosal capillaries into, and through, the epithelium to enter the airway lumen. The airway epithelium is a rich source of the cytokines/chemokines that recruit both neutrophils and macrophages into the airspaces. Many of these cytokines/chemokines are overexpressed in COPD [52,53]. IL-6, IL-1β, TNF-α, growth-related gene-α (Gro-α)/keratinocyte-derived chemokine (KC, CXCL1), MCP-1, and IL-8 are increased in the sputum in COPD patients, and the bronchiolar epithelium overexpresses MCP-1, its receptor CCR2, macrophage inflammatory protein (MIP-1α), and IL-8. The degree of airflow limitation correlates with the expression of IL-8, MIP-1α, MCP-1, and CCR2 on the airway epithelium [54], although IL-8 expression does not correlate with the numbers of neutrophils in the airspaces in smokers [50].

Neutrophils may play a role in the pathogenesis of COPD by releasing reactive oxygen species (ROS) and serum proteinases, including neutrophil elastase, cathepsin G, and proteinase 3, and matrix metalloproteinase (MMP)-8 and -9. These proteases may contribute to alveolar destruction and are also potent stimuli of mucus secretion (see later discussion, "Proteases/Antiprotease"). Relationships have been shown between circulating neutrophils and the decline in FEV$_1$ [55]. Similarly, neutrophil numbers in bronchial biopsy specimens and induced sputum are related to disease severity [56] and the rate of decline in lung function [57].

Macrophages

Macrophages are another key component of the inflammation found in COPD. The number of macrophages in the airways, lung parenchyma, and BALF of patients who have COPD is increased 5 to 10 fold. Macrophage numbers in the airways correlate with the severity of COPD [58]. Cigarette smoke activates macrophages to release inflammatory mediators, including TNF-α, IL-8, and other CXC chemokines, leukotriene B$_4$, and ROS. Macrophages also secrete proteases, including MMP-2; MMP-9; MMP-12; cathepsins K, L, and S; and neutrophil elastase, taken up from neutrophils. Macrophages from COPD patients are more activated, secrete more inflammatory proteins, and have greater elasteolitic activity compared with macrophages from normal smokers, and their activity is further enhanced by exposure to cigarette smoke [59]. Increased numbers of macrophages in the lungs of COPD patients and smokers may result from increased recruitment of monocytes from the circulation in response to monocyte chemoattractant chemokines such as MCP-1, which have been shown to be increased in the sputum and BALF of patients who have COPD [60]. CXC chemokines also act as chemoattractants to monocytes. The concentration of GRO-α is increased markedly in the sputum and BALF from patients who have COPD. Furthermore, monocytes from patients who have COPD show a greater chemotactic response to GRO-α than cells from normal smokers and nonsmokers [61].

Dendritic cells

Dendritic cells are also present in increased numbers in the airways and alveolar walls of smokers [62]. The role of dendritic cells in COPD is not yet defined, but they are likely to have an important role in the innate and adaptive immune responses in COPD.

Airway epithelial cells

Cigarette smoke activates airway epithelial cells to produce inflammatory mediators, including TNF-α, IL-1β, granulocyte macrophage colony-stimulating factor, and IL-8, which may in turn augment or perpetuate the inflammatory response. The epithelium in the small airways may also be an important source of transforming growth factor (TGF)-β, adding to the induction of local fibrosis [63]. Epithelial cells can also secrete antioxidants, antiproteases, and transport immunoglobulins, and thus may be involved in adaptive immunity. Cigarette smoke may impair these innate and adaptive immune responses of the airway epithelium and increase the likelihood of infection.

Finally, the expression of many of the inflammatory mediators implicated in the inflammatory response in the lungs in COPD is controlled by the transcription factor, nuclear factor (NF)-κB. NF-κB is up-regulated in alveolar macrophages [64] in patients who have COPD and in airway cells [27] in patients who have mild to moderate COPD, in comparison with control nonsmokers. Up-regulation of NF-κB in lung cells in COPD may be a key molecular mechanism, involved in the ongoing inflammatory process in the airways.

Cytokines and chemokines

The cytokines, the receptors, and the functions involved in COPD are shown in Table 2 [65–69]. In patients who have severe emphysema, lymphocytes in the lungs strongly express TH1 cytokines and secrete high levels of IFN-g, CCR5, and CXCR3, and, in addition, show increased expression of CXCR3 ligands, monokine induced by INF-γ, and IP-10 [70]. All of these findings indicate a polarization of alveolar lymphocytes toward the TH1 phenotype in severe emphysema. On treatment with IP-10, alveolar macrophages in culture express MMP-12 protein, which can also be detected in alveolar macrophages in emphysematous lungs [70]. These studies suggest that the lymphocytic infiltrate, which has been shown to occur in emphysema, may be linked to the observed increased chemokines in emphysema and the activation of MMP-12 [70]. Further evidence for a role of cytokines/chemokines in the pathogenesis of emphysema has been shown in animal studies where inducible and lung- specific overexpression of the prototypic TH1 cytokine IFN-g [71] or the TH2 cytokine IL-13 [72] resulted

in emphysema associated with an inflammatory response and a variable degree of fibrosis and increased MMP and cathepsin expression. In IL-13 overexpressing mice, MMP-9 and MMP-12 are responsible for the emphysema phenotype, because combined MMP-9 and 12 knock-out mice were partially protected against emphysema, which resulted from lung overexpression of IL-13 [73]. In addition, inhalation of cathepsins led to enhanced protection against emphysema [74].

Additional studies have demonstrated that mice lacking the CCR6 receptor of MIP-3 α/CCL20 show reduced cigarette smoke–induced emphysema and a decrease in dendritic cells, CD8+ T cells, and neutrophils in the lungs [75]. These CCR6 knock-out mice demonstrate lower levels of TNF-α and do not show an increase in MCP-1 in bronchoalveolar lavage (BAL), suggesting that the MCP-1-CCR2 inter action was affected by CCR6 deficiency.

TNF-α has also been implicated in cigarette smoke–induced emphysema. Increased levels of TNF-α are present in the airways of cigarette smokers [45]. Animals that overexpress TNF-α show evidence of emphysema and an exaggerated alveolar inflammatory response [76], whereas tumor necrosis factor (TNF) receptor knock-out mice demonstrate significant protection against cigarette smoke–induced emphysema [77]. Enhanced TNF-α expression can be implicated in many of the pathologic changes seen in COPD. With respect to emphysema, TNF-α stimulates metalloproteinase (MMP) synthesis by alveolar macrophages [53]. Cultured macrophages exposed to cigarette smoke extract release TNF-α, and, in addition, circulating TNF-α–soluble receptors p55 and p75 are significantly increased in COPD patients, compared with healthy controls [78]. It appears that TNF-α p55, rather than p75, is a critical factor in the development of cigarette smoke–induced emphysema [79]. Absence of TNF-α receptor type 2 in animal studies was associated with reduced inflammatory responses in terms of neutrophil, macrophage, and CD4 and CD8 cell influx, and protected against cigarette smoke emphysema [73]. TNF-α may also have a role in alveolar cell apoptosis. Induction of alveolar wall apoptosis, particularly of type II epithelial cells, appears to depend on the activation of both TNF-α receptors.

IL-1β may also play a role in the development of emphysema. In animal models, lung-specific induction of human IL-1β resulted in emphysema [80], whereas inhibition with IL-1β antibody

Table 2
Variation of inflammatory cells and markers of inflammation in the central and peripheral airways

Cell type	Central airways						Peripheral airways (<3 mm diameter)			
	Neutrophils	CD68	CD4	CD8	IL-4	IL-5	Neutrophils	CD68	CD4	CD8
Mild/moderate COPD	→ [33]	→ [33]	→ [33]	→ [33]	↓ [65]	↑ [65]	→ [35,66,68,69]	↑ [66,67] → [35,68,69]	→ [35,66,68,69]	↑ [35] → [66–69]
Chronic bronchitis with normal FEV₁	—	—	—	—	↑ [65]	↑ [65]	—	—	—	—
Control smokers	→ [33]	→ [33]	→ [33]	→ [33]	→ [65]	→ [65]	→ [35,66,68,69]	→ [35,66–69]	→ [35,66–69]	→ [35,66–69]

Numbers close to the arrows indicate references.
↑ significantly increased values in comparison with that indicated by →.
→ basal values or values nonsignificantly changed.
↓ significantly decreased values in comparison with that indicated by →.
Abbreviation: FEV₁, forced expiratory volume in 1 second.
Data from Di Stefano A, Caramori G, Ricciardolo FL, et al. Cellular and molecular mechanisms in chronic obstructive pulmonary disease: an overview. Clin Exp Allergy 2004;34(8):1156–67.

reduced alveolar macrophage influx into the air-spaces following cigarette smoke exposure [81]. Furthermore, double IL-1 receptor and TNF-α receptor knock-out mice are protected against elastase-induced emphysema [82] and are protected against alveolar cell apoptosis caused by elastase instillation.

In general, with increasing severity of COPD comes a further enhancement of the inflammatory response. Compared with mild to moderate disease, the expression of inflammatory proteins such as MIP-1α, a chemokine involved in the activation of mononuclear cells and granulocytes, is further increased. The number of neutrophils and macrophages is also further increased in severe disease, and T lymphocytes (CD3$^+$ cells) are decreased. The cellular type in severe disease appears to be shifting toward cells with a phagocytic and proteolytic role in the bronchial tissues (see Tables 1 and 2; Table 3).

Effects of smoking cessation on airway inflammation

The effects of smoking cessation on airway inflammation have been studied in patients who have COPD largely in cross-sectional studies and, to a limited extent, in bronchial biopsy or lung tissue specimens from smokers and ex-smokers with chronic bronchitis or COPD [50,83–85]. Bronchial biopsies from patients who had COPD who currently did not smoke had increased numbers of inflammatory cells [83]. A further study showed that ex-smokers with COPD tended to have lower numbers of mast cells than smokers [84]. In patients who had chronic bronchitis or mild to moderate COPD, one study [85] found no differences between smokers and ex-smokers in the numbers of neutrophils, eosinophils, macrophages, and lymphocytes; in the cytokines TNF-α and IL-1; in the IL2 receptor; or in the expression of the very late activation antigen VLA-1, ICAM-1, and selectin adhesion molecules in bronchial biopsies. However, macrophage numbers, expression of IL-2 receptor, VLA-1, and ICAM-1 were higher in both smokers and ex-smokers who had COPD than in non-smokers. Thus, the current evidence suggests that in patients who have COPD, inflammation seems to persist in lung tissue after smoking cessation. A recent longitudinal study showed that inflammation was not only sustained but was increased in some aspects among those who had stopped smoking [20]. One potential explanation is that the persistent airway inflammation in patients who have COPD may relate to repair of tissue damage in the airways.

Inflammation, airway remodeling, and airflow limitation

The peripheral airways (bronchioles <2 mm in diameter) are the major site of increased airway resistance in COPD [3,11,86]. The main pathologic lesions in the peripheral airways include an increased number of inflammatory cells and structural changes, such as epithelial goblet cell metaplasia, airway wall fibrosis, and smooth muscle hypertrophy [24]. The increase in the thickness of the airway wall from inflammation, fibrosis, and smooth muscle hypertrophy will encroach upon the lumen, thus reducing airway diameter. It may also result in uncoupling between airways and the surrounding lung parenchyma, thereby reducing the elastic force that opposes bronchiolar smooth muscle contraction and promoting airway closure. Airway wall inflammation can also contribute to the destruction of alveolar–bronchiolar

Table 3
Variation of inflammatory cells in the lung parenchyma

	Neutrophils	CD68	CD3	CD4	CD8	Eosinophils
Mild/moderate COPD	→ [42,83]	→ [83]	↑ [42]	→ [42,83]	↑ [42,83]	→ [83]
Smokers with normal FEV$_1$	→ [42,83,86]	↑ [86] → [83]	↑ [86] → [42]	→ [42,83]	→ [42,83]	→ [83]
Control nonsmokers	↑ [86] → [42,83]	→ [83,96]	→ [42,86]	→ [42,83]	→ [42,83]	→ [83]

Numbers close to the arrows indicate references.
↑ significantly increased values in comparison with that indicated by →.
→ basal values or values nonsignificantly changed.
↓ significantly decreased values in comparison with that indicated by →.
Data from Di Stefano A, Caramori G, Ricciardolo FL, et al. Cellular and molecular mechanisms in chronic obstructive pulmonary disease: an overview. Clin Exp Allergy 2004;34(8):1156–67.

attachments, producing deformation and narrowing of the airway lumen. This suggestion is supported by the observation that, in smokers, the destruction of alveolar attachments correlates with the degree of inflammation in peripheral airways [87].

The airflow limitation in smokers may also result from the increased goblet cell metaplasia and subsequent hyperplasia in the small airways of smokers [24]. This hyperplasia may contribute to the increased peripheral airway resistance as a result of the production of mucus at a site at which this does not normally occur, leading to a marked increase in the surface tension of the airway-lining fluid and to instability of the peripheral airways, facilitating their early closure during expiration.

The increase in goblet cells in the peripheral airway epithelium of smokers is associated with an increased number of neutrophils [24]. Because neutrophil elastase is a potent secretagogue [88], the co-location of neutrophils and goblet cells within the epithelium may be relevant to the increased discharge of mucus by the increased number of goblet cells in COPD.

Increased numbers of neutrophils are also found within the bronchiolar smooth muscle of smokers who have COPD [34], which suggests a possible interaction between neutrophils and airway smooth muscle in the pathogenesis of smoking-induced airflow limitation by alteration of the normal structure–function relationships.

In smokers who have COPD, $CD8^+$ T lymphocytes are increased not only in the central airways but also in the peripheral airways and lung parenchyma [35,89]. Traditionally, the major activity of $CD8^+$ cytotoxic T cells has been considered to be the rapid resolution of acute viral infections, which are a frequent occurrence in patients who have COPD. The observation that people with frequent respiratory infections in childhood are more prone to develop COPD [90] supports the role of current and latent viral infections in this disease [38,91]. In response to repeated or persistent viral infection, it is possible that an excessive recruitment of $CD8^+$ T lymphocytes may occur, which damages the lungs in susceptible smokers, possibly through the release of TNF-α and perforins [31,92,93]. Conversely, it is also possible that $CD8^+$ T lymphocytes are able to damage the lung directly, even in the absence of viral infection, as shown by experimental studies that demonstrated recognition of a lung "autoantigen" by T cytotoxic cells [94]. It has been hypothesized

recently that the $CD8^+$ cytotoxic T cell and the accumulation of other inflammatory cells may also occur in response to an autoantigen [40].

A comparison of the central and peripheral airways shows an increase in the total inflammatory cells in the peripheral airways (<2 mm diameter) in patients who have chronic bronchitis with normal lung function, compared with control smokers (see Table 2). Some studies have shown an increase in total inflammation and an increase in $CD8^+$ cells in the peripheral airways of patients who have mild or moderate COPD in comparison with control smokers [35].

Recent studies that have assessed tissue obtained from lung volume reduction surgery in patients who have severe COPD and have shown an increase in total leukocytes and in $CD4^+$ and $CD8^+$ lymphocytes in the peripheral airways and the lung parenchyma [23]. In contrast, smokers with normal lung function show an increased number of macrophages and T lymphocytes in lung parenchyma, compared with control nonsmokers, with no changes in $CD4^+$ and $CD8^+$ cells. Patients who have mild to moderate COPD show an increase in $CD8^+$ cells in the alveolar septa, compared with control nonsmokers [89,95], and no change in the numbers of neutrophils, macrophages, or $CD4^+$ cells.

The inflammatory response in the peripheral airways may play a role in the fibrosis that characterizes the small airways and may contribute to airflow limitation in patients who have moderate to severe COPD [11,96,97].

As the disease progresses, small airways develop increased thickness and enhanced inflammatory infiltrate by neutrophils, macrophages, T lymphocytes ($CD4^+$ and $CD8^+$ T cells), and B-lymphocytes. Lymphoid follicles also accumulate within the walls of the bronchioles, and the lumens of these airways are more often obliterated by mucus [13,98]. A number of mechanisms have been proposed to link inflammation and small airway remodeling. Fibroblast growth factor (FGF) and FGF receptor (FGFR) signaling appear to be associated with the airway vascular remodeling in chronic bronchitis. Studies of lung tissue from COPD show that FGF-1 and its receptor FGFR-1 are detected by immunohistochemistry in the vascular and airway smooth muscle and airway epithelial cells [99]. FGF-1 or FGF-2 increase the mRNA levels of FGFR-1 and induce cellular proliferation of cultured human airway epithelial smooth muscle cells [100]. Smokers who have COPD show increased expression of FGF in central airways, predominantly caused by enhanced expression in the bronchial glands, suggesting that FGF may also have a role in promoting mucus hypersecretion in smokers [101].

The pattern of cytokine profile and chemokine receptor expression has been investigated in the peripheral airways in COPD. As discussed earlier, CD8[+] T cells in the peripheral airways in COPD are associated with INF-γ, and express CXCR3 [102], a chemokine receptor thought to be preferentially expressed on TH1 cells. Moreover, CXCR3 expression is associated with the expression in the epithelium of its ligand CXCL10, which suggests that the CXCR3/CXCL10 axis may be involved in the recruitment of TH1 cells into the peripheral airways of smokers with COPD. Recently, CXCR3 has been found on lymphocytes isolated from smokers who have COPD [70]. These studies also showed that the interaction of CXCL10 with CXCR3 drives the release of macrophage metalloelastase (MMP)-12 from macrophages. MMP-12 is a potent elastolytic enzyme that can cause lung tissue destruction. These data suggest a possible mechanism through which T helper1 lymphocytes can drive the progression of small airway and emphysematous destruction, thus relating the inflammation in peripheral airways to the surrounding alveoli. Very recent studies suggest differences in gene expression in the small airways and surrounding lung parenchyma, which may cause fibrosis in the small airways, but alveolar cell loss in the lung parenchyma, resulting in emphysematous destruction [103].

Mucus hypersecretion

Mucus forms a film, coating the airway epithelium. Under the action of the coordinated movement of cilia, the mucus layer is propelled from the periphery of the lung to the upper airways. The main constituents of the mucus layer are mucus glycoproteins (mucins), water, and peptides. Mucus plays a key role in the clearance of foreign material and infectious agents, and has important antioxidant properties. In chronic bronchitis, mucus in the airways is increased, resulting from increased production of mucins and increased secretion from goblet cells. In healthy subjects, at least 12 human mucin genes are expressed in the lower respiratory tract.

Mucus production and secretion in COPD is regulated by multiple cellular and molecular mechanisms. Goblet cells express MUC5AC and 2, whereas glandular mucosal cells express MUC5B, 8, and 19 [104]. Expression of MUC5B has been shown to be enhanced in the bronchiolar epithelium of COPD patients [105]. A number of stimuli, such as neutrophil elastase, lipopolysaccharides (LPS), IL-1β, TNF-α, cigarette smoke, and oxidative stress, cause goblet cell metaplasia and mucus hypersecretion (Fig. 4) [106].

Neutrophil elastase increases MUC5AC mRNA levels by enhancing mRNA stability [107]. Instillation of pancreatic elastase in animal lungs induces MUC5AC mRNA and protein expression and results in goblet cell metaplasia 8 days after instillation. LPS also induces MUC5AC expression in animal models, which is associated with neutrophil infiltration [108], and increased expression of MMP-9 [109]. LPS, TNF-α, and IL-1β-induced MUC5AC synthesis is mediated by a number of signaling cascades including IKKβ, NF-κB [110], mitogen, and stress-activated protein kinase-1, leading to activation of the cyclic adenosine monophosphate (cAMP)-response element by the cAMP-response element binding protein by way of the extracellular signal-regulated kinase (ERK) and p38 mitogen-activated protein (MAP) kinase pathways (see Fig. 4) [111].

Signaling pathways initiated by epidermal growth factor receptor (EGFR) phosphorylation, which can be induced by cigarette smoke–derived oxidative stress, epidermal growth factor (EGF), transforming growth factor alpha (TGF-α), or heparin-binding epidermal growth factor also play an important role in mucin production in human airway epithelial cells. ROS resulting in hyaluronan augmentation can activate the serine protease tissue kallikrein, which can then cleave the transmembrane precursor of EGF. EGF-EGFR–dependent stimulation of Ras MAPK/ERK kinase (MEK-ERK) seems to have a central role in goblet cell hyperplasia and increased MUC5AC gene expression [112,113]. Cigarette smoke produces ROS also resulting in vascular endothelial growth factor receptor (VEGFR) activation and mucus production by activation of the TNF-α–converting enzyme (TACE), resulting in loss of TGF-α in airway epithelial cells [8]. Acrolein, a component of cigarette smoke, can also induce MUC5AC expression created by ligand/dependent activation of EGFR and mediated by TACE and MMP-9 [114]. In addition, ROS derived from cigarette smoke can activate c-Jun N-terminal kinase by way of an src-dependant signaling cascade. This downstream signaling can trigger transcriptional regulation of the

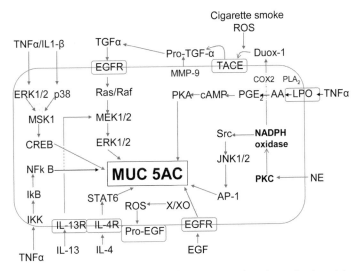

Fig. 4. The signal transduction mechanisms involved in the regulation of mucin production. AA, arachidonate; AP-1, activator protein-1; COX2, cyclooxygenase-2; CREB, cAMP-response element-binding protein; Duox1, dual oxidase 1fd; EGF, epidermal growth factor; EGFR, epidermal growth factor receptor; IκB, inhibitor of κB; IKK (IκB kinase); IL-1b, interleukin-1β; JNK1/2, c-Jun NH2-terminal kinase 1/2; LPO, lipoxygenase; MEK1/2, ERK kinase 1/2; MSK1, mitogen- and stress-activated protein kinase 1; NADPH, nicotinamide adrenine dinucleotide phosphate; NE, neutrophil elastase; NF-κB, nuclear factor-κB; PGE2, prostaglandin E2; PKA, protein kinase A; PKC, protein kinase C; PLA2, phospholipase A2; STAT6, signal transducers and activators of transcription 6; TACE, TNF-α–converting enzyme; TGF-α, transforming growth factor-α; X/XO, xanthine/xanthine oxidase.

MUC5AC, mediated by binding of activator protein 1 response element by JunD and Fra-2 [115]. Moreover, cigarette smoke extract has been shown to synergize with LPS or TNF-α in the induction of MUC5AC expression, suggesting a potential amplification by cigarette smoke and inflammatory stimuli relevant to the pathogenesis of COPD [116]. A number of transgenic mice experiments have begun to unravel the complex interplay among inflammation, oxidative stress, and growth factors in the development of mucus hyperplasia. These studies suggest that CD4+ TH2 cells and the cytokine network, including IL-4, IL-10, and IL-13, play a crucial role in the development of goblet cell hyperplasia/metaplasia [72,117,118]. Mice that overexpress IL13 also show increased expression of MUC5AC, 1 and 4 [119,120].

Proteases/antiproteases

A large body of literature has been amassed to test the hypothesis that a protease/antiprotease imbalance, leading to the breakdown of connective tissue components, particularly elastin, is the critical mechanism in the pathogenesis of emphysema in smokers. This concept developed from studies showing the development of early-onset emphysema in patients deficient in the major ant elastase α1-AT [121] and from animal studies showing the development of emphysema in response to the instillation of proteolytic enzymes [82,122–130]. Pallid mice that have decreased α1-AT levels develop emphysema earlier on exposure to cigarette smoke than mice with normal levels [131,132]. Furthermore, mice lacking neutrophil elastase are protected from chronic cigarette smoke–induced emphysema [133].

Elastin is an important target for proteolytic enzymes, and its destruction results in loss of elasticity in the lung parenchyma. Elastin is the principal component of elastic fibers and is secreted from several cell types as a precursor, tropoelastin. These tropoelastin molecules become aligned in the extracellular space on microfibrils. Under the action of lysyl oxidase, the lysine residues in tropoelastin are modified, which causes the tropoelastin monomers to cross-link and form larger, insoluble elastin polymers. Because the cross-links, known as desmosines, are unique to elastin, they have been used as a marker of elastin degradation. Desmosine and elastin peptides are elevated in smokers and patients who have COPD [134]. However, the specificity of measurements of these peptides in urine is controversial, particularly as a reflection of lung elastin degradation alone, because of the extreme durability of lung elastin. Elastin turnover is minimal in normal subjects; thus, breakdown products should not be detectable. Nevertheless, studies indicate that the annual rate of decline in FEV_1 in a group of smokers correlated positively with urine levels of desmosine [135]. The validity of the use of desmosine or elastin peptides as markers of elastolysis remains unresolved.

Together with the destruction of elastin, inactivation of antiproteases is central to the protease/antiprotease imbalance hypothesis. Early studies showed that the function of α_1-AT was reduced by around 40% in smokers, compared with nonsmokers [136]. This "functional α_1-AT deficiency" was thought to result from inactivation of α_1-AT by oxidants in cigarette smoke. However, most of the α_1-AT in cigarette smokers remains active and is therefore still capable of protecting against the increased protease burden. Only a transient and nonsignificant fall in α_1-AT activity in BALF occurs, 1 hour after smoking [137]. Thus, studies assessing the function of α_1-AT in either chronic or acute cigarette smoking have not been definitive. The hypothesis that the major event is an imbalance between an increased elastase burden in the lungs and a "functional deficiency" of α_1-AT, due to its inactivation, is an oversimplification.

As discussed earlier, the number of neutrophils and macrophages in the airspaces in chronic cigarette smokers is increased, which may increase the elastase burden because of enhanced degranulation and therefore release of elastase from activated neutrophils. Some evidence supports this, because neutrophils isolated from patients who have emphysema show greater elastase-induced fibronectin degradation in vitro than cells from control subjects matched for age and smoking history [138].

Other studies have invoked a contributory role for other antiproteases, such as antileukoprotease, or more subtle changes (eg, a decrease in the association rate constant of α_1-AT for neutrophil elastase), which may contribute to elastin degradation.

Some evidence also supports the concept that an abnormality in elastin synthesis and repair may be involved in the pathogenesis of emphysema. In animal models involving intratracheal instillation of elastases, lung elastin is depleted within hours to a few days [139], followed by increased elastin synthesis over a period of weeks. However, in areas of emphysema in these models, alveolar elastic fibers have an abnormal appearance [140] and resemble the aberrant elastic fibers in human emphysema [141]. Thus, although elastin synthesis following injury may restore the elastin content of the lungs, it does not restore normal lung architecture in these experimental models.

In an animal model of elastase-induced emphysema, treatment with retinoic acid restored normal alveolar architecture [142]. These studies in adult male rats (which, in contrast to humans, have continued lung growth throughout their adult lives) have to be verified, but they provide some intriguing evidence that the destructive process in emphysema, which was always considered irreversible, may be capable of repair.

In addition to serine proteases, cysteine proteases (cathepsins) may have a role in COPD. Cathepsin C was induced in mice by overexpression of INF-γ, which resulted in emphysema [71]. Cathepsin inhibitors have also been shown to reduce emphysema induced by overexpression of IL-13 in mouse lung [72]. Moreover, cathepsin-L has been detected in BALF from patients who have emphysema [143], and alveolar macrophages in patients who have COPD secrete more cysteine proteases than macrophages from normal smokers or nonsmokers [144].

Matrix metalloproteases (MMPs) are a group of at least 20 proteolytic enzymes that have a role in tissue remodeling and repair associated with normal development and inflammation by degrading collagen, laminin, and elastin. They are characterized in distinct subclasses, depending on their substrates' specificity, amino acid similarity, and identifiable sequence molecules. The subclasses are collagenases (MMP-1, -8, -13), gelatinases (MMP-2, -9), stromelysin S (MMP-3, -10, -11), membrane-type MMP-14 to MMP-25), matrilysin (MMP-7), and macrophage metalloelastase (MMP-12) [145]. The major inhibitors of MMPs are alpha-2 macroglobulin and the tissue inhibitor of the metalloproteases (TIMP) family. The TIMP family comprises four structurally related members, TIMP-1, 2, 3, and 4.

Evidence is substantial for a role of MMPs in the pathogenesis of COPD (Fig. 5) [146]. Several studies have shown increased expression of several MMPs in the lungs of COPD patients. MMP-12 protein has been observed in sputum, BAL, bronchial biopsies, and peripheral lung tissue in patients who have severe emphysema [147,148]. Increased concentrations of MMP-1 and MMP-9 are present in BALF from patients who have

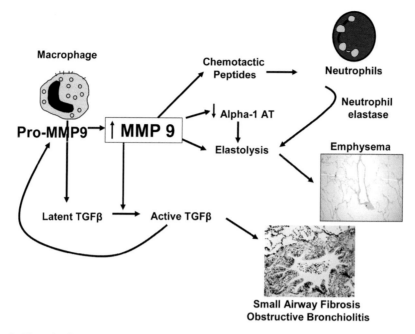

Fig. 5. The role of MMP-9 in interaction between small airway fibrosis and emphysema in COPD.

COPD [149,150], and the lung parenchyma of patients who have emphysema shows increased activity of MMP-9 [151,152]. MMP-1 expression is also increased in the lungs of patients who have emphysema, particularly in type II pneumocytes [153]. MMP-12 mRNA can be induced by exposure of human bronchial epithelial cells to cigarette smoke extract or cytokine mix (TNF-α and INF-γ) [154,155]. Alveolar macrophages from smokers express more MMP-9 than those from normal subjects [59], and patients who have COPD have an even greater increase [58].

Considerable evidence from experimental models of emphysema links MMP-12 and the development of emphysema. Increased MMP-12 macroglobulin was present in alveolar macrophages after smoke exposure in C57BL/6 mice [156], and chronic smoke exposure for 1 to 6 months results in significant increases in MMP-12 mRNA and protein expression in the lungs of C57BL/6 mice, without change in TIMP-1 and -2, indicating an increase in the MMP-12/TIMP ratio [41,156]. Animal models have shown that cigarette smoke–induced emphysema does not occur in mice lacking MMP-12 [157]. In such mice, emphysema induced by IL-13 or INF-γ expression is also reduced [72] and is associated with a marked reduction in monocyte recruitment to the lungs.

MMPs are also known to activate the latent form of TGF-β to its active form. Mice lacking the integrin α-V-β-6 fail to activate TGF-β, and these animals do not develop age-related emphysema, which can be overcome by overexpression of TGF-β1 [158]. These data suggest that TGF-β1 may down-regulate MMP-12 under normal conditions and that the absence of TGF-β results in excessive MMP-12 production and emphysema.

The remodeling of the extracellular matrix may itself modulate alveolar inflammation, because fragmentation of elastin by MMP-12 acts as a chemoattractant for monocytes through an interaction with the elastin-binding protein [124]. Other breakdown products of the extracellular matrix also have proinflammatory effects, such as the collagen-derived peptide N-acetyl pro-gly-pro (PGP), which has been shown to cause neutrophil influx into the lungs and depends on the activation of the chemokine receptor CXCR2 [159]. PGP levels have been shown to be significantly increased in COPD patients, compared with control subjects [159]. Thus, the degradation products of the extracellular matrix may be important proinflammatory mediators in the pathogenesis of COPD.

Although MMP-9 and -2 both degrade elastin and are expressed in COPD lungs, the role of these MMPs in the pathogenesis of COPD remains unclear. Mice lacking MMP-9 are not protected against emphysema caused by cigarette smoke, but are protected from small-airway fibrosis [73]. TGF-β is activated by MMP-9, and this mechanism could provide a link between enhanced elastolytic activity by MMP-9 and the simultaneous production of fibrosis by activation of TGF-β.

Lack of other antiproteases, other than α_1-AT may also have a role in the pathogenesis of emphysema. TIMP-3–null mice develop spontaneous alveolar enlargement [160–162]. Cigarette exposure of male BALB/c mice produced an increase in the MMP-12 /TIMP-2 ratio [163]. An increase in MMP-9 and a decrease in TIMP-1 have been reported in the emphysematous lung of the senescence mouse that lacks the age- protective protein Klotho [164]. Alveolar macrophages from patients who have COPD have a blunted response to stimuli for the release of tissue inhibitor of metalloproteinase-1 [58], which would favor increased elastolysis. Taken together, existing data do suggest that a protease/antiprotease imbalance likely plays an important role in the pathogenesis of COPD, but the full spectrum of molecules and processes involved still remains unclear. It is likely to result from a complex set of processes that may differ among individual patients with different genetic backgrounds and phenotypes of COPD.

Oxidants/antioxidants

Oxidative stress

The lungs are unique compared with other organs in that they are directly exposed to high levels of oxygen. In addition, because of its direct contact with the environment, the respiratory epithelium is a major target for oxidative injury from oxidants generated either exogenously (inhaled oxidants such as cigarette smoke or air pollutants), or endogenously (from phagocytes and other cell types). As a result, the lungs require efficient enzymatic and nonenzymatic antioxidant systems to protect the airways against exogenous and endogenous oxidants. If the balance between oxidants and antioxidants shifts in favor of the former, owing to an excess of oxidants or a depletion of antioxidants, oxidative stress occurs.

Because cigarette smoke contains 10^{17} oxidant-molecules per puff [165], and is the major etiologic factor in the pathogenesis of COPD, it has been proposed that an imbalance occurs in some smokers, resulting in oxidative stress that has a role in many of the pathogenic mechanisms in COPD [166]. Both reactive oxygen and reactive nitrogen species (ROS and RNS, respectively) contribute to the oxidative stress that occurs in COPD. Evidence is now considerable of increased oxidative stress in smokers and in patients who have COPD [167,168].

Cigarette smoke contains free radicals in the gas and the tar phases [169].The gas phase has an estimated 10^{15} free radicals per puff, including ROS, epoxides, peroxides, nitric oxide (NO), nitrogen dioxide, and peroxynitrite. The tar phase has more stable ROS (10^{18}/g), including phenol and semiquinone and other, more reactive, ROS, such as hydrogen peroxide and hydroxyl ions [165,169]. Short-lived radicals in the gas phase of cigarette smoke may be quenched immediately in the lung epithelial lining fluid; however, redox reactions in cigarette smoke condensate may produce ROS for a considerable time.

The oxidant burden in lungs may be further enhanced in smokers by the increased numbers of neutrophils and macrophages in the alveolar space [170]. Oxidants in cigarette smoke can stimulate alveolar macrophages to produce ROS and to release a number of mediators, some of which attract neutrophils and other inflammatory cells into the lungs. Neutrophils and macrophages, which migrate in increased numbers into the lungs of cigarette smokers, particularly those with airways obstruction, can generate ROS by way of the reduced nicotinamide adrenine dinucleotide phosphate oxidase system. Circulating neutrophils from cigarette smokers and patients who have exacerbations of COPD release more $O_2^{\bullet-}$ [171]. Cigarette smoking is associated with increased content of myeloperoxidase in neutrophils [172,173], which correlates with the degree of airflow limitation [172–174] and suggests that neutrophil myeloperoxidase-mediated oxidative stress plays a role in lung inflammation.

In vitro studies have shown that alveolar leukocytes from cigarette smokers spontaneously release increased amounts of oxidants, such as $O_2^{\bullet-}$ and H_2O_2, compared with those from nonsmokers [175–177]. Exposure to cigarette smoke in vitro has also been shown to increase the oxidative metabolism of alveolar macrophages [178]. Subpopulations of alveolar macrophages with a higher granular density appear to be more prevalent in the lungs of smokers and are likely to be responsible for the increased $O_2^{\bullet-}$ production by smokers' macrophages [178,179]. The generation of ROS in epithelial lining fluid may be further enhanced by the presence of increased amounts of free iron in the airspaces in smokers [180,181], which is relevant to COPD because the intracellular iron content of alveolar macrophages is increased in cigarette smokers and is increased further in those who develop chronic bronchitis, compared with nonsmokers [182]. In addition, macrophages obtained from smokers release more free iron in vitro than those obtained from nonsmokers [183].

Previous epidemiologic studies have shown an inverse relationship between circulating neutrophil numbers and FEV_1 [184]. A similar relationship has also been shown between the change in peripheral blood neutrophil count and the change in airflow limitation over time [185]. Moreover, an association exists between $O_2^{\bullet-}$ release by peripheral blood neutrophils and bronchial hyperresponsiveness in patients who have COPD, suggesting a role for systemic ROS in the pathogenesis of the airway abnormalities in COPD [186]. Another study has shown a negative relationship between peripheral blood neutrophil luminol-enhanced chemiluminescence, as a measure of the release of ROS, and measurements of airflow limitation in young cigarette smokers [187].

Studies have also shown that circulating neutrophils from patients who have COPD show upregulation of their surface adhesion molecules, which may also be an oxidant-mediated effect [188]. Activation may be even more pronounced in neutrophils that are sequestered in the pulmonary microcirculation in smokers and in patients who have COPD, because these cells release more ROS than circulating neutrophils in animal models of lung inflammation [189]. Thus, sequestered neutrophils may be a source of ROS, and may have a role in inducing endothelial adhesion molecule expression in COPD.

Additionally, xanthine oxidase activity has been shown to be increased in cell-free BAL fluid and plasma from COPD patients, compared with normal subjects, and has been associated with increased $O_2^{\bullet-}$ and lipid peroxide levels [190–192]. Cigarette smoking increases the formation of RNS and results in nitration and oxidation of plasma proteins. β-unsaturated aldehydes (acrolein, acetaldehyde, and crotonaldehyde), which are abundantly present in cigarette smoke, are likely to react with protein-sulfhydryl and $-NH_2$ groups, leading to the formation of a protein-bound aldehyde functional group capable of

converting tyrosine to 3-nitrotyrosine and dityrosine [193]. NO- and peroxynitrite ($ONOO^-$)-mediated formation of 3-nitrotyrosine in plasma and free catalytic iron levels in epithelial lining fluid are elevated in chronic smokers [194–196]. Furthermore, levels of nitrotyrosine and inducible NO synthase (iNOS) were higher in airway inflammatory cells obtained by induced sputum from patients who had COPD, compared with those who had asthma [194] and the levels of nitrotyrosine were negatively correlated with the degree of airflow limitation.

It has been shown that increased levels of NO and reduced peroxynitrite inhibitory activity were present in induced sputum from patients who had COPD [197]. Steroid therapy was shown to decrease the increased level of RNS in patients who had COPD, and the reduction in nitrotyrosine and iNOS immunoreactivity in sputum cells was correlated with an improvement in FEV_1 [198]. These studies suggest that an increased RNS- and ROS-mediated protein nitration, and lipid peroxidation, may play a role in the inflammatory response that occurs in these patients.

Considerable evidence exists for increased oxidative stress in the lungs of COPD patients. Numerous studies have shown that markers of oxidative stress are increased in the lungs of COPD patients compared with healthy subjects, but also compared with smokers with a similar smoking history who have not developed COPD [199].

Smokers and patients who have COPD have higher levels of H_2O_2 in exhaled breath condensate, a direct measurement of airspace oxidative burden, than ex-smokers with COPD or, indeed, nonsmokers [200,201]. Increased $NO^{\bullet}$ in breath occurs in some studies in patients who have COPD, but the levels are not as high as those reported in asthma [202–205]. The rapid reaction of $NO^{\bullet}$ with $O_2^{\bullet-}$ to produce $ONOO^-$, or the thiols to produce nitrosothiols, may alter breath $NO^{\bullet}$ levels. Nitrosothiol levels have been shown to be high in breath condensate in smokers and in COPD patients, compared with nonsmoking subjects [206]. $ONOO^-$ formed by the reaction of $NO^{\bullet}$ with $O_2^{\bullet-}$ can cause nitration of tyrosine to produce nitrotyrosine [194]. Nitrotyrosine levels are elevated in sputum leukocytes of patients who have COPD and these levels are correlated negatively with FEV_1 as a measure of airflow limitation [195].

Exhaled carbon monoxide as a measure of the response of heme oxygenase to oxidative stress has been shown to be elevated in the exhaled breath of patients who have COPD, compared with normal subjects [202]. Lipid peroxidation products, such as thiobarbituric acid-reacting substances or malondialdehyde, are elevated in sputum in COPD patients, and correlate negatively with the FEV_1 [203,204]. Levels of 8-isoprostane produced by nonenzymatic lipid peroxidation of arachidonic acid [207] are elevated in COPD patients compared with normal subjects and smokers who have not developed the disease, and have been shown to correlate with the degree of airflow limitation [208].

Lipid peroxides can interact with enzymatic or nonenzymatic antioxidants and can decompose by reacting with metal ions or iron-containing proteins, thereby forming hydrocarbon gases and unsaturated aldehydes [209]. COPD patients show an increased level of ethane in breath compared with control subjects, and ethane levels correlate negatively with lung function [210,211].

A highly reactive lipid peroxidation end product, 4-hydroxy-2-nonenal, can act as a chemoattractant for neutrophils [212] and is also involved in numerous cellular functions such as cell proliferation, inhibition [213], T-cell apoptosis [214], and activation of various signaling pathways [215,216]. It has also been shown to activate the synthesis of the antioxidant glutathione (GSH) by induction of the glutamate cysteine lygase (GCL) gene and various proinflammatory genes such as IL-8, MCP-1, EGF, and MUC5AC [216], and it reacts quickly with extracellular proteins to form adducts. These adducts have been shown to be present in greater quantities in airway epithelial and endothelial cells in the lungs of COPD patients, compared with smokers with a similar smoking history who have not developed the disease [217].

Other markers of oxidative stress, such as 8-OHG and 4-hydroxy-nonenal, have been shown to have increased expression associated with emphysematous lesions in the lungs [218].

Antioxidants

The lungs contain abundant antioxidants to counteract the effects of oxidants. Antioxidants can be broadly grouped as nonenzymatic antioxidants such as GSH, vitamin C, and urea, and enzymatic antioxidant systems such as superoxide dismutase, catalases, and peroxidases [219]. A further enzymatic group is involved in recycling the first level of antioxidants, and includes

hemoxygenases and reductases, including peroxyredoxin, thioredoxins, and glutaredoxins [220,221]. GSH is the most abundant nonprotein thiol in the epithelial lining fluid and is one of the most important antioxidants in the lung. GSH is synthesized by GCL, which is localized in the cytosol. GCL is expressed prominently in human bronchial epithelial cells and, to some extent, in alveolar macrophages [222]. GSH controls the expression of several critical enzymes involved in free-radical detoxification, including superoxide dismutases, GSH peroxidase, thioreductase, and GCL [221,222]. Increased levels of total GSH and oxidized GSH have been shown in supernatants of the processed sputum of patients who have moderate to severe COPD compared with healthy nonsmokers [223]. GSH is increased in the BAL in healthy smokers and in stable patients who have moderate COPD [176,224]. The finding of higher levels of GSH in smokers and in patients who have stable COPD may be an adaptive response against oxidative stress. These responses are likely to be mediated by GCL, the enzyme that regulates GSH synthesis, because the mRNA heavy chain catalytic subunit of GCL was increased in the bronchial and alveolar epithelial cells in patients who had COPD [225]. Other groups have reported that the GCL heavy chain was diminished in the bronchial epithelial cells and alveolar macrophages of COPD patients [226], suggesting differential responses of GCL in different lung sites. Other antioxidant enzymes have also been shown to be increased in COPD patients. Manganese superoxide dismutase (SOD) showed an increased expression in the airways of patients who had COPD [227,228], again likely as a response to increased oxidative stress [229].

Oxidative stress can potentially play a role in the pathogenesis of COPD through many mechanisms (Fig. 6) [230,231]. It has been proposed that a relative "deficiency" of antiproteases such as α_1-AT, resulting from inactivation by oxidants, creates a protease/antiprotease imbalance in the lungs. This proposal forms the basis of the protease/antiprotease theory of the pathogenesis of emphysema. Inactivation of α_1-AT by oxidants occurs as a critical methionine residue in its active site. This finding has been demonstrated in vitro as a result of oxidants in cigarette smoke or oxidants released from inflammatory leukocytes, resulting in a marked reduction in the α_1-AT inhibitory capacity [229,232]. However, as noted previously, the acute effects of cigarette smoke

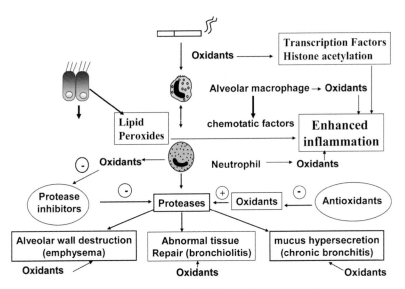

Fig. 6. The role of oxidants in pathogenic mechanisms in COPD. Oxidants released from cigarette smoke or from alveolar macrophages and neutrophils cause the release of chemotactic factors from epithelial cells, increasing leukocyte influx into the lungs. Lipid peroxidation products resulting from oxidant effects on the cell membrane act as chemotactic factors, and work together with other oxidant-mediated transcription factor, histone acetylation, or decreased deacetylation to enhance inflammation. Oxidants can inhibit antiproteases, leading to protease imbalance and alveolar wall destruction and emphysema. Oxidants may also activate proteases, and may also cause direct injury to alveolar walls, resulting in apoptosis. Oxidants are involved in abnormal tissue repair and in mucus hypersecretion.

on the functional activity of α_1-AT in vivo show only a transient and nonsignificant fall in the antiprotease activity in BAL 1 hour after smoking [137]. Thus, the hypothesis of oxidant-mediated protease/antiprotease imbalance as a relevant pathogenic mechanism in COPD remains unproven.

Oxidative stress may also have a direct effect on the epithelium, causing increased epithelial permeability. Injury to the epithelium is an important early event following exposure to cigarette smoke. This effect has been shown both in vivo and by in vitro experiments to result from oxidative injury to the epithelium. Extra- and intracellular GSH appears to be critical to the maintenance of epithelial integrity following exposure to cigarette smoke [233]. Studies show that the increased epithelial permeability of epithelial cell monolayers in vitro, and in rat lungs in vivo following exposure to cigarette smoke condensate, is associated with profound changes in the homeostasis of the antioxidant GSH [176,233–235]. Similar results to these in vitro and animal studies were shown in human studies demonstrating increased epithelial permeability in chronic smokers compared with nonsmokers, with a further increase in epithelial permeability following acute

smoking [176]. Thus, cigarette smoke has a detrimental effect on alveolar epithelial cell function which is, in part, oxidant-mediated, because antioxidants provide protection against this injurious event.

Moreover, components of the lung matrix (eg, elastin and collagen) can be directly damaged by oxidants in cigarette smoke. Furthermore, cigarette smoke can interfere with elastin synthesis and repair, potentially leading to the development of emphysema.

Another major site of free radical attack is on polyunsaturated fatty acids in cell membranes producing lipid peroxidation, a process that may continue as a chain reaction to generate hydroperoxides and long-lived aldehydes. Levels of products of lipid peroxidation are significantly increased in plasma and BALF in healthy smokers and in patients who have acute exacerbations of COPD, compared with healthy nonsmokers [171,176,236,237].

Several studies demonstrate increased levels of oxidants in exhaled air or breath condensates [238]. Patients who have COPD have an increased concentration of H_2O_2 in exhaled breath condensate [200]. Concentrations of lipid peroxidation products in exhaled breath condensate are increased even in patients who are ex-smokers [208,239]. Furthermore, evidence indicates that oxidative stress can cause increased lipid peroxidation in lung tissue in COPD patients, compared with smokers who have a similar smoking history but have not developed the disease [217]. In that study, the level of lipid peroxidation correlated with the degree of airflow limitation.

The major antioxidants in respiratory tract lining fluid include mucin, reduced GSH, uric acid, protein (largely albumin), and ascorbic acid [240]. Information on respiratory epithelial antioxidant defenses in smokers is limited, and even more limited on those in COPD patients. Although, as noted, studies have shown that GSH is elevated in BALF from chronic smokers [176], GSH may not be present in sufficient quantities to deal with the excessive oxidant burden during acute smoking, because cigarette smoke exposure depletes GSH in a dose- and time-dependent manner [241].

Reduced levels of vitamin E are present in the BALF of smokers, compared with nonsmokers [242]. By contrast, other studies found a marginal increase in vitamin C in the BALF of smokers, compared with nonsmokers [243]. The apparent discrepancy may be due to different smoking histories in chronic smokers, particularly the time of the last cigarette in relation to the sampling of BALF. Expression of GSH peroxidase and superoxide dismutase, another antioxidant enzyme, is elevated in the lungs of rats exposed to cigarette smoke [222,244].

The critical role of oxidative stress in the pathogenesis of emphysema has recently been emphasized by experiments in animals with increased susceptibility to oxidative stress. The master antioxidant transcription factor Nrf2 can be activated by oxidants, and translates to the nucleus of cells binding to an antioxidant response element located in the DNA promoter region of several antioxidant genes, such as hemoxygenase-1, GSH reductase, GSH peroxidase, and GCL. Nrf2, therefore, activates critical cellular pathways that protect against oxidative injury or inflammation, injury/immunity, and apoptosis. Mice lacking Nrf2 are highly susceptible to cigarette smoke [245,246] and demonstrate enhanced inflammatory response and increased neutrophil elastase activity in BAL, associated with increased markers of oxidative stress, increased apoptosis of alveolar cells [246], and decreased antiproteases such as secretory leukoprotease inhibitor [245], when compared with wild-type mice. These Nrf2-null mice also show

enhanced development of emphysema following instillation of elastase [125].

Oxidants may also be involved in mucus hypersecretion in chronic bronchitis. Oxidant-generating systems such as xanthine/xanthine oxidase have been shown to cause airway epithelial cell mucus secretion. Oxidants are also involved in the signaling pathways for EGF, which has an important role in mucus production [113]. Hydrogen peroxide and superoxide have also been shown to cause increased mucus secretion [247] and significant impairment of ciliary function after short-term exposure in low concentrations [248]. These effects may have important implications in the pathogenesis of chronic bronchitic element in COPD.

Mechanisms by which inflammation may be enhanced in chronic obstructive pulmonary disease

Latent viral infection

Possible mechanisms related to the abnormal regulation of inflammation in COPD are shown in Fig. 7. Studies have suggested that susceptibility to COPD may be related to latent adenoviral infection (see Fig. 7). These studies have demonstrated the ability of adenoviral E1A proteins, which associate with DNA, to enhance the binding of a number of transcription factors to their nuclear consensus sites, to activate subsequently various genes [249]. The E1A protein occurs more commonly in the lungs of smokers who have COPD than in smokers who have not developed the disease [250]. Furthermore, it has been shown in an animal model that latent adenoviral infection increases the inflammation that follows exposure to cigarette smoke [251]. Transfection of an E1A-type human epithelial cell line results in increased activation of NF-κB, and consequently, increased release of IL-8 in response to cell activation and increased production of TGF-β, suggesting a molecular mechanism for the amplification of inflammatory response [252,253].

Transcription factor activation

Many different pathways are activated during the inflammatory response; however, studies have focused on NF-κB as a crucial controlling factor in the inflammatory response in COPD because it is activated by many stimuli known to be increased in COPD lungs, including cytokines such as IL-1β and TNF-α, oxidative stress, viruses, and environmental particles [254]. NF-κB is expressed

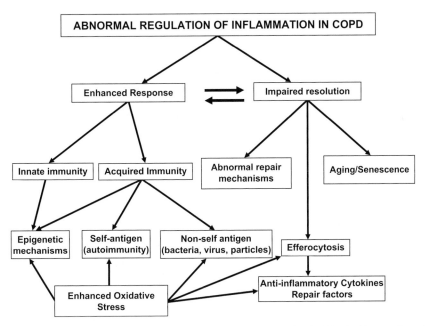

Fig. 7. Possible mechanisms related to the abnormal regulation of inflammation in COPD. Abnormal regulation of inflammation in COPD can result from either an enhanced response, impaired resolution, or an interaction between these two. Augmented inflammatory responses can result from enhanced innate or acquired immunity. Enhanced innate immunity may result from abnormal epigenetic mechanisms triggered by enhanced oxidative stress and from enhanced acquired immunity as a result of self (antigens and particles), nonself (bacteria, viruses, particles), or self-antigen–backed-up immunity. Impaired resolution can result from impaired efferocytosis, abnormal repair mechanisms, or aging/senescence. Efferocytosis reduces anti-inflammatory cytokine and repair factor release. Oxidative stress is involved in autoimmunity, efferocytosis, and impairment of repair.

ubiquitously within cells and controls induction of inflammatory genes. It also enhances other cell- and signaling-specific transcription factors. NF-κB also stimulates cell survival by means of enhanced expression of the prosurvival Bcl-2 family and cell proliferation–related genes (c-MYC, cyclin D1) [254]. NF-κB exists as a heterodimeric complex usually of p50 and p65/RelA subunits [255]. In unstimulated cells, it is found in the cytoplasm in an inactive form associated with an inhibitor protein (inhibitor of κB [IκB]), which masks the nuclear translocation signal and prevents NF-κB from entering the nucleus. On cell stimulation, NF-κB alpha is rapidly phosphorylated, which targets the inhibitor protein for ubiquitination and degradation in the proteasome. The activated Nf-κB dimer can then translocate to the nucleus and activate target genes by binding to high affinity κB elements and their promoters [255]. In addition to this classic pathway of NF-κB activation, an alternative pathway responds to certain members of the TNF family and involves upstream kinase NF-κB inducing kinase,

which activates IκB, leading to phosphorylation and processing of p100, which is degraded to p52 by the proteasome. IκB alpha levels have been shown to be significantly decreased, whereas NF-κB DNA binding was significantly increased in healthy smokers and current smokers with moderate COPD compared with healthy non-smokers [256]. The degree of DNA NF-κB binding was similar in ex-smokers with COPD and in healthy smokers. The study suggested that ongoing cigarette smoking may increase NF-κB DNA binding in individuals with or without COPD.

A further study, however, showed that macrophage expression of NF-κB and activator protein 1 was decreased in BAL leukocytes from smokers and patients who had severe exacerbations of COPD, when compared with nonsmokers [224]. The mechanism of NF-κB activation in cigarette smoking is still debated.

Histone acetylation/deacetylation

Gene activation by transcription factors depends on a number of factors, among which is the

DNA remodeling by the nuclear histone acetyla-tion/deacetylation balance, which depends on the activities of histone acetyl-transferases and his-tone deacetylases (HDACs) [170]. In the resting cell, DNA is coiled around a nucleosome core comprising the histones H2A, H2B, H3, and H4. This configuration suppresses the accessibility of transcription factors such as Nf-κB to their cog-nate DNA sequences. Acetylastion of the lysine residues in the internal tails of the core histones results in uncoiling of the DNA, making the chro-matin less condensed and increasing the accessibil-ity of transcription factors and RNA polymerase to the transcriptional machinery and hence in-creased gene transcription. Deacetylation is under the influence of HDACs and results in rewinding of the DNA around the histone proteins, decreas-ing gene transcription.

Macrophages of cigarette smokers show a de-crease in HDAC activity [257], as has also been shown in the lungs of smoke-exposed animals [258]. Exposure of human alveolar epithelial cells and macrophage-like cells to cigarette smoke ex-tract produced reduced HDAC activity and pro-tein [259,260]. In rats exposed to cigarette smoke, HDAC2 activity and protein expression were significantly decreased after 3 days of expo-sure, whereas histone-3 phosphoacetylation and histone-4 acetylation increased at 8 weeks of exposure [258]. These changes were associated with nitrotyrosine, 4-hydroxynonenal, and alde-hyde-modified HDAC proteins, resulting in decreased HDAC activity.

Studies of resected lung indicate that HDAC activity is also reduced in lung tissue in COPD, associated with lower HDAC 2, 5, and 8 mRNA levels, and expression of HDAC 2 protein [256,261]. This decrease in HDACs increased with disease severity and was associated with an increase in histone-4 acetylation at the IL-8 pro-moter and increased IL-8 mRNA expression. Thus, collectively, reduction in HDACs may be another mechanism by which inflammation may be amplified in the airways and lung parenchyma of patients who have COPD, by way of dysregula-tion of transcription factor activation pathways.

Evidence indicates that smoking cessation does not resolve the inflammatory response in the airways, particularly in advanced COPD. Molec-ular mechanisms such as transcription factor activation and chromatin remodeling, perhaps as a result of increased oxidative stress, might be one mechanism responsible for perpetuating the in-flammatory process (see Fig. 7) [262].

Apoptosis and emphysema

As explained earlier, the traditional paradigm for the alveolar wall destruction in emphysema has been that increased inflammatory response results in a protease/antiprotease imbalance. It has been suggested that a central feature of emphysema (ie, loss of alveolar cells) is caused by increased cell apoptosis [263,264].

Studies over the past 5 years have documented that increased lung cell apoptosis occurs in emphysematous lungs, predominantly involving endothelial cells in the alveolar walls, compared with normal or non-COPD smokers' lungs [265]. Experimental emphysema in animals can be pro-duced by decreased vascular endothelial growth factor (VEGF) or VEGF signaling [263,266], and studies in human lungs demonstrated de-creased expression of VEGF and VEGFR 2 ex-pression in association with emphysema [265]. This finding led to the concept of an alveolar maintenance program that was required for struc-tural preservation of the lungs. Cigarette smoke was thought to cause destruction of this mainte-nance program, thus causing emphysema [267]. Several experimental models have supported this hypothesis. Rat lungs treated with a VEGFR blocker developed apoptosis-dependent emphy-sema [263]. Similarly, emphysema also developed in animals in which the VEGF gene was depleted in the lungs [266]. Alveolar septal cell apoptosis has been confirmed also in COPD lungs and has been shown to correlate with a decrease in alveo-lar surface area [268]. Other support comes from studies in strains of mice with low lung levels of VEGF, where enhanced alveolar apoptosis and emphysema occur on exposure to cigarette smoke [269]. Firm evidence that apoptosis could initiate alveolar wall destruction and alveolar enlarge-ment is provided by studies in which active cas-pase 3 was instilled in animals, thus causing acute apoptosis and alveolar enlargement, a fea-ture that was reversible 1 week after the initial cas-pase instillation [270]. Experimental studies also showed that a broad spectrum caspase inhibitor prevented VEGFR-blockade–induced emphy-sema [263] and that oxidative stress was involved in these processes such that an antioxidant treat-ment [218] but also strategies to increase plasma levels of α₁-AT [271] prevented apoptosis and em-physema. The interaction between apoptosis and its interaction with lung elastolysis has been shown by the fact that lung cell apoptosis was re-quired for cigarette smoke–induced mouse emphysema, and the cathepsin S was mechanistically upstream of lung cell apoptosis and alveolar enlargement [74]. Apoptotic cells also have been shown to release intracellular proteases, oxidants, and inflammatory mediators and also express several caspases on their cell surface [272]. The precise pathways for cigarette smoke–induced emphysema have not been determined, although evidence indicates increased expression of Bax in COPD lungs, suggesting that cigarette smoke–induced emphysema may activate this pathway of apoptosis [268].

The effect of alveolar cell death by apoptosis on alveolar structure depends on the lungs' ability to undergo cell proliferation. No clear picture exists on the balance of apoptosis versus cell proliferation in COPD patients. One study has shown that patients who had emphysema had higher rates of both apoptosis and cell proliferation than healthy smokers or nonsmokers [273]. In another study, no correlation was shown between apoptosis and cell proliferation [268]. However, a further study has reported an increase in apoptosis, but not in cell proliferation, in emphysematous lungs [274].

The ability of the lungs to clear apoptotic cells, efferocytosis, may also play a role in the balance between apoptosis and cell proliferation [272]. Some evidence suggests that efferocytosis may be impaired in COPD patients. Specifically, efferocytosis of apoptotic airway epithelial cells by macrophages from COPD patients is significantly decreased, when compared with control macrophages [275].

Inadequate repair mechanisms

Inadequate repair may be another important mechanism that contributes to the development of emphysema [276]. Cigarette smoke extract has been shown to impair significantly human airway epithelial cell chemotaxis, proliferation, and contraction of these cells plated onto three-dimensional gels in vitro as a model of extracellular matrix remodeling [277]. Studies have also shown that the impairment of function of these cells was associated with inhibition of TGF-β and fibronectin synthesis. TGF-β inhibits cellular proliferation and also regulates cellular differentiation in extracellular matrix production. Thus, reduced activity of TGF-β may result in destruction of the alveolar structure. Animal studies have shown that regulation of TGF-β signaling is critical in repair processes and in lung development [278–280].

Human studies have shown that the expression of TGF-β1 and TGF-β1 receptor is significantly reduced in COPD patients, when compared with control subjects [281]. Cigarette smoke also has profound systemic effects on the bone marrow affecting circulating precursor cells. Circulating endothelial cell progenitor cells (EPCs) from chronic smokers have altered functional properties [282]. The numbers of EPCs that adhere to cultured endothelial cells in response to TNF is lower in smokers than in control subjects. These changes were associated with a higher formation of ROS and lower serum antioxidant and nitrite in smokers' EPCs. In patients who had moderate to severe COPD, $CD34^+$ or $AC133^+$ or circulating hemopoietic endothelial cells were reduced in number, compared with controls, and showed decreased function as assessed by a decrease in their ability to form colonies [283]. In these patients, exercise capacity and FEV_1 correlated inversely with the $CD34^+$ cell counts. The role of circulating progenitor cells in lung repair in emphysema remains unclear.

Acquired immunity

It has been suggested that abnormalities in the acquired immune system could contribute to the persistence of inflammation in COPD [40]. As mentioned, some evidence suggests that airway inflammation persists in COPD patients after smoking cessation [284]. Moreover, at later stages of the disease (GOLD stage III and IV), lymphoid follicles develop in the airways and T lymphocyte clusters occur in the lung parenchyma and airway mucosa in patients who have COPD [13,89]. These findings suggest an enhanced acquired immune response to an antigen. These antigens can be either self or nonself antigens. Foreign (nonself) antigens may result from infections with various organisms in COPD [285]. Persistent infection (either bacterial or viral) without full recovery may contribute to the development of foreign antigens, which fuel the inflammatory response. It is also possible that components of cigarette smoke causing lung tissue damage might result in novel antigens being presented to antigen-presenting cells that result in antibodies against lung cells. Experimental studies have supported the hypothesis that autoimmunity may contribute to the development of emphysema. Xenogeneic human umbilical endothelial cells (HUVECs) or human pulmonary artery smooth muscle cells injected into rats produced antibodies against these cells. However, only rats injected with HUVECs developed pulmonary emphysema [286]. Emphysema could also be produced in naive animals after passive transfer of $CD4^+$ T cells of serum from emphysematous animals [286]. This model of autoimmune emphysema also confirmed the central role of lung cell apoptosis in the alveolar destruction. Recently, additional support for the hypothesis of an autoimmune component for the pathogenesis of emphysema has come from studies where oligoclonal $CD4^+$ T cells were found in patients who had severe emphysema in contrast to control lungs [287], suggesting a response to antigen in the COPD patients. T and B lymphocyte responses to elastin peptide have been demonstrated in T and B cells obtained from emphysematous subjects compared with controls and asthmatics [288]. Collectively, these data suggest that autoimmunity to self or nonself antigens may be a mechanism of the persistent inflammatory response in COPD, leading ultimately to the pathologic changes of emphysema.

Aging senescence and emphysema

Age is an important independent risk factor for cigarette smoke–induced COPD. With age comes progressive airspace enlargement in the lungs; this enlargement is considered to be a nondestructive process, compared with the alveolar wall destruction that occurs in smokers' emphysema. Studies have suggested markers of enhanced aging in emphysematous lungs and in COPD patients. Mononuclear cells from patients who have COPD have decreased telomere length (a marker of cell senescence), when compared with normal individuals [289]. Other studies have shown that alveolar epithelial and endothelial cells of emphysematous patients show enhanced expression of markers of cell senescence, including p16 InK 4a and p21 CIP 1/WAF 1/Sdi1, and have telomere shortening, when compared with smokers without emphysema or with normal individuals [290]. Lung fibroblasts from emphysematous patients also show an increase in senescence markers [291]. Senescence cells show increased cytokine/chemokine production and enhanced matrix protease activity, which could result in tissue destruction [292]. Oxidative stress from mitochondrial free radical generation is thought to be a central feature in the pathophysiologic changes of aging [293]. Cigarette smoke can cause cellular senescence in human alveolar epithelial cells;

this effect can be prevented by the antioxidant N-acetylcysteine [294].

A link between aging and cigarette smoke emphysema has been studied in animal models of premature aging. Senescence-accelerated mice develop premature aging and also lung airspace enlargement [295]. Exposure of these senescence-accelerated mice to cigarette smoke showed enhanced alveolar enlargement, compared with those who were not exposed [295]. The Klotho protein is an alpha glycosidase associated with protection against aging [296,297]. Klotho-deficient mice develop premature airspace enlargement very soon after birth [298]. The senescence marker protein-30 (SMP-30) has been studied in animals in which this protein has been knocked out. These animals develop age-related changes in the lungs, including alveolar enlargement resembling emphysema [299,300]. The development of emphysema in SMP-30 knock-out mice is associated with increased markers of oxidative stress [301]. When these mice were exposed to cigarette smoke, marked alveolar enlargement with further enhanced expression of markers of oxidative stress and alveolar cell apoptosis occurred [301]. This occurrence demonstrates a synergistic effect of cigarette smoke and SMP-30 deficiency, which might contribute to enhanced alveolar destruction.

Summary

No single mechanism can account for the complex pathology in COPD. It is likely that interactions occur among different mechanisms, such as interactions among inflammation, protease/antiprotease imbalance, oxidative stress, and apoptosis as destructive processes in emphysema. Better understanding of the relative importance of these different pathogenic mechanisms and the processes that amplify and perpetuate them will come from proof-of-concept therapeutic intervention studies.

References

[1] Celli BR, MacNee W. Standards for the diagnosis and treatment of patients with COPD: a summary of the ATS/ERS position paper. Eur Respir J 2004;23(6):932–46.
[2] Fletcher C, Peto R. The natural history of chronic airflow obstruction. Br Med J 1977;1(6077):1645–8.
[3] Hogg JC. Pathophysiology of airflow limitation in chronic obstructive pulmonary disease. Lancet 2004;364(9435):709–21.

[4] Jeffery PK. Comparison of the structural and inflammatory features of COPD and asthma. Giles F. Filley Lecture. Chest 2000;117(5 Suppl 1): 251S–60S.

[5] Vestbo J, Lange P. Can GOLD stage 0 provide information of prognostic value in chronic obstructive pulmonary disease? Am J Respir Crit Care Med 2002;166(3):329–32.

[6] Vestbo J, Prescott E, Lange P. Association of chronic mucus hypersecretion with FEV1 decline and chronic obstructive pulmonary disease morbidity. Copenhagen City Heart Study Group. Am J Respir Crit Care Med 1996;153(5):1530–5.

[7] Sommerhoff CP, Nadel JA, Basbaum CB, et al. Neutrophil elastase and cathepsin G stimulate secretion from cultured bovine airway gland serous cells. J Clin Invest 1990;85(3):682–9.

[8] Shao MX, Nakanaga T, Nadel JA. Cigarette smoke induces MUC5AC mucin overproduction via tumor necrosis factor-alpha-converting enzyme in human airway epithelial (NCI-H292) cells. Am J Physiol Lung Cell Mol Physiol 2004;287(2): L420–7.

[9] Snider GL, Kleinerman J, Thurlbeck WM, et al. The definition of emphysema: report of a National Heart Lung and Blood Institute, Division of Lung Diseases workshop. Am Rev Respir Dis 1985;132: 182–5.

[10] Kim WD, Eidelman DH, Izquierdo JL, et al. Centrilobular and panlobular emphysema in smokers. Two distinct morphologic and functional entities. Am Rev Respir Dis 1991;144(6):1385–90.

[11] Hogg JC, Macklem PT, Thurlbeck WM. Site and nature of airway obstruction in chronic obstructive lung disease. N Engl J Med 1968;278(25):1355–60.

[12] Niewoehner DE, Kleinerman J, Rice DB. Pathologic changes in the peripheral airways of young cigarette smokers. N Engl J Med 1974;291(15): 755–8.

[13] Hogg JC, Chu F, Utokaparch S, et al. The nature of small-airway obstruction in chronic obstructive pulmonary disease. N Engl J Med 2004;350(26): 2645–53.

[14] Saetta M, Di Stefano A, Maestrelli P, et al. Activated T-lymphocytes and macrophages in bronchial mucosa of subjects with chronic bronchitis. Am Rev Respir Dis 1993;147(2):301–6.

[15] Vaart van der H, Postma DS, Timens W, et al. Acute effects of cigarette smoke on inflammation and oxidative stress: a review. Thorax 2004;59(8): 713–21.

[16] Cosio MG, Majo J, Cosio MG. Inflammation of the airways and lung parenchyma in COPD: role of T cells. Chest 2002;121(Suppl 5):160S–5S.

[17] Willemse BW, Postma DS, Timens W, et al. The impact of smoking cessation on respiratory symptoms, lung function, airway hyperresponsiveness and inflammation. Eur Respir J 2004;23(3): 464–76.

[18] Wright JL, Hobson JE, Wiggs B, et al. Airway inflammation and peribronchiolar attachments in the lungs of nonsmokers, current and ex-smokers. Lung 1988;166(5):277–86.

[19] Mullen JB, Wright JL, Wiggs BR, et al. Structure of central airways in current smokers and ex-smokers with and without mucus hypersecretion: relationship to lung function. Thorax 1987;42(11): 843–8.

[20] Willemse BW, ten Hacken NH, Rutgers B, et al. Effect of 1-year smoking cessation on airway inflammation in COPD and asymptomatic smokers. Eur Respir J 2005;26(5):835–45.

[21] Saetta M, Turato G, Luppi F. Inflammation in the pathogenesis of chronic obstructive pulmonary disease. In: Voelkel NF, MacNee W, editors. Chronic obstructive lung disease. Ontario (Canada): BC Decker; 2002. p. 114–26.

[22] O'Shaughnessy TC, Ansari TW, Barnes N, et al. Reticular basement membrane thickness in moderately severe asthma and smokers' chronic bronchitis with and without airflow obstruction. Am J Respir Crit Care Med 1996;153:A879.

[23] Di Stefano A, Caramori G, Ricciardolo FL, et al. Cellular and molecular mechanisms in chronic obstructive pulmonary disease: an overview. Clin Exp Allergy 2004;34(8):1156–67.

[24] Saetta M, Turato G, Baraldo S, et al. Goblet cell hyperplasia and epithelial inflammation in peripheral airways of smokers with both symptoms of chronic bronchitis and chronic airflow limitation. Am J Respir Crit Care Med 2000;161(3 Pt 1): 1016–21.

[25] Lams BE, Sousa AR, Rees PJ, et al. Subepithelial immunopathology of the large airways in smokers with and without chronic obstructive pulmonary disease. Eur Respir J 2000;15(3):512–6.

[26] Ollerenshaw SL, Woolcock AJ. Characteristics of the inflammation in biopsies from large airways of subjects with asthma and subjects with chronic airflow limitation. Am Rev Respir Dis 1992; 145(4 Pt 1):922–7.

[27] Di Stefano A, Caramori G, Oates T, et al. Increased expression of nuclear factor-kappa B in bronchial biopsies from smokers and patients with COPD. Eur Respir J 2002;20(3):556–63.

[28] Di Stefano A, Capelli A, Lusuardi M, et al. Decreased T lymphocyte infiltration in bronchial biopsies of subjects with severe chronic obstructive pulmonary disease. Clin Exp Allergy 2001;31(6): 893–902.

[29] O'Shaughnessy TC, Ansari TW, Barnes NC, et al. Inflammation in bronchial biopsies of subjects with chronic bronchitis: inverse relationship of CD8+ T lymphocytes with FEV1. Am J Respir Crit Care Med 1997;155(3):852–7.

[30] Zhu J, Qiu YS, Majumdar S, et al. Exacerbations of bronchitis: bronchial eosinophilia and gene expression for interleukin-4, interleukin-5, and eosinophil

chemoattractants. Am J Respir Crit Care Med 2001;164(1):109–16.

[31] Chrysofakis G, Tzanakis N, Kyriakoy D, et al. Perforin expression and cytotoxic activity of sputum CD8+ lymphocytes in patients with COPD. Chest 2004;125(1):71–6.

[32] Tzanakis N, Chrysofakis G, Tsoumakidou M, et al. Induced sputum CD8+ T-lymphocyte subpopulations in chronic obstructive pulmonary disease. Respir Med 2004;98(1):57–65.

[33] Saetta M, Turato G, Facchini FM, et al. Inflammatory cells in the bronchial glands of smokers with chronic bronchitis. Am J Respir Crit Care Med 1997;156(5):1633–9.

[34] Baraldo S, Turato G, Badin C, et al. Neutrophilic infiltration within the airway smooth muscle in patients with COPD. Thorax 2004;59(4):308–12.

[35] Saetta M, Di Stefano A, Turato G, et al. CD8+ T-lymphocytes in peripheral airways of smokers with chronic obstructive pulmonary disease. Am J Respir Crit Care Med 1998;157(3 Pt 1):822–6.

[36] Kim WD, Kim WS, Koh Y, et al. Abnormal peripheral blood T-lymphocyte subsets in a subgroup of patients with COPD. Chest 2002;122(2):437–44.

[37] Majori M, Corradi M, Caminati A, et al. Predominant TH1 cytokine pattern in peripheral blood from subjects with chronic obstructive pulmonary disease. J Allergy Clin Immunol 1999;103(3 Pt 1):458–62.

[38] Retamales I, Elliott WM, Meshi B, et al. Amplification of inflammation in emphysema and its association with latent adenoviral infection. Am J Respir Crit Care Med 2001;164(3):469–73.

[39] Bruder D, Srikiatkhachorn A, Enelow RI. Cellular immunity and lung injury in respiratory virus infection. Viral Immunol 2006;19(2):147–55.

[40] Agusti A, MacNee W, Donaldson K, et al. Hypothesis: does COPD have an autoimmune component? Thorax 2003;58(10):832–4.

[41] Bracke K, Cataldo D, Maes T, et al. Matrix metalloproteinase-12 and cathepsin D expression in pulmonary macrophages and dendritic cells of cigarette smoke-exposed mice. Int Arch Allergy Immunol 2005;138(2):169–79.

[42] Majo J, Ghezzo H, Cosio MG. Lymphocyte population and apoptosis in the lungs of smokers and their relation to emphysema. Eur Respir J 2001;17(5):946–53.

[43] Yasuda N, Gotoh K, Minatoguchi S, et al. An increase of soluble Fas, an inhibitor of apoptosis, associated with progression of COPD. Respir Med 1998;92(8):993–9.

[44] Takabatake N, Nakamura H, Inoue S, et al. Circulating levels of soluble Fas ligand and soluble Fas in patients with chronic obstructive pulmonary disease. Respir Med 2000;94(12):1215–20.

[45] Keatings VM, Collins PD, Scott DM, et al. Differences in interleukin-8 and tumor-necrosis-factor-alpha in induced sputum from patients with chronic obstructive pulmonary disease or asthma. Am J Respir Crit Care Med 1996;153:530–4.

[46] MacNee W, Wiggs B, Belzberg AS, et al. The effect of cigarette smoking on neutrophil kinetics in human lungs. N Engl J Med 1989;321(14):924–8.

[47] Terashima T, Wiggs B, English D, et al. Phagocytosis of small carbon particles (PM10) by alveolar macrophages stimulates the release of polymorphonuclear leukocytes from bone marrow. Am J Respir Crit Care Med 1997;155(4):1441–7.

[48] Takanashi S, Hasegawa Y, Kanehira Y, et al. Interleukin-10 level in sputum is reduced in bronchial asthma, COPD and in smokers. Eur Respir J 1999;14(2):309–14.

[49] Pilette C, Godding V, Kiss R, et al. Reduced epithelial expression of secretory component in small airways correlates with airflow obstruction in chronic obstructive pulmonary disease. Am J Respir Crit Care Med 2001;163(1):185–94.

[50] De Boer WI, Sont JK, van Schadewijk A, et al. Monocyte chemoattractant protein 1, interleukin 8, and chronic airways inflammation in COPD. J Pathol 2000;190(5):619–26.

[51] Di Stefano A, Maestrelli P, Roggeri A, et al. Upregulation of adhesion molecules in the bronchial mucosa of subjects with chronic obstructive bronchitis. Am J Respir Crit Care Med 1994;149(3 Pt 1):803–10.

[52] Chung KF. Cytokines in chronic obstructive pulmonary disease. Eur Respir J Suppl 2001;34:50s–9s.

[53] Chung KF. Cytokines as targets in chronic obstructive pulmonary disease. Curr Drug Targets 2006;7(6):675–81.

[54] Gompertz S, O'Brien C, Bayley DL, et al. Changes in bronchial inflammation during acute exacerbations of chronic bronchitis. Eur Respir J 2001;17(6):1112–9.

[55] Sparrow D, Glynn RJ, Cohen M, et al. The relationship of the peripheral leukocyte count and cigarette smoking to pulmonary function among adult men. Chest 1984;86(3):383–6.

[56] Di Stefano A, Capelli A, Lusuardi M, et al. Severity of airflow limitation is associated with severity of airway inflammation in smokers. Am J Respir Crit Care Med 1998;158(4):1277–85.

[57] Stanescu D, Sanna A, Veriter C, et al. Airways obstruction, chronic expectoration, and rapid decline of FEV1 in smokers are associated with increased levels of sputum neutrophils. Thorax 1996;51(3):267–71.

[58] Russell RE, Culpitt SV, DeMatos C, et al. Release and activity of matrix metalloproteinase-9 and tissue inhibitor of metalloproteinase-1 by alveolar macrophages from patients with chronic obstructive pulmonary disease. Am J Respir Cell Mol Biol 2002;26(5):602–9.

[59] Lim S, Roche N, Oliver BG, et al. Balance of matrix metalloprotease-9 and tissue inhibitor of

metalloprotease-1 from alveolar macrophages in cigarette smokers. Regulation by interleukin-10. Am J Respir Crit Care Med 2000;162(4 Pt 1): 1355–60.

[60] Capelli A, Di Stefano A, Gnemmi I, et al. Increased MCP-1 and MIP-1beta in bronchoalveolar lavage fluid of chronic bronchitics. Eur Respir J 1999; 14(1):160–5.

[61] Traves SL, Smith SJ, Barnes PJ, et al. Increased migration of monocytes from COPD patients towards GRO-alpha is not mediated by an increase in CSCR2 receptor expression. Am J Respir Crit Care Med 2003;165:A824.

[62] Soler P, Moreau A, Basset F, et al. Cigarette smoking-induced changes in the number and differentiated state of pulmonary dendritic cells/Langerhans cells. Am Rev Respir Dis 1989;139(5):1112–7.

[63] Takizawa H, Tanaka M, Takami K, et al. Increased expression of transforming growth factor-beta1 in small airway epithelium from tobacco smokers and patients with chronic obstructive pulmonary disease (COPD). Am J Respir Crit Care Med 2001;163(6):1476–83.

[64] Caramori G, Romagnoli M, Casolari P, et al. Nuclear localisation of p65 in sputum macrophages but not in sputum neutrophils during COPD exacerbations. Thorax 2003;58(4):348–51.

[65] Zhu J, Majumdar S, Qiu Y, et al. Interleukin-4 and interleukin-5 gene expression and inflammation in the mucus-secreting glands and subepithelial tissue of smokers with chronic bronchitis. Lack of relationship with CD8(+) cells. Am J Respir Crit Care Med 2001;164(12):2220–8.

[66] Grashoff WF, Sont JK, Sterk PJ, et al. Chronic obstructive pulmonary disease: role of bronchiolar mast cells and macrophages. Am J Pathol 1997; 151(6):1785–90.

[67] De Boer WI, van Schadewijk A, Sont JK, et al. Transforming growth factor beta1 and recruitment of macrophages and mast cells in airways in chronic obstructive pulmonary disease. Am J Respir Crit Care Med 1998;158(6):1951–7.

[68] Lams BE, Sousa AR, Rees PJ, et al. Immunopathology of the small-airway submucosa in smokers with and without chronic obstructive pulmonary disease. Am J Respir Crit Care Med 1998; 158(5 Pt 1):1518–23.

[69] Bosken CH, Hards J, Gatter K, et al. Characterization of the inflammatory reaction in the peripheral airways of cigarette smokers using immunocytochemistry. Am Rev Respir Dis 1992;145(4 Pt 1): 911–7.

[70] Grumelli S, Corry DB, Song LZ, et al. An immune basis for lung parenchymal destruction in chronic obstructive pulmonary disease and emphysema. PLoS Med 2004;1(1):e8.

[71] Wang Z, Zheng T, Zhu Z, et al. Interferon gamma induction of pulmonary emphysema in the adult murine lung. J Exp Med 2000;192(11):1587–600.

[72] Zheng T, Zhu Z, Wang Z, et al. Inducible targeting of IL-13 to the adult lung causes matrix metalloproteinase- and cathepsin-dependent emphysema. J Clin Invest 2000;106(9):1081–93.

[73] Lanone S, Zheng T, Zhu Z, et al. Overlapping and enzyme-specific contributions of matrix metalloproteinases-9 and -12 in IL-13-induced inflammation and remodeling. J Clin Invest 2002;110(4): 463–74.

[74] Zheng T, Kang MJ, Crothers K, et al. Role of cathepsin S-dependent epithelial cell apoptosis in IFN-gamma-induced alveolar remodeling and pulmonary emphysema. J Immunol 2005;174(12): 8106–15.

[75] Bracke KR, D'hulst AI, Maes T, et al. Cigarette smoke-induced pulmonary inflammation and emphysema are attenuated in CCR6-deficient mice. J Immunol 2006;177(7):4350–9.

[76] Fujita M, Shannon JM, Irvin CG, et al. Overexpression of tumor necrosis factor-alpha produces an increase in lung volumes and pulmonary hypertension. Am J Physiol Lung Cell Mol Physiol 2001; 280(1):L39–49.

[77] Churg A, Wang RD, Tai H, et al. Tumor necrosis factor-alpha drives 70% of cigarette smoke-induced emphysema in the mouse. Am J Respir Crit Care Med 2004;170(5):492–8.

[78] Vernooy JH, Kucukaycan M, Jacobs JA, et al. Local and systemic inflammation in patients with chronic obstructive pulmonary disease: soluble tumor necrosis factor receptors are increased in sputum. Am J Respir Crit Care Med 2002;166(9): 1218–24.

[79] D'hulst AI, Bracke KR, Maes T, et al. Role of tumour necrosis factor-alpha receptor p75 in cigarette smoke-induced pulmonary inflammation and emphysema. Eur Respir J 2006;28(1): 102–12.

[80] Lappalainen U, Whitsett JA, Wert SE, et al. Interleukin-1beta causes pulmonary inflammation, emphysema, and airway remodeling in the adult murine lung. Am J Respir Cell Mol Biol 2005; 32(4):311–8.

[81] Castro P, Legora-Machado A, Cardilo-Reis L, et al. Inhibition of interleukin-1beta reduces mouse lung inflammation induced by exposure to cigarette smoke. Eur J Pharmacol 2004;498(1–3):279–86.

[82] Lucey EC, Keane J, Kuang PP, et al. Severity of elastase-induced emphysema is decreased in tumor necrosis factor-alpha and interleukin-1beta receptor-deficient mice. Lab Invest 2002;82(1):79–85.

[83] Rutgers SR, Postma DS, ten Hacken NH, et al. Ongoing airway inflammation in patients with COPD who do not currently smoke. Thorax 2000;55(1): 12–8.

[84] Pesci A, Rossi GA, Bertorelli G, et al. Mast cells in the airway lumen and bronchial mucosa of patients with chronic bronchitis. Am J Respir Crit Care Med 1994;149(5):1311–6.

[85] Turato G, Di Stefano A, Maestrelli P, et al. Effect of smoking cessation on airway inflammation in chronic bronchitis. Am J Respir Crit Care Med 1995;152(4 Pt 1):1262–7.

[86] Cosio M, Ghezzo H, Hogg JC, et al. The relationship between structural changes in small airways and pulmonary-function tests. N Engl J Med 1978;298(23):1277–81.

[87] Saetta M, Ghezzo H, Kim WD, et al. Loss of alveolar attachments in smokers. A morphometric correlate of lung function impairment. Am Rev Respir Dis 1985;132(4):894–900.

[88] Nadel JA. Role of mast cell and neutrophil proteases in airway secretion. Am Rev Respir Dis 1991;144(3 Pt 2):S48–51.

[89] Saetta M, Baraldo S, Corbino L, et al. CD8+ve cells in the lungs of smokers with chronic obstructive pulmonary disease. Am J Respir Crit Care Med 1999;160(2):711–7.

[90] Paoletti P, Prediletto R, Carrozzi L, et al. Effects of childhood and adolescence-adulthood respiratory infections in a general population. Eur Respir J 1989;2(5):428–36.

[91] Matsuse T, Hayashi S, Kuwano K, et al. Latent adenoviral infection in the pathogenesis of chronic airways obstruction. Am Rev Respir Dis 1992; 146(1):177–84.

[92] Liu AN, Mohammed AZ, Rice WR, et al. Perforin-independent CD8(+) T-cell-mediated cytotoxicity of alveolar epithelial cells is preferentially mediated by tumor necrosis factor-alpha: relative insensitivity to Fas ligand. Am J Respir Cell Mol Biol 1999;20(5):849–58.

[93] Zhao MQ, Amir MK, Rice WR, et al. Type II pneumocyte-CD8+ T-cell interactions. Relationship between target cell cytotoxicity and activation. Am J Respir Cell Mol Biol 2001;25(3): 362–9.

[94] Enelow RI, Mohammed AZ, Stoler MH, et al. Structural and functional consequences of alveolar cell recognition by CD8(+) T lymphocytes in experimental lung disease. J Clin Invest 1998;102(9): 1653–61.

[95] Finkelstein R, Fraser RS, Ghezzo H, et al. Alveolar inflammation and its relation to emphysema in smokers. Am J Respir Crit Care Med 1995; 152(5 Pt 1):1666–72.

[96] Adesina AM, Vallyathan V, McQuillen EN, et al. Bronchiolar inflammation and fibrosis associated with smoking. A morphologic cross-sectional population analysis. Am Rev Respir Dis 1991;143(1): 144–9.

[97] Matsuba K, Wright JL, Wiggs BR, et al. The changes in airways structure associated with reduced forced expiratory volume in one second. Eur Respir J 1989;2(9):834–9.

[98] Hogg J. Peripheral lung remodelling in asthma and chronic obstructive pulmonary disease. Eur Respir J 2004;24(6):893–4.

[99] Kranenburg AR, De Boer WI, van Krieken JH, et al. Enhanced expression of fibroblast growth factors and receptor FGFR-1 during vascular remodeling in chronic obstructive pulmonary disease. Am J Respir Cell Mol Biol 2002;27(5):517–25.

[100] Kranenburg AR, Willems-Widyastuti A, Mooi WJ, et al. Chronic obstructive pulmonary disease is associated with enhanced bronchial expression of FGF-1, FGF-2, and FGFR-1. J Pathol 2005; 206(1):28–38.

[101] Guddo F, Vignola AM, Saetta M, et al. Upregulation of basic fibroblast growth factor in smokers with chronic bronchitis. Eur Respir J 2006;27(5): 957–63.

[102] Saetta M, Mariani M, Panina-Bordignon P, et al. Increased expression of the chemokine receptor CXCR3 and its ligand CXCL10 in peripheral airways of smokers with chronic obstructive pulmonary disease. Am J Respir Crit Care Med 2002; 165(10):1404–9.

[103] McDonough JE, Gosselink JV, Javadifard A, et al. Correlation between gene expression in airways to morphometry and the remodeling of the peripheral lung in COPD. Am J Respir Crit Care Med 2007; 175:A553.

[104] Rose MC, Voynow JA. Respiratory tract mucin genes and mucin glycoproteins in health and disease. Physiol Rev 2006;86(1):245–78.

[105] Caramori G, Di Gregorio C, Carlstedt I, et al. Mucin expression in peripheral airways of patients with chronic obstructive pulmonary disease. Histopathology 2004;45(5):477–84.

[106] Voynow JA, Gendler SJ, Rose MC. Regulation of mucin genes in chronic inflammatory airway diseases. Am J Respir Cell Mol Biol 2006;34(6):661–5.

[107] Voynow JA, Young LR, Wang Y, et al. Neutrophil elastase increases MUC5AC mRNA and protein expression in respiratory epithelial cells. Am J Physiol 1999;276(5 Pt 1):L835–43.

[108] Yanagihara K, Seki M, Cheng PW. Lipopolysaccharide induces mucus cell metaplasia in mouse lung. Am J Respir Cell Mol Biol 2001;24(1):66–73.

[109] Kim JH, Lee SY, Bak SM, et al. Effects of matrix metalloproteinase inhibitor on LPS-induced goblet cell metaplasia. Am J Physiol Lung Cell Mol Physiol 2004;287(1):L127–33.

[110] Lora JM, Zhang DM, Liao SM, et al. Tumor necrosis factor-alpha triggers mucus production in airway epithelium through an IkappaB kinase beta-dependent mechanism. J Biol Chem 2005; 280(43):36510–7.

[111] Song KS, Lee WJ, Chung KC, et al. Interleukin-1 beta and tumor necrosis factor-alpha induce MUC5AC overexpression through a mechanism involving ERK/p38 mitogen-activated protein kinases-MSK1-CREB activation in human airway epithelial cells. J Biol Chem 2003;278(26):23243–50.

[112] Casalino-Matsuda SM, Monzon ME, Conner GE, et al. Role of hyaluronan and reactive oxygen

species in tissue kallikrein-mediated epidermal growth factor receptor activation in human airways. J Biol Chem 2004;279(20):21606–16.

[113] Casalino-Matsuda SM, Monzon ME, Forteza RM. Epidermal growth factor receptor activation by epidermal growth factor mediates oxidant-induced goblet cell metaplasia in human airway epithelium. Am J Respir Cell Mol Biol 2006;34(5): 581–91.

[114] Deshmukh HS, Case LM, Wesselkamper SC, et al. Metalloproteinases mediate mucin 5AC expression by epidermal growth factor receptor activation. Am J Respir Crit Care Med 2005;171(4):305–14.

[115] Gensch E, Gallup M, Sucher A, et al. Tobacco smoke control of mucin production in lung cells requires oxygen radicals AP-1 and JNK. J Biol Chem 2004;279(37):39085–93.

[116] Baginski TK, Dabbagh K, Satjawatcharaphong C, et al. Cigarette smoke synergistically enhances respiratory mucin induction by proinflammatory stimuli. Am J Respir Cell Mol Biol 2006;35(2): 165–74.

[117] Lee CG, Homer RJ, Cohn L, et al. Transgenic overexpression of interleukin (IL)-10 in the lung causes mucus metaplasia, tissue inflammation, and airway remodeling via IL-13-dependent and -independent pathways. J Biol Chem 2002;277(38):35466–74.

[118] Ma B, Blackburn MR, Lee CG, et al. Adenosine metabolism and murine strain-specific IL-4-induced inflammation, emphysema, and fibrosis. J Clin Invest 2006;116(5):1274–83.

[119] Chen Q, Rabach L, Noble P, et al. IL-11 receptor alpha in the pathogenesis of IL-13-induced inflammation and remodeling. J Immunol 2005;174(4): 2305–13.

[120] Lee PJ, Zhang X, Shan P, et al. ERK1/2 mitogen-activated protein kinase selectively mediates IL-13-induced lung inflammation and remodeling in vivo. J Clin Invest 2006;116(1):163–73.

[121] Stoller JK, Aboussouan LS. Alpha1-antitrypsin deficiency. Lancet 2005;365(9478):2225–36.

[122] Foronjy RF, Mirochnitchenko O, Propokenko O, et al. Superoxide dismutase expression attenuates cigarette smoke- or elastase-generated emphysema in mice. Am J Respir Crit Care Med 2006;173(6): 623–31.

[123] Hayes JA, Korthy A, Snider GL. The pathology of elastase-induced panacinar emphysema in hamsters. J Pathol 1975;117(1):1–14.

[124] Houghton AM, Quintero PA, Perkins DL, et al. Elastin fragments drive disease progression in a murine model of emphysema. J Clin Invest 2006; 116(3):753–9.

[125] Ishii Y, Itoh K, Morishima Y, et al. Transcription factor Nrf2 plays a pivotal role in protection against elastase-induced pulmonary inflammation and emphysema. J Immunol 2005;175(10):6968–75.

[126] Ishizawa K, Kubo H, Yamada M, et al. Bone marrow-derived cells contribute to lung regeneration after elastase-induced pulmonary emphysema. FEBS Lett 2004;556(1–3):249–52.

[127] Ishizawa K, Kubo H, Yamada M, et al. Hepatocyte growth factor induces angiogenesis in injured lungs through mobilizing endothelial progenitor cells. Biochem Biophys Res Commun 2004;324(1): 276–80.

[128] Kaplan PD, Kuhn C, Pierce JA. The induction of emphysema with elastase. I. The evolution of the lesion and the influence of serum. J Lab Clin Med 1973;82(3):349–56.

[129] Shigemura N, Sawa Y, Mizuno S, et al. Induction of compensatory lung growth in pulmonary emphysema improves surgical outcomes in rats. Am J Respir Crit Care Med 2005;171(11): 1237–45.

[130] Shigemura N, Sawa Y, Mizuno S, et al. Amelioration of pulmonary emphysema by in vivo gene transfection with hepatocyte growth factor in rats. Circulation 2005;111(11):1407–14.

[131] Cavarra E, Bartalesi B, Lucattelli M, et al. Effects of cigarette smoke in mice with different levels of alpha(1)-proteinase inhibitor and sensitivity to oxidants. Am J Respir Crit Care Med 2001;164(5): 886–90.

[132] Takubo Y, Guerassimov A, Ghezzo H, et al. Alpha1-antitrypsin determines the pattern of emphysema and function in tobacco smoke-exposed mice: parallels with human disease. Am J Respir Crit Care Med 2002;166(12 Pt 1):1596–603.

[133] Shapiro SD, Goldstein NM, Houghton AM, et al. Neutrophil elastase contributes to cigarette smoke-induced emphysema in mice. Am J Pathol 2003;163(6):2329–35.

[134] Harel S, Janoff A, Yu SY, et al. Desmosine radioimmunoassay for measuring elastin degradation in vivo. Am Rev Respir Dis 1980;122(5): 769–73.

[135] Gottlieb DJ, Stone PJ, Sparrow D, et al. Urinary desmosine excretion in smokers with and without rapid decline of lung function: the Normative Aging Study. Am J Respir Crit Care Med 1996; 154(5):1290–5.

[136] Gadek JE, Fells GA, Crystal RG. Cigarette smoking induces functional antiprotease deficiency in the lower respiratory tract of humans. Science 1979; 206(4424):1315–6.

[137] Abboud RT, Fera T, Richter A, et al. Acute effect of smoking on the functional activity of alpha1-protease inhibitor in bronchoalveolar lavage fluid. Am Rev Respir Dis 1985;131(1):79–85.

[138] Burnett D, Chamba A, Hill SL, et al. Neutrophils from subjects with chronic obstructive lung disease show enhanced chemotaxis and extracellular proteolysis. Lancet 1987;2(8567):1043–6.

[139] Goldstein RA, Starcher BC. Urinary excretion of elastin peptides containing desmosin after intratracheal injection of elastase in hamsters. J Clin Invest 1978;61(5):1286–90.

[140] Kuhn C, Yu SY, Chraplyvy M, et al. The induction of emphysema with elastase. II. Changes in connective tissue. Lab Invest 1976;34(4):372–80.

[141] Fukuda Y, Masuda Y, Ishizaki M, et al. Morphogenesis of abnormal elastic fibers in lungs of patients with panacinar and centriacinar emphysema. Hum Pathol 1989;20(7):652–9.

[142] Massaro GD, Massaro D. Retinoic acid treatment abrogates elastase-induced pulmonary emphysema in rats. Nat Med 1997;3(6):675–7.

[143] Takeyabu K, Betsuyaku T, Nishimura M, et al. Cysteine proteinases and cystatin C in bronchoalveolar lavage fluid from subjects with subclinical emphysema. Eur Respir J 1998;12(5):1033–9.

[144] Russell RE, Thorley A, Culpitt SV, et al. Alveolar macrophage-mediated elastolysis: roles of matrix metalloproteinases, cysteine, and serine proteases. Am J Physiol Lung Cell Mol Physiol 2002;283(4):L867–73.

[145] Lagente V, Manoury B, Nenan S, et al. Role of matrix metalloproteinases in the development of airway inflammation and remodeling. Braz J Med Biol Res 2005;38(10):1521–30.

[146] Atkinson JJ, Senior RM. Matrix metalloproteinase-9 in lung remodeling. Am J Respir Cell Mol Biol 2003;28(1):12–24.

[147] Demedts IK, Morel-Montero A, Lebecque S, et al. Elevated MMP-12 protein levels in induced sputum from patients with COPD. Thorax 2006;61(3):196–201.

[148] Molet S, Belleguic C, Lena H, et al. Increase in macrophage elastase (MMP-12) in lungs from patients with chronic obstructive pulmonary disease. Inflamm Res 2005;54(1):31–6.

[149] Culpitt SV, Maziak W, Loukidis S, et al. Effect of high dose inhaled steroid on cells, cytokines, and proteases in induced sputum in chronic obstructive pulmonary disease. Am J Respir Crit Care Med 1999;160(5 Pt 1):1635–9.

[150] Finlay GA, O'Driscoll LR, Russell KJ, et al. Matrix metalloproteinase expression and production by alveolar macrophages in emphysema. Am J Respir Crit Care Med 1997;156(1):240–7.

[151] Betsuyaku T, Nishimura M, Takeyabu K, et al. Neutrophil granule proteins in bronchoalveolar lavage fluid from subjects with subclinical emphysema. Am J Respir Crit Care Med 1999;159(6):1985–91.

[152] Ohnishi K, Takagi M, Kurokawa Y, et al. Matrix metalloproteinase-mediated extracellular matrix protein degradation in human pulmonary emphysema. Lab Invest 1998;78(9):1077–87.

[153] Imai K, Dalal SS, Chen ES, et al. Human collagenase (matrix metalloproteinase-1) expression in the lungs of patients with emphysema. Am J Respir Crit Care Med 2001;163(3 Pt 1):786–91.

[154] Lavigne MC, Eppihimer MJ. Cigarette smoke condensate induces MMP-12 gene expression in airway-like epithelia. Biochem Biophys Res Commun 2005;330(1):194–203.

[155] Lavigne MC, Thakker P, Gunn J, et al. Human bronchial epithelial cells express and secrete MMP-12. Biochem Biophys Res Commun 2004;324(2):534–46.

[156] Valenca SS, da Hora K, Castro P, et al. Emphysema and metalloelastase expression in mouse lung induced by cigarette smoke. Toxicol Pathol 2004;32(3):351–6.

[157] Hautamaki RD, Kobayashi DK, Senior RM, et al. Requirement for macrophage elastase for cigarette smoke-induced emphysema in mice. Science 1997;277(5334):2002–4.

[158] Morris DG, Huang X, Kaminski N, et al. Loss of integrin alpha(v)beta6-mediated TGF-beta activation causes Mmp12-dependent emphysema. Nature 2003;422(6928):169–73.

[159] Weathington NM, van Houwelingen AH, Noerager BD, et al. A novel peptide CXCR ligand derived from extracellular matrix degradation during airway inflammation. Nat Med 2006;12(3):317–23.

[160] Leco KJ, Waterhouse P, Sanchez OH, et al. Spontaneous air space enlargement in the lungs of mice lacking tissue inhibitor of metalloproteinases-3 (TIMP-3). J Clin Invest 2001;108(6):817–29.

[161] Martin EL, Moyer BZ, Pape MC, et al. Negative impact of tissue inhibitor of metalloproteinase-3 null mutation on lung structure and function in response to sepsis. Am J Physiol Lung Cell Mol Physiol 2003;285(6):L1222–32.

[162] Martin EL, McCaig LA, Moyer BZ, et al. Differential response of TIMP-3 null mice to the lung insults of sepsis, mechanical ventilation, and hyperoxia. Am J Physiol Lung Cell Mol Physiol 2005;289(2):L244–51.

[163] da Hora K, Valenca SS, Porto LC. Immunohistochemical study of tumor necrosis factor-alpha, matrix metalloproteinase-12, and tissue inhibitor of metalloproteinase-2 on alveolar macrophages of BALB/c mice exposed to short-term cigarette smoke. Exp Lung Res 2005;31(8):759–70.

[164] Funada Y, Nishimura Y, Yokoyama M. Imbalance of matrix metalloproteinase-9 and tissue inhibitor of matrix metalloproteinase-1 is associated with pulmonary emphysema in Klotho mice. Kobe J Med Sci 2004;50(3–4):59–67.

[165] Church DF, Pryor WA. Free-radical chemistry of cigarette smoke and its toxicological implications. Environ Health Perspect 1985;64:111–26.

[166] Rahman I, MacNee W. Role of oxidants/antioxidants in smoking-induced lung diseases. Free Radic Biol Med 1996;21(5):669–81.

[167] MacNee W. Oxidants and COPD. Curr Drug Targets Inflamm Allergy 2005;4(6):627–41.

[168] MacNee W. Oxidative stress and lung inflammation in airways disease. Eur J Pharmacol 2001;429(1–3):195–207.

[169] Pryor WA, Stone K. Oxidants in cigarette smoke. Radicals, hydrogen peroxide, peroxynitrate, and peroxynitrite. Ann N Y Acad Sci 1993;686:12–27.

[170] Rahman I, Biswas SK, Kode A. Oxidant and anti-oxidant balance in the airways and airway diseases. Eur J Pharmacol 2006;533(1–3):222–39.

[171] Rahman I, Morrison D, Donaldson K, et al. Systemic oxidative stress in asthma, COPD, and smokers. Am J Respir Crit Care Med 1996; 154(4 Pt 1):1055–60.

[172] Aaron SD, Angel JB, Lunau M, et al. Granulocyte inflammatory markers and airway infection during acute exacerbation of chronic obstructive pulmonary disease. Am J Respir Crit Care Med 2001; 163(2):349–55.

[173] Fiorini G, Crespi S, Rinaldi M, et al. Serum ECP and MPO are increased during exacerbations of chronic bronchitis with airway obstruction. Biomed Pharmacother 2000;54(5):274–8.

[174] Gompertz S, Bayley DL, Hill SL, et al. Relationship between airway inflammation and the frequency of exacerbations in patients with smoking related COPD. Thorax 2001;56(1):36–41.

[175] Schaberg T, Haller H, Rau M, et al. Superoxide anion release induced by platelet-activating factor is increased in human alveolar macrophages from smokers. Eur Respir J 1992;5(4):387–93.

[176] Morrison D, Rahman I, Lannan S, et al. Epithelial permeability, inflammation, and oxidant stress in the air spaces of smokers. Am J Respir Crit Care Med 1999;159(2):473–9.

[177] Nakashima H, Ando M, Sugimoto M, et al. Receptor-mediated O2- release by alveolar macrophages and peripheral blood monocytes from smokers and nonsmokers. Priming and triggering effects of monomeric IgG, concanavalin A, N-formyl-methionyl-leucyl-phenylalanine, phorbol myristate acetate, and cytochalasin D. Am Rev Respir Dis 1987;136(2):310–5.

[178] Drath DB, Karnovsky ML, Huber GL. The effects of experimental exposure to tobacco smoke on the oxidative metabolism of alveolar macrophages. J Reticuloendothel Soc 1979;25(6):597–604.

[179] Schaberg T, Klein U, Rau M, et al. Subpopulations of alveolar macrophages in smokers and nonsmokers: relation to the expression of CD11/CD18 molecules and superoxide anion production. Am J Respir Crit Care Med 1995;151(5):1551–8.

[180] Mateos F, Brock JH, Perez-Arellano JL. Iron metabolism in the lower respiratory tract. Thorax 1998;53(7):594–600.

[181] Lapenna D, de Gioia S, Mezzetti A, et al. Cigarette smoke, ferritin, and lipid peroxidation. Am J Respir Crit Care Med 1995;151(2 Pt 1):431–5.

[182] Thompson AB, Bohling T, Heires A, et al. Lower respiratory tract iron burden is increased in association with cigarette smoking. J Lab Clin Med 1991; 117(6):493–9.

[183] Wesselius LJ, Nelson ME, Skikne BS. Increased release of ferritin and iron by iron-loaded alveolar macrophages in cigarette smokers. Am J Respir Crit Care Med 1994;150(3):690–5.

[184] Chan-Yeung M, Lam S, Koener S. Clinical features and natural history of occupational asthma due to western red cedar (Thuja plicata). Am J Med 1982; 72(3):411–5.

[185] Chan-Yeung M, Abboud R, Buncio AD, et al. Peripheral leucocyte count and longitudinal decline in lung function. Thorax 1988;43(6):462–6.

[186] Postma DS, Renkema TE, Noordhoek JA, et al. Association between nonspecific bronchial hyper-reactivity and superoxide anion production by polymorphonuclear leukocytes in chronic air-flow obstruction. Am Rev Respir Dis 1988;137(1): 57–61.

[187] Richards GA, Theron AJ, Van der Merwe CA, et al. Spirometric abnormalities in young smokers correlate with increased chemiluminescence responses of activated blood phagocytes. Am Rev Respir Dis 1989;139(1):181–7.

[188] Noguera A, Busquets X, Sauleda J, et al. Expression of adhesion molecules and G proteins in circulating neutrophils in chronic obstructive pulmonary disease. Am J Respir Crit Care Med 1998;158(5 Pt 1):1664–8.

[189] Brown DM, Drost E, Donaldson K, et al. Deformability and CD11/CD18 expression of sequestered neutrophils in normal and inflamed lungs. Am J Respir Cell Mol Biol 1995;13(5):531–9.

[190] Pinamonti S, Muzzoli M, Chicca MC, et al. Xanthine oxidase activity in bronchoalveolar lavage fluid from patients with chronic obstructive pulmonary disease. Free Radic Biol Med 1996;21(2): 147–55.

[191] Heunks LM, Vina J, van Herwaarden CL, et al. Xanthine oxidase is involved in exercise-induced oxidative stress in chronic obstructive pulmonary disease. Am J Physiol 1999;277(6 Pt 2): R1697–704.

[192] Pinamonti S, Leis M, Barbieri A, et al. Detection of xanthine oxidase activity products by EPR and HPLC in bronchoalveolar lavage fluid from patients with chronic obstructive pulmonary disease. Free Radic Biol Med 1998;25(7): 771–9.

[193] Eiserich JP, van d V, Handelman GJ, et al. Dietary antioxidants and cigarette smoke-induced biomolecular damage: a complex interaction. Am J Clin Nutr 1995;62(Suppl 6):1490S–500S.

[194] Petruzzelli S, Puntoni R, Mimotti P, et al. Plasma 3-nitrotyrosine in cigarette smokers. Am J Respir Crit Care Med 1997;156(6):1902–7.

[195] Ichinose M, Sugiura H, Yamagata S, et al. Increase in reactive nitrogen species production in chronic obstructive pulmonary disease airways. Am J Respir Crit Care Med 2000;162(2 Pt 1): 701–6.

[196] Pignatelli B, Li CQ, Boffetta P, et al. Nitrated and oxidized plasma proteins in smokers and lung cancer patients. Cancer Res 2001;61(2):778–84.

[197] Kanazawa H, Shiraishi S, Hirata K, et al. Imbalance between levels of nitrogen oxides and peroxynitrite inhibitory activity in chronic obstructive pulmonary disease. Thorax 2003;58(2):106–9.

[198] Sugiura H, Ichinose M, Yamagata S, et al. Correlation between change in pulmonary function and suppression of reactive nitrogen species production following steroid treatment in COPD. Thorax 2003;58(4):299–305.

[199] MacNee W. Oxidants/antioxidants and COPD. Chest 2000;117(5 Suppl 1):303S–17S.

[200] Dekhuijzen PN, Aben KK, Dekker I, et al. Increased exhalation of hydrogen peroxide in patients with stable and unstable chronic obstructive pulmonary disease. Am J Respir Crit Care Med 1996;154(3 Pt 1):813–6.

[201] Nowak D, Kasielski M, Pietras T, et al. Cigarette smoking does not increase hydrogen peroxide levels in expired breath condensate of patients with stable COPD. Monaldi Arch Chest Dis 1998;53(3):268–73.

[202] Montuschi P, Kharitonov SA, Barnes PJ. Exhaled carbon monoxide and nitric oxide in COPD. Chest 2001;120(2):496–501.

[203] Nowak D, Kasielski M, Antczak A, et al. Increased content of thiobarbituric acid-reactive substances and hydrogen peroxide in the expired breath condensate of patients with stable chronic obstructive pulmonary disease: no significant effect of cigarette smoking. Respir Med 1999;93(6):389–96.

[204] Corradi M, Rubinstein I, Andreoli R, et al. Aldehydes in exhaled breath condensate of patients with chronic obstructive pulmonary disease. Am J Respir Crit Care Med 2003;167(10):1380–6.

[205] Delen FM, Sippel JM, Osborne ML, et al. Increased exhaled nitric oxide in chronic bronchitis: comparison with asthma and COPD. Chest 2000;117(3):695–701.

[206] Corradi M, Montuschi P, Donnelly LE, et al. Increased nitrosothiols in exhaled breath condensate in inflammatory airway diseases. Am J Respir Crit Care Med 2001;163(4):854–8.

[207] Lawson JA, Rokach J, FitzGerald GA. Isoprostanes: formation, analysis and use as indices of lipid peroxidation in vivo. J Biol Chem 1999;274(35):24441–4.

[208] Montuschi P, Collins JV, Ciabattoni G, et al. Exhaled 8-isoprostane as an in vivo biomarker of lung oxidative stress in patients with COPD and healthy smokers. Am J Respir Crit Care Med 2000;162(3 Pt 1):1175–7.

[209] Paredi P, Kharitonov SA, Barnes PJ. Elevation of exhaled ethane concentration in asthma. Am J Respir Crit Care Med 2000;162(4 Pt 1):1450–4.

[210] Paredi P, Kharitonov SA, Leak D, et al. Exhaled ethane, a marker of lipid peroxidation, is elevated in chronic obstructive pulmonary disease. Am J Respir Crit Care Med 2000;162(2 Pt 1):369–73.

[211] Habib MP, Clements NC, Garewal HS. Cigarette smoking and ethane exhalation in humans. Am J Respir Crit Care Med 1995;151(5):1368–72.

[212] Schaur RJ, Dussing G, Kink E, et al. The lipid peroxidation product 4-hydroxynonenal is formed by–and is able to attract–rat neutrophils in vivo. Free Radic Res 1994;20(6):365–73.

[213] Liu W, Akhand AA, Kato M, et al. 4-Hydroxynonenal triggers an epidermal growth factor receptor-linked signal pathway for growth inhibition. J Cell Sci 1999;112(Pt 14):2409–17.

[214] Liu W, Kato M, Akhand AA, et al. 4-Hydroxynonenal induces a cellular redox status-related activation of the caspase cascade for apoptotic cell death. J Cell Sci 2000;113(Pt 4):635–41.

[215] Uchida K, Shiraishi M, Naito Y, et al. Activation of stress signaling pathways by the end product of lipid peroxidation. 4-Hydroxy-2-nonenal is a potential inducer of intracellular peroxide production. J Biol Chem 1999;274(4):2234–42.

[216] Parola M, Bellomo G, Robino G, et al. 4-Hydroxynonenal as a biological signal: molecular basis and pathophysiological implications. Antioxid Redox Signal 1999;1(3):255–84.

[217] Rahman I, van Schadewijk AA, Crowther AJ, et al. 4-Hydroxy-2-nonenal, a specific lipid peroxidation product, is elevated in lungs of patients with chronic obstructive pulmonary disease. Am J Respir Crit Care Med 2002;166(4):490–5.

[218] Tuder RM, Zhen L, Cho CY, et al. Oxidative stress and apoptosis interact and cause emphysema due to vascular endothelial growth factor receptor blockade. Am J Respir Cell Mol Biol 2003;29(1):88–97.

[219] Gutteridge JM. Biological origin of free radicals, and mechanisms of antioxidant protection. Chem Biol Interact 1994;91(2–3):133–40.

[220] Rahman I, Yang SR, Biswas SK. Current concepts of redox signaling in the lungs. Antioxid Redox Signal 2006;8(3–4):681–9.

[221] Rahman I, Kilty I. Antioxidant therapeutic targets in COPD. Curr Drug Targets 2006;7(6):707–20.

[222] Rahman I, MacNee W. Regulation of redox glutathione levels and gene transcription in lung inflammation: therapeutic approaches. Free Radic Biol Med 2000;28(9):1405–20.

[223] Beeh KM, Beier J, Koppenhoefer N, et al. Increased glutathione disulfide and nitrosothiols in sputum supernatant of patients with stable COPD. Chest 2004;126(4):1116–22.

[224] Drost EM, Skwarski KM, Sauleda J, et al. Oxidative stress and airway inflammation in severe exacerbations of COPD. Thorax 2005;60(4):293–300.

[225] Rahman I, van Schadewijk AA, Hiemstra PS, et al. Localization of gamma-glutamylcysteine synthetase messenger RNA expression in lungs of smokers and patients with chronic obstructive

pulmonary disease. Free Radic Biol Med 2000; 28(6):920–5.

[226] Harju T, Kaarteenaho-Wiik R, Soini Y, et al. Diminished immunoreactivity of gamma-glutamylcysteine synthetase in the airways of smokers' lung. Am J Respir Crit Care Med 2002;166(5): 754–9.

[227] Kinnula VL, Crapo JD. Superoxide dismutases in the lung and human lung diseases. Am J Respir Crit Care Med 2003;167(12):1600–19.

[228] Harju T, Kaarteenaho-Wiik R, Sirvio R, et al. Manganese superoxide dismutase is increased in the airways of smokers' lungs. Eur Respir J 2004; 24(5):765–71.

[229] Cross CE, van d V, O'Neill CA, et al. Oxidants, antioxidants, and respiratory tract lining fluids. Environ Health Perspect 1994;102(Suppl 10):185–91.

[230] Repine JE, Bast A, Lankhorst I. Oxidative stress in chronic obstructive pulmonary disease. Oxidative Stress Study Group. Am J Respir Crit Care Med 1997;156(2 Pt 1):341–57.

[231] MacNee W. Oxidative stress and chronic obstructive pulmonary disease. Eur Respir Monograph 2006;38:100–29.

[232] Aoshiba K, Yasuda K, Yasui S, et al. Serine proteases increase oxidative stress in lung cells. Am J Physiol Lung Cell Mol Physiol 2001;281(3): L556–64.

[233] Rahman I, Li XY, Donaldson K, et al. Cigarette smoke, glutathione metabolism and epithelial permeability in rat lungs. Biochem Soc Trans 1995; 23(2):235S.

[234] Li XY, Rahman I, Donaldson K, et al. Mechanisms of cigarette smoke induced increased airspace permeability. Thorax 1996;51(5):465–71.

[235] Li XY, Donaldson K, Rahman I, et al. An investigation of the role of glutathione in increased epithelial permeability induced by cigarette smoke in vivo and in vitro. Am J Respir Crit Care Med 1994; 149(6):1518–25.

[236] Lannan S, Donaldson K, Brown D, et al. Effect of cigarette smoke and its condensates on alveolar epithelial cell injury in vitro. Am J Physiol 1994; 266(1 Pt 1):L92–100.

[237] Morrow JD, Frei B, Longmire AW, et al. Increase in circulating products of lipid peroxidation (F2-isoprostanes) in smokers. Smoking as a cause of oxidative damage. N Engl J Med 1995;332(18): 1198–203.

[238] Kharitonov SA, Barnes PJ. Exhaled biomarkers. Chest 2006;130(5):1541–6.

[239] Kinnula VL, Ilumets H, Myllarniemi M, et al. 8-Isoprostane as a marker of oxidative stress in nonsymptomatic cigarette smokers and COPD. Eur Respir J 2007;29(1):51–5.

[240] Cantin AM, Fells GA, Hubbard RC, et al. Antioxidant macromolecules in the epithelial lining fluid of the normal human lower respiratory tract. J Clin Invest 1990;86(3):962–71.

[241] Rahman I, Li XY, Donaldson K, et al. Glutathione homeostasis in alveolar epithelial cells in vitro and lung in vivo under oxidative stress. Am J Physiol 1995;269(3 Pt 1):L285–92.

[242] Pacht ER, Kaseki H, Mohammed JR, et al. Deficiency of vitamin E in the alveolar fluid of cigarette smokers. Influence on alveolar macrophage cytotoxicity. J Clin Invest 1986;77(3):789–96.

[243] Bui MH, Sauty A, Collet F, et al. Dietary vitamin C intake and concentrations in the body fluids and cells of male smokers and nonsmokers. J Nutr 1992;122(2):312–6.

[244] Gilks CB, Price K, Wright JL, et al. Antioxidant gene expression in rat lung after exposure to cigarette smoke. Am J Pathol 1998;152(1):269–78.

[245] Iizuka T, Ishii Y, Itoh K, et al. Nrf2-deficient mice are highly susceptible to cigarette smoke-induced emphysema. Genes Cells 2005;10(12):1113–25.

[246] Rangasamy T, Cho CY, Thimmulappa RK, et al. Genetic ablation of Nrf2 enhances susceptibility to cigarette smoke-induced emphysema in mice. J Clin Invest 2004;114(9):1248–59.

[247] Adler KB, Holden-Stauffer WJ, Repine JE. Oxygen metabolites stimulate release of high-molecular-weight glycoconjugates by cell and organ cultures of rodent respiratory epithelium via an arachidonic acid-dependent mechanism. J Clin Invest 1990; 85(1):75–85.

[248] Feldman C, Anderson R, Kanthakumar K, et al. Oxidant-mediated ciliary dysfunction in human respiratory epithelium. Free Radic Biol Med 1994; 17(1):1–10.

[249] Keicho N, Elliott WM, Hogg JC, et al. Adenovirus E1A upregulates interleukin-8 expression induced by endotoxin in pulmonary epithelial cells. Am J Physiol 1997;272(6 Pt 1):L1046–52.

[250] Elliott WM, Hayashi S, Hogg JC. Immunodetection of adenoviral E1A proteins in human lung-tissue. Am J Respir Cell Mol Biol 1995;12:642–8.

[251] Vitalis TZ, Kern I, Croome A, et al. The effect of latent adenovirus 5 infection on cigarette smoke-induced lung inflammation. Eur Respir J 1998; 11(3):664–9.

[252] Gilmour PS, Rahman I, Hayashi S, et al. Adenoviral E1A primes alveolar epithelial cells to PM(10)-induced transcription of interleukin-8. Am J Physiol Lung Cell Mol Physiol 2001;281(3): L598–606.

[253] Higashimoto Y, Elliott WM, Behzad AR, et al. Inflammatory mediator mRNA expression by adenovirus E1A-transfected bronchial epithelial cells. Am J Respir Crit Care Med 2002;166(2): 200–7.

[254] Rahman I, Adcock IM. Oxidative stress and redox regulation of lung inflammation in COPD. Eur Respir J 2006;28(1):219–42.

[255] Bonizzi G, Karin M. The two NF-kappaB activation pathways and their role in innate and adaptive immunity. Trends Immunol 2004;25(6):280–8.

[256] Szulakowski P, Crowther AJ, Jimenez LA, et al. The effect of smoking on the transcriptional regulation of lung inflammation in patients with chronic obstructive pulmonary disease. Am J Respir Crit Care Med 2006;174(1):41–50.

[257] Cosio BG, Tsaprouni L, Ito K, et al. Theophylline restores histone deacetylase activity and steroid responses in COPD macrophages. J Exp Med 2004; 200(5):689–95.

[258] Marwick JA, Kirkham PA, Stevenson CS, et al. Cigarette smoke alters chromatin remodeling and induces proinflammatory genes in rat lungs. Am J Respir Cell Mol Biol 2004;31(6):633–42.

[259] Moodie FM, Marwick JA, Anderson CS, et al. Oxidative stress and cigarette smoke alter chromatin remodeling but differentially regulate NF-kappaB activation and proinflammatory cytokine release in alveolar epithelial cells. FASEB J 2004;18(15): 1897–9.

[260] Yang SR, Chida AS, Bauter MR, et al. Cigarette smoke induces proinflammatory cytokine release by activation of NF-kappaB and posttranslational modifications of histone deacetylase in macrophages. Am J Physiol Lung Cell Mol Physiol 2006;291(1):L46–57.

[261] Ito K, Ito M, Elliott WM, et al. Decreased histone deacetylase activity in chronic obstructive pulmonary disease. N Engl J Med 2005;352(19):1967–76.

[262] Adcock IM, Ford P, Barnes PJ, et al. Epigenetics and airways disease. Respir Res 2006;7(1):21.

[263] Kasahara Y, Tuder RM, Taraseviciene-Stewart L, et al. Inhibition of VEGF receptors causes lung cell apoptosis and emphysema. J Clin Invest 2000; 106(11):1311–9.

[264] Aoshiba K, Nagai A. [Apoptosis in chronic obstructive pulmonary disease]. Nippon Rinsho 1999;57(9):1972–5.

[265] Kasahara Y, Tuder RM, Cool CD, et al. Endothelial cell death and decreased expression of vascular endothelial growth factor and vascular endothelial growth factor receptor 2 in emphysema. Am J Respir Crit Care Med 2001;163(3 Pt 1): 737–44.

[266] Tang K, Rossiter HB, Wagner PD, et al. Lung-targeted VEGF inactivation leads to an emphysema phenotype in mice. J Appl Physiol 2004; 97(4):1559–66.

[267] Tuder RM, Voelkel NF. Pathology of chronic bronchitis and emphysema. In: Voelkel NF, MacNee W, editors. Chronic obstructive lung disease. London: BC Decker; 2001. p. 90–113.

[268] Imai K, Mercer BA, Schulman LL, et al. Correlation of lung surface area to apoptosis and proliferation in human emphysema. Eur Respir J 2005; 25(2):250–8.

[269] Bartalesi B, Cavarra E, Fineschi S, et al. Different lung responses to cigarette smoke in two strains of mice sensitive to oxidants. Eur Respir J 2005; 25(1):15–22.

[270] Aoshiba K, Yokohori N, Nagai A. Alveolar wall apoptosis causes lung destruction and emphysematous changes. Am J Respir Cell Mol Biol 2003; 28(5):555–62.

[271] Petrache I, Fijalkowska I, Zhen L, et al. A novel antiapoptotic role for alpha1-antitrypsin in the prevention of pulmonary emphysema. Am J Respir Crit Care Med 2006;173(11):1222–8.

[272] Vandivier RW, Henson PM, Douglas IS. Burying the dead: the impact of failed apoptotic cell removal (efferocytosis) on chronic inflammatory lung disease. Chest 2006;129(6):1673–82.

[273] Yokohori N, Aoshiba K, Nagai A. Increased levels of cell death and proliferation in alveolar wall cells in patients with pulmonary emphysema. Chest 2004;125(2):626–32.

[274] Calabrese F, Giacometti C, Beghe B, et al. Marked alveolar apoptosis/proliferation imbalance in end-stage emphysema. Respir Res 2005;6:14.

[275] Hodge S, Hodge G, Scicchitano R, et al. Alveolar macrophages from subjects with chronic obstructive pulmonary disease are deficient in their ability to phagocytose apoptotic airway epithelial cells. Immunol Cell Biol 2003;81(4): 289–96.

[276] Rennard SI. Inflammation and repair processes in chronic obstructive pulmonary disease. Am J Respir Crit Care Med 1999;160(5 Pt 2):S12–6.

[277] Wang H, Liu X, Umino T, et al. Cigarette smoke inhibits human bronchial epithelial cell repair processes. Am J Respir Cell Mol Biol 2001;25(6): 772–9.

[278] Koli K, Wempe F, Sterner-Kock A, et al. Disruption of LTBP-4 function reduces TGF-beta activation and enhances BMP-4 signaling in the lung. J Cell Biol 2004;167(1):123–33.

[279] Bonniaud P, Kolb M, Galt T, et al. Smad3 null mice develop airspace enlargement and are resistant to TGF-beta-mediated pulmonary fibrosis. J Immunol 2004;173(3):2099–108.

[280] Chen H, Sun J, Buckley S, et al. Abnormal mouse lung alveolarization caused by Smad3 deficiency is a developmental antecedent of centrilobular emphysema. Am J Physiol Lung Cell Mol Physiol 2005;288(4):L683–91.

[281] Zandvoort A, Postma DS, Jonker MR, et al. Altered expression of the Smad signalling pathway: implications for COPD pathogenesis. Eur Respir J 2006;28(3):533–41.

[282] Michaud SE, Dussault S, Haddad P, et al. Circulating endothelial progenitor cells from healthy smokers exhibit impaired functional activities. Atherosclerosis 2006;187(2):423–32.

[283] Palange P, Testa U, Huertas A, et al. Circulating haemopoietic and endothelial progenitor cells are decreased in COPD. Eur Respir J 2006;27(3): 529–41.

[284] Hogg JC. Why does airway inflammation persist after the smoking stops? Thorax 2006;61(2):96–7.

[285] Monso E, Ruiz J, Rosell A, et al. Bacterial infection in chronic obstructive pulmonary disease. A study of stable and exacerbated outpatients using the protected specimen brush. Am J Respir Crit Care Med 1995;152(4 Pt 1):1316–20.

[286] Taraseviciene-Stewart L, Scerbavicius R, Choe KH, et al. An animal model of autoimmune emphysema. Am J Respir Crit Care Med 2005;171(7):734–42.

[287] Sullivan AK, Simonian PL, Falta MT, et al. Oligoclonal CD4+ T cells in the lungs of patients with severe emphysema. Am J Respir Crit Care Med 2005; 172(5):590–6.

[288] Lee SH, Goswami S, Grudo A, et al. Antielastin autoimmunity in tobacco smoking-induced emphysema. Nat Med 2007;13(5):567–9.

[289] Morla M, Busquets X, Pons J, et al. Telomere shortening in smokers with and without COPD. Eur Respir J 2006;27(3):525–8.

[290] Tsuji T, Aoshiba K, Nagai A. Alveolar cell senescence in patients with pulmonary emphysema. Am J Respir Crit Care Med 2006;174(8): 886–93.

[291] Muller KC, Welker L, Paasch K, et al. Lung fibroblasts from patients with emphysema show markers of senescence in vitro. Respir Res 2006;7:32.

[292] Tuder RM, Yoshida T, Arap W, et al. State of the art. Cellular and molecular mechanisms of alveolar destruction in emphysema: an evolutionary perspective. Proc Am Thorac Soc 2006;3(6): 503–10.

[293] Balaban RS, Nemoto S, Finkel T. Mitochondria, oxidants, and aging. Cell 2005;120(4):483–95.

[294] Tsuji T, Aoshiba K, Nagai A. Cigarette smoke induces senescence in alveolar epithelial cells. Am J Respir Cell Mol Biol 2004;31(6):643–9.

[295] Teramoto S, Uejima Y, Oka T, et al. Effects of chronic cigarette smoke inhalation on the development of senile lung in senescence-accelerated mouse. Res Exp Med (Berl) 1997;197(1):1–11.

[296] Arking DE, Krebsova A, Macek M Sr, et al. Association of human aging with a functional variant of Klotho. Proc Natl Acad Sci USA 2002;99(2): 856–61.

[297] Kuro-o M, Matsumura Y, Aizawa H, et al. Mutation of the mouse Klotho gene leads to a syndrome resembling ageing. Nature 1997;390(6655):45–51.

[298] Suga T, Kurabayashi M, Sando Y, et al. Disruption of the Klotho gene causes pulmonary emphysema in mice. Defect in maintenance of pulmonary integrity during postnatal life. Am J Respir Cell Mol Biol 2000;22(1):26–33.

[299] Ishigami A, Fujita T, Handa S, et al. Senescence marker protein-30 knockout mouse liver is highly susceptible to tumor necrosis factor-alpha- and Fas-mediated apoptosis. Am J Pathol 2002; 161(4):1273–81.

[300] Mori T, Ishigami A, Seyama K, et al. Senescence marker protein-30 knockout mouse as a novel murine model of senile lung. Pathol Int 2004;54(3): 167–73.

[301] Sato T, Seyama K, Sato Y, et al. Senescence marker protein-30 protects mice lungs from oxidative stress, aging, and smoking. Am J Respir Crit Care Med 2006;174(5):530–7.

ELSEVIER
SAUNDERS

CLINICS
IN CHEST
MEDICINE

Clin Chest Med 28 (2007) 515–524

Predictors of Mortality in Chronic Obstructive Pulmonary Disease

Claudia G. Cote, MD[a,b],*, Bartolome R. Celli, MD[c,d]

[a]University of South Florida, Tampa, FL, USA
[b]Pulmonary Rehabilitation Program, Bay Pines Veterans Administration Health Care System,
111 A - PO BOX 5005, Bay Pines, FL 33744, USA
[c]Tufts University Medical School, Boston, MA, USA
[d]Division of Pulmonary and Critical Care Medicine, Caritas Saint Elizabeth's Medical Center,
736 Cambridge Street, Boston, MA 02135, USA

Chronic obstructive pulmonary disease (COPD) is a major cause of morbidity and mortality in adults and currently represents the fourth leading cause of death in the world [1]. It has become a major and growing health problem, with a mortality rate that continues to increase [2–5]. COPD is the only leading cause of death showing increases in prevalence worldwide, and it is expected that by the year 2020, COPD will become the third leading cause of death and the number one cause of disability in adults [2].

In the United States, the age-adjusted (2005 United States standard population) mortality rates for COPD showed an increase from 25.6 per 100,000 population in 1979 to 43.5 per 100,000 population in 2005 [6]. Age-adjusted mortality rates in males have slowly declined over the last few years (55.8 per 100,000 population in 2000 to 52.3 per 100,000 population in 2003). For females, however, the rates have remained unchanged (37.4 per 100,000 population in 2000 to 37.8 per 100,000 population in 2003) [7]. Additionally, for the last 3 consecutive years, COPD mortality in women has surpassed that of men, claiming the lives of 63,000 women in contrast to 59,000 men [6]. The staggering rates for smoking cessation is responsible for the alarming epidemic of COPD and the increase in mortality rates seen among females [3].

Although COPD is characterized primarily by the presence of airflow limitation owing to chronic bronchitis, emphysema, or both, a myriad of systemic manifestations that accompany this disease effectively can signal an increased risk for mortality. Recognizing these manifestations provides a more comprehensive assessment of disease severity and helps elucidate prognosis. Several factors, including forced expiratory volume in 1 second (FEV_1), airway hyper-responsiveness, severity of dyspnea, gas exchange disturbances, lung hyperinflation, pulmonary hypertension, malnutrition-impaired exercise capacity and health-related quality of life, anemia, and other comorbidities have been identified as individual predictors of mortality in COPD. This article reviews these individual predictors for mortality. It also discusses the ability of an integrated, multidimensional tool to more broadly characterize COPD severity, assess response to therapeutic interventions and exacerbations, and predict mortality.

Predictors of mortality in chronic obstructive pulmonary disease

Forced expiratory volume in 1 second

Spirometry first was introduced in the late 1800s, and with its application to patients with obstructive lung disease, the FEV_1 expressed as a percentage of the forced vital capacity (FVC)

* Corresponding author. Bay Pines VA Health Care System, 111 A - PO BOX 5005, Bay Pines, FL 33744.
    E-mail address: claudia.cote@med.va.gov (C.G. Cote).

0272-5231/07/$ - see front matter. Published by Elsevier Inc.
doi:10.1016/j.ccm.2007.05.002

has been used as the standard measurement of air-flow limitation, and therefore, of disease severity in COPD [3]. The landmark study of Fletcher and Peto [8], published in 1976, identified a relationship between airflow obstruction and survival in a study of over 2700 British men initially tested from 1954 to 1961, and followed for 20 to 25 years. The investigators found that in patients who had COPD, the risk of death was correlated strongly with the initial degree of measured FEV_1 [8]. These findings then were expanded by Anthonisen and colleagues [9] during the Intermittent Positive Pressure Breathing (IPPB) trial, which identified both age and FEV_1 as independent and accurate predictors of mortality among 985 patients who had COPD, followed over 3 years. Numerous studies since have confirmed and further described the relationship between FEV_1, all-cause mortality and cause-specific mortality [10–13]. Most recently, Mannino and colleagues [14] described a report from the National Health and Nutrition Examination Survey (NHA-NESI). The primary outcome was death, and the main predictor of interest was baseline lung function. Among 5542 adults followed for 22 years in the United States, 1301 deaths were found. The authors found a higher risk of death among patients who had moderate or severe COPD identified by their baseline spirometry data [15]. These results once again validate the importance of the FEV_1 as a prognostic indicator in COPD.

Airway hyper-responsiveness

The importance of airway hyper-responsiveness (AHR) in obstructive lung diseases is defined better for asthma than for COPD. In the Dutch study from Orie and colleagues [16], histamine challenge airway hyper-responsiveness was evaluated in approximately 2000 patients, then followed for over 20 years. In a mortality analysis of this patient cohort, Hospers and colleagues [17] found that increased AHR predicted mortality for COPD after adjusting for gender, age, smoking history, and numerous confounders. The number of COPD deaths was very small (21), and more studies are needed to better define the relationship between AHR and mortality in COPD.

Dyspnea

Dyspnea is the cardinal, most disabling symptom of COPD [18] and the primary reason for patients to seek medical attention [19,20]. The perception of breathlessness differs from patient to patient, as it responds to the interaction of respiratory mechanics including airflow limitation and other cognitive and nonvolitional neuronal processes. Importantly, the correlation of breathlessness and FEV_1 has been noted to be weak [21]. Numerous studies have identified dyspnea as an independent predictor of mortality in this disease. In a prospective, multicenter, 5-year trial, dyspnea was measured by the Medical Research Council Dyspnea Scale (MRC) in a cohort of 227 patients who had COPD [22]. These investigators found that survival rate was predicted better by dyspnea ($P < .001$) and that this outcome was not significantly related to the severity of COPD according to staging by FEV_1 percent of predicted value. These findings were confirmed in a much larger cohort of 625 patients with COPD. In this cohort, dyspnea also was measured with the MMRC, and patients were followed over time [23]. The measurement of dyspnea therefore should be an integral part of the evaluation of patients who have COPD, when assessing the risk for premature mortality in this disease.

Hypoxemia

The presence of hypoxemia ($PaO_2 < 55$ mm Hg or $SaO_2 < 88\%$) while the patient is breathing room air long has been known to predict mortality in COPD. Conversely, the correction of gas exchange derangement results in better survival. In 1970, Neff and Petty [24] first published a 30% to 40% reduction in mortality among a group of hypoxic COPD patients given continuous oxygen supplementation. The most important evidence supporting its use, however, was derived from two large controlled trials evaluating the effect of supplemental oxygen on hypoxemic patients with COPD. The first trial, conducted by the British Medical Research Council [25], randomized patients to receive 15 hours of continuous oxygen or room air. The study found a significant reduction in mortality among patients given oxygen supplementation during a follow-up period of 5 years. The Nocturnal Oxygen Therapy Trial (NOTT) [26] compared 12 hours of oxygen supplementation with 24 hours of oxygen supplementation. Mortality among patients given continuous oxygen for 24 hours was 50% less than mortality among those given oxygen for only 12 hours. These data show that survival in hypoxemic patients who have COPD is proportional to the number of hours of oxygen supplementation.

Hypercapnia

Hypercapnia is usually found in patients who have advanced COPD and reflects both the severe ventilation–perfusion inequality and the inability of the patient to increase ventilation to maintain an adequate elimination of carbon dioxide.

The presence of chronic hypercapnia usually is associated with a negative prognostic value for survival in COPD [27–29]. Hypercapnia commonly is associated with hypoxemia, and it has been difficult to elucidate which gas exchange derangement carries the most ominous prognosis. In a cohort of hypoxemic COPD patients receiving long-term oxygen therapy (LTOT) in Japan [30] 4552 patients were followed between 1985 and 1993. During the follow-up period, 1611 patients died (5-year survival 39.5%). The authors found the cumulative survival curves for the hypoxemic, hypercapnic COPD patients to be quite similar to those of hypoxemic, normocapnic patients. Cox's proportional hazards models identified age, gender, PaO_2, and percent of vital capacity as independent predictors for survival, but no statistical significance was found for $PaCO_2$ or FEV_1/FVC to predict this outcome.

Static hyperinflation

The presence of lung hyperinflation is a frequent occurrence in patients who have COPD, and it is getting increased recognition as an important manifestation of the disease. It is recognized easily on the physical examination by the barrel-shaped chest seen in patients who have emphysema, and results from destruction of lung parenchyma, loss of lung elastic recoil, and increase in resting lung volume. The resting inspiratory capacity (IC) performed during pulmonary function testing reflects the end-expiratory lung volume. Schols and colleagues [31] reviewed data from 603 patients and used IC expressed as a percentage of normal, as an index of hyperinflation. The authors did not find IC to predict mortality in this cohort. In another prospective study [22], however, hyperinflation expressed as the residual volume (RV)/total lung capacity (TLC) proved to be a powerful predictor of mortality in patients who had COPD. A recent study proposes the inspiratory fraction, or IC/TLC, as a measurement of functional reserve. In this study of 689 patients (95% males) who had COPD, IC/TLC was found to be an important independent predictor of increased mortality after

34 months of follow-up. The increase in mortality became critical for an IC/TLC ratio below 25% (critical hyperinflation) [32].

Pulmonary hypertension

Pulmonary hypertension (PH) is defined as a pulmonary artery mean pressure (Ppa) at rest, equal or greater than 20 mm Hg. Although it generally is recognized that PH is common in COPD, when present, it is usually mild to moderate in severity [33,34]. In a recent retrospective study of 998 patients undergoing right heart catheterization between 1990 and 2002, only 11 patients were identified as having severe PH as the result of COPD. The authors reported an increased mortality rate among these patients when compared with a control group of 30 patients who had COPD with similar degree of airflow limitation but no evidence of severe PH [35]. It generally is accepted that the presence of pulmonary PH in COPD correlates with the presence of chronic hypoxemia [36–38]. Conversely, studies have shown that treatment with long term oxygen therapy reverses the progression of PH in a high percentage of hypoxemic COPD patients, although complete normalization is seen infrequently. In earlier studies by Weitzenblum and colleagues [36], Ppa was measured by three consecutive right heart catheterizations in a small group of COPD patients affected by hypoxemia (mean PaO_2 50 plus or minus 6.6 mmHg). From the baseline measurement T0 to T1 (47 plus or minus 28 months), hypoxemia worsened from 59 plus or minus 9 to 50 plus or minus 6, and Ppa worsened from 23 plus or minus 6 to 28 plus or minus 7 mmHg in patients not receiving LTOT. Patients then were prescribed O_2 for 15 to 18 h/d, and a third measurement was obtained after 31 plus or minus 18 months. The investigators found a significant decrease in Ppa among 12 out of 16 patients (28 plus or minus 7 to 23.9 plus or minus 6 mm Hg ($P < .005$), which suggested modulation of PH after correction of hypoxemia. Not all hypoxemic patients show this beneficial effect. Other studies have shown that not all hypoxemic patients respond with a decrease in Ppa after oxygen administration. In a study by Ashutosh and colleagues [37], the response of the Ppa to the administration of 28% oxygen for 24 hours was measured among 28 patients who had COPD. Seventeen patients responded with a decrease in Ppa greater than 5 mm Hg, and 11 did not. More importantly, the investigators found an

88% 2-year survival among responders versus 22% among nonresponders. These findings suggest that LTOT attenuates the development of more severe PH over time, and by doing so, decreases mortality in COPD. The natural history of PH in COPD was studied by Kessler and colleagues [38]. One hundred thirty-one COPD patients with mild to moderate hypoxemia not meeting criteria for LTOT were followed for 6.8 years with two right heart catheterizations. During the first measurement T0, all patients had normal Ppa less than 20 mm Hg. The patients underwent a steady-state 40 W exercise test, and Ppa after exercise also was measured. Seventy-six patients (group 2) were noted to develop exercise-induced PH (Ppa greater than 30 mm Hg). On average, these patients had higher resting Ppa than 55 patients (group 1) who did not have PH during exercise (16 plus or minus 3 versus 14 plus or minus 2 mm Hg, $P = .001$). During the second catheterization, Ppa had changed to 19 plus or minus 7 and 16 plus or minus 5 mm Hg, respectively ($P = .01$). Thirty-three patients developed resting Ppa, nine from group 1 and 24 from group 2. These patients had significantly higher Ppa at rest and with exercise at T0, and lower resting and exercise PaO_2 when compared with those who did not develop PH. The authors found that higher resting and exercise Ppa at baseline predicted the development of PH over a 6-year period. The development of PH is rather slow in patients with mild to moderate hypoxemic COPD not meeting criteria for LTOT.

Malnutrition

Nutritional depletion is a prevalent finding among patients who have COPD, in particular those who have advanced disease. The prevalence of weight loss in stable COPD is in the range of 20%, and it increases to 35% among those who are hospitalized [39,40]. Several studies have found that the body mass index (BMI) is an independent risk factor for COPD mortality [41–43]. Landbo and colleagues [42], in The Copenhagen City Heart Study, found BMI to be an independent predictor of all-cause and respiratory mortality among COPD patients with FEV_1 less than 50% predicted. The impact of weight change on survival in COPD also was examined retrospectively by Schols and colleagues [31] in 400 COPD patients who participated in a pulmonary rehabilitation program. A low BMI (less than 25 kg/m²) was associated with a significant increase in the risk for

mortality ($P < .001$). In a prospective post hoc analysis of 203 COPD patients who received nutritional support, weight gain (greater than 2 kg/8 wks) was a significant predictor of survival [31]. Studies using more complex tests to evaluate nutrition, such as midthigh [44] and midarm [45] muscle cross-sectional area obtained by CT also have shown significant association between malnutrition and mortality in COPD, with a predictive value that is superior to that of BMI. Taken together, the evidence suggests that weight loss can be considered an independent risk factor for mortality in patients who have COPD.

Exercise capacity

Exercise intolerance afflicts many patients who have COPD and is likely multifactorial. Exercise capacity reflects the respiratory and nonrespiratory expressions of the disease and the integrated activities of the pulmonary and cardiovascular systems. The peak oxygen uptake (peak VO_2) determined during a cardiopulmonary exercise test (CPX) has been shown to predict survival in COPD patients undergoing lung resection [46,47], and to be a better predictor of survival than FEV_1 and health status [48]. In a study by Epstein and colleagues [49], COPD patients who were unable to perform a CPX were 11 times more likely to die following lung resection than those able to complete the test independent of the achieved peak VO_2. The 6-minute walk distance (6MWD) is a simple field test that also has been correlated with mortality in COPD patients in various settings, including postpulmonary rehabilitation [50], and following lung-volume–reduction surgery (LVRS) [51,52]. Gerardi and colleagues [50] reported on predictors of survival in a group of severe COPD patients graduating from a pulmonary rehabilitation program. In this rather homogeneous group of patients who had a uniformly low FEV_1, the 6MWD was a better predictor of survival, and FEV_1 failed to predict this outcome. In a study by Pinto-Plata and colleagues [53], exercise capacity was tested with the 6MWD in 198 patients with severe COPD followed for 2 years. In this patient cohort, survival increased progressively with increases in the 6MWD, when distances were divided into discrete 100 m increments. Those patients unable to walk 100 m had a mortality rate approaching 90% at 1 year. On the other hand, COPD patients with similar degree of airflow limitation who were able to walk more than 400 m had significantly higher survival ($P < .0001$). The investigators also found that the 6MWD test was a better predictor of mortality than FEV_1 and BMI. In this study, the decline in 6MWD occurred independently of changes in FEV_1, indicating that both tests measure different domains of the disease and could be considered complementary.

Health status

Health Related Quality of Life (HRQoL) is an important patient-reported health outcome in COPD. HRQoL has been defined as: "The extents to which one's usual or expected physical, emotional, and social well-being are affected by a medical condition or its treatment" [54]. To this effect, COPD is a disease that has a profound impact on patients' HRQoL, even among those with relatively modest airflow limitation [55]. Importantly, a weak association between HRQoL and the main respiratory defect that characterizes COPD, FEV_1, long has been described. This poor correlation reflects the marked heterogeneity and complexity of this disease. Domingo-Salvany and colleagues [56] were first to describe an association between measurements of HRQoL and mortality in COPD. In their study, 321 male patients were tested with both generic and disease-specific HRQoL instruments. The patients were followed for a mean 4.8 years, and mortality was documented. The investigators found that survival was shorter among patients who had worse quality- of-life scores. The predictive value of HRQoL has been confirmed in several studies [57,58]. Using univariate analysis, HRQoL also was identified as a predictor of mortality in a study of 609 patients with severe emphysema enrolled in the National Emphysema Treatment Trial (NETT) [58].

Anemia

Anemia is a common comorbidity in many chronic diseases, and its importance in COPD is gaining interest. Recent reports suggests that anemia in patients who have COPD may be more prevalent than expected and could be associated with increased mortality [59–61]. The reported prevalence of anemia in COPD ranges from 10% to 15% in patients suffering from severe forms of the disease. In a study of 2524 COPD patients who were prescribed long-term oxygen therapy, 12.6% of males and 8.2% of females were identified as anemic [60]. Recently, in a retrospective analysis of prospectively collected data of a cohort of 683 COPD patients [23,61], anemia was found in 17% of the cohort in contrast to polycythemia, which was present in only 6% of the patients (and when present carried no clinical relevance). The investigators found that anemic patients had significantly higher dyspnea, lower 6MWD, and shorter median survival (49 versus 74 months) when compared with nonanemic COPD patients. These differences remained significant when controlling for the relevant demographic, physiologic, and disease covariates in regression analyses, where anemia was an independent predictor of outcomes. The relationship between anemia and mortality in COPD, and the possible effect that its correction may have on survival, need to be confirmed by prospective and controlled clinical trials.

Comorbidities

Tobacco use is without doubt the most important etiologic factor behind the development of COPD [62]. Cigarette smoking induces a state of systemic inflammation characterized by the intense interaction and accumulation of cells capable of creating a marked oxidant-antioxidant imbalance that results in cellular injury [63]. Miller and colleagues [64] reported that the numbers of circulating CD8+ T-cells were increased, and CD4+ T-cells decreased in heavy smokers. This abnormality was reversible upon discontinuation of smoking. A low CD4+/CD8+ ratio is a characteristic of the systemic inflammation seen in COPD, and it is controlled genetically [65]. It is possible then, that in genetically predisposed smokers, tobacco initiates a state of generalized, chronic inflammation. A comorbidity is defined as a disease that coexists with the primary disease of interest. Because the toxic effects of tobacco extend to other organ systems, it is no surprise that the most common comorbid conditions associated with COPD are cardiovascular disease and cancer [66]. In a study by Soriano and colleagues [67] from the UK General Practice Research Database, 2699 patients who had COPD were identified. Compared with controls, COPD patients had a significantly higher comorbidity burden, in particular cardiovascular diseases, osteoporosis, and cataracts. The association with mortality was described by Almagro and colleagues [68], in a study of hospitalized COPD patients who had their comorbidities measured by the Charlson index [69]. The authors found that a higher score in the Charlson index was an independent predictor of mortality among these patients, $(P < .001)$. This independent predictive value of comorbidities in COPD also has been demonstrated by others [23–32].

Multidimensional mortality risk assessment in chronic obstructive pulmonary disease

Since the early studies of Fletcher and Peto [8], FEV_1 has been used to define the severity of the disease and its prognosis. For many years now, FEV_1 and age have been considered as the most important prognostic indicators in this disease. Unfortunately, both of them are, for the most part, irreversible. On the other hand, most studies done to evaluate the effectiveness of therapies in COPD have focused on this physiologic outcome, and the failure of most therapies to significantly increase or delay the rate of decline of FEV_1 has led to nihilism. The evidence presented in this article, however, suggests that multiple factors other than FEV_1 also are associated with mortality in COPD. Some of these factors include: hypoxemia, the timed walking distance, BMI, dyspnea, hyperinflation, malnutrition, pulmonary hypertension, comorbidities, anemia, and health status. These factors are reflections of the systemic involvement of COPD, and many of them are amenable to treatment [51,58,70–74]. As such, sole reliance on FEV_1 during the evaluation of a patient with COPD would lead to an incomplete assessment of disease severity. It is then reasonable that a composite index that incorporates the most important predictors of mortality, reflecting not only impairment in lung function, but also systemic consequences of the disease, may provide a more comprehensively way to evaluate COPD. In a pioneer study by Celli and colleagues [23], 207 patients who had COPD were enrolled prospectively, and the predictive value of numerous variables was evaluated. These variables included: age, gender, smoking history in pack per year, FVC, FEV_1, dyspnea measured with the MMRC, BMI, functional residual capacity, inspiratory capacity, hematocrit, and albumin level. The independent association with mortality at 1 year was evaluated with stepwise forward logistic-regression analysis. The authors identified four variables that predicted an elevated risk for death: BMI (B), degree of airflow obstruction (O) as measured by FEV_1, dyspnea as measured

by the MRC dyspnea scale (D), and exercise capacity (E) as measured by the 6MWD test. These variables were incorporated into a multidimensional scale, the BODE index, that ranged from 0 (least risk) to 10 (highest risk) (Table 1). The BODE index then was validated prospectively in a separate cohort of 625 predominantly male patients with COPD who were evaluated every 6 months for at least 2 years, or until death. The authors found that each quartile increase in the BODE index score yielded an increase in the risk for mortality. Those patients who had a BODE index in the quartile 4 (BODE index score of 7 to 10) had a mortality rate of 80% at 52 months. The results of this study indicated that the BODE index was a much better predictor of mortality than any of the individual variables alone.

The predictive value of BODE has been tested by other investigators [75–77]. In a study by Ong and colleagues [75], 127 COPD patients were recruited and tested with the BODE index. The patients were followed for up to 2 years, and the number of hospital admissions and mortality were documented. The investigators found the median BODE score to be lower among survivors than among nonsurvivors (4 versus 6, respectively, $P = .003$) and a significant effect of the BODE scores on mortality (hazard ratio, 1.30; 95% confidence interval [CI], 1.08 to 1, 56; $P = .006$). The investigators used Poisson regression analysis to evaluate the effect of BODE scores on hospitalizations and found BODE to also be a predictor of this outcome.

Furthermore, in a retrospective clinical study of 186 patients who had severe emphysema, Imfeld and colleagues [76] tested the predictive value of BODE following LVRS. The investigators found that the postoperative BODE, but

Table 1
Calculation of the BODE index

Variable	BODE score			
	0	1	2	3
FEV_1, % predicted	≥65	50–65	35–49	≤35
Dyspnea: MRC	0–1	2	3	4
6MWD meters	≥350	250–349	150–249	≤149
BMI	>21	≤21	—	—

Points from each variable are added according to the threshold value measured for each one. The value ranges from 0 to a maximum of 10.

Abbreviations: BMI, body mass index; FEV_1, forced expiratory volume in 1 second; MRC, Medical Research Council; 6MWD, 6-minute walk distance test.

not the preoperative BODE, predicted survival. Most patients undergoing LVRS showed an improvement in BODE index following the intervention from 7.2 (quartile 4), to 4.0 (quartile 2) ($P < .001$). Those patients having the most improvement in BODE had the best 5-year survival (HR, 0.497; 95% CI, 0.375 to 0.659; $P < .001$). The investigators found that the BODE index was able to predict the risk of death (0.74) better than FEV_1 (0.63).

The capacity of patients to significantly modify their BODE index after LVRS suggests that the BODE index can be used not only as a surrogate of mortality but as a tool for disease modification. To this effect, other interventions also have proven to be able to modify BODE. Pulmonary rehabilitation (PR) is known to improve several of the surrogate markers for mortality in COPD, namely dyspnea, health status, and exercise capacity. Based on this observation, it was hypothesized that PR would be able to modify the severity of COPD and the risk for mortality, as measured by the BODE index [77]. In this study, of the 246 patients who qualified for and were offered rehabilitation, 116 accepted and completed the 8-week, three times weekly rehabilitation program; 130 declined participation. The change in BODE scores were compared between rehabilitated patients and non-PR participants. The patients had severe COPD both by FEV_1 and by the BODE index scores. Seventy-five percent of patients belonged to the third and fourth quartiles. Patients were followed for more than 2 years or until death. Approximately 30% of the patients who graduated from PR joined a maintenance program and exercised three times weekly for the entire 2-year period. Following PR, 71% of the participating patients improved their BODE index scores by at least 1 point; of these, 25% improved by 2 points.

After graduation from PR, the BODE index decreased significantly from 5.07 to 4.18. This resulted in a shift from the third quartile to second quartile, and their initially predicted mortality of 20% to 30% changed to an observed mortality of 11.2%. Patients who declined PR had a worse BODE index at entry of 6.94 (approaching BODE fourth quartile), and in this group, there was almost a 20% worsening of BODE index over time. This group of patients had the highest mortality rate (50%). For patients who responded to PR, defined as an improvement in the BODE index score of at least 1 point, BODE index scores improved by a statistically significant 25% at 3 months, compared with the patients who did not respond to rehabilitation. These improvements in BODE index scores were maintained for a full 2 years after the start of pulmonary rehabilitation, while patients who did not participate in pulmonary rehabilitation displayed an 18% deterioration in BODE index scores. These results support the concept that the BODE index can be a useful tool to assess disease modification.

Patients who have advanced COPD experience frequent exacerbations and hospitalizations, which usually are associated with poor outcomes and worsening of the FEV_1 [78].

In a study assessing the impact of exacerbations on several patient-centered outcomes [79] and BODE, this multidimensional index proved to be a more sensitive tool than FEV_1 alone to reflect progression of disease over a 2-year follow-up period. In this study, 205 patients were recruited and evaluated with the BODE index at baseline while stable, during the exacerbation event and every 6 months thereafter. The authors presented data on the impact of exacerbations on FEV_1, 6MWD, MMRC, BMI, and BODE. One hundred thirty patients experienced exacerbations, and 75 patients remained exacerbation free for the duration of the study. Exacerbators showed a worsening of BODE index of 1.38 points during the exacerbation event, and although there was a partial improvement, the BODE index at 24 months remained 1.09 points above baseline. On the contrary, nonexacerbators showed a negligible increase in BODE at 2 years (0.07 points), which differed significantly from that of the exacerbators ($P < .001$). Taken together, the response of patients to exacerbations, LVRS and PR, can be captured as changes in the BODE index, not only reflecting changes on disease severity, but changes in outcome, suggesting that the BODE index can be used as both surrogate marker for mortality and as a tool to assess disease modification.

Summary

Although FEV_1 remains the most important physiologic indicator of the severity of airflow obstruction in COPD, its predictive value is weak above 50% [8] of its predicted value, and once patients reach very low values of FEV_1, other markers of mortality in COPD become more accurate. Chief among these predictors of mortality are dyspnea, exercise capacity, and BMI.

Evidence also exists for markers such as health status, anemia, hypoxemia, comorbidities, and hyperinflation, among others. Simple to use, the validated multidimensional BODE index encompasses the predictive validity of the best of these potential surrogates into a single measure of disease severity and survival. The BODE index or other multidimensional staging tools that capture the multisystemic manifestations of COPD may prove to be a valuable, not only in assessing severity and progression of disease, but also in evaluating the response to medical interventions.

References

[1] Murray CJL, Lopez AD. Mortality by cause for eight regions of the world: global burden of disease study. Lancet 1997;349:1269–76.

[2] World Health Organization. Global initiative for chronic obstructive lung disease. Geneva (Switzerland): World Health Organization; 2002.

[3] Pauwels RA, Buist AS, Calverley PM, et al. Global strategy for the diagnosis, management, and prevention of chronic obstructive pulmonary disease. NHLBI/WHO global initiative for chronic obstructive lung disease (GOLD) workshop summary. Am J Respir Crit Care Med 2001;163:1256–76.

[4] Mannino DM, Homa DM, Akinbami LJ, et al. Chronic obstructive pulmonary disease surveillance–United States, 1971–2000. MMWR Surveill Summ 2002;51:1–16.

[5] Pauwels R. Global initiative for chronic obstructive lung diseases (GOLD): time to act. Eur Respir J 2001;18:901–2.

[6] National center for Health Statistics. Report of final mortality statistics; 2003. Available at: http://www.nlm.nih.gov/medlineplus/healthstatistics.html.

[7] National Heart Lung and Blood Institute. Morbidity and mortality chartbook, 2004. Division epidemiology, NHLBI. Available at: www.nhlbi.gov 2004. Accessed January 2007.

[8] Fletcher C, Peto R. The natural history of chronic airflow obstruction. Br Med J 1977;1:1645–8.

[9] Anthonisen NR, Wright EC, Hodgkin JE. Prognosis in chronic obstructive pulmonary disease. Am Rev Respir Dis 1986;133:14–20.

[10] Beaty TH, Cohen BH, Newill CA, et al. Impaired pulmonary function as a risk factor for mortality. Am J Epidemiol 1982;116:102–13.

[11] Hole DJ, Watt GCM, Davey-Smith G, et al. Impaired lung function and mortality risk in men and women: findings from the Renfrew and Paisley prospective population study. BMJ 1996;313:711–5.

[12] Bang KM, Gergen PJ, Kramer R, et al. The effect of pulmonary impairment on all-cause mortality in national–cohort. Chest 1993;103:536–40.

[13] Schunemann HJ, Dorn J, Grant BJ, et al. Pulmonary function is a long-term predictor of mortality in the general population. Chest 2000;118:656–64.

[14] National Center for Health Statistics. Plan and operation of the NHANES I augmentation survey of adults 25–74 years, United States, 1974–1975. Washington, DC: National Center for Health Statistics; 1973.

[15] Mannino DM, Buist AS, Petty TL, et al. Lung function and mortality in the United States: data from the first national health and nutrition examination survey follow up study. Thorax 2003;58: 388–93.

[16] Orie NGM, VanderLende Reds. Bronchitis III. In: Proceedings of the Third International Symposium on Bronchitis. Assen (the Netherlands): 115 Royal Van Gorcum; 1970.

[17] Hospers JJ, Postma DS, Rijcken B, et al. Histamine airway hyper-responsiveness and mortality from chronic obstructive pulmonary disease: a cohort study. Lancet 2000;356:1313–7.

[18] American Thoracic Society. Dyspnea: mechanisms, assessment, and management: a consensus statement. Am J Respir Crit Care Med 1999;159:321–40.

[19] Celli BR, MacNee W. Standards for the diagnosis and treatment of COPD. Eur Respir J 2004;23: 932–46.

[20] Mahler DA, Weinburg DH, Wells CK, et al. The measurement of dyspnea: contents, interobserver agreement, and physiologic correlates of two new clinical indexes. Chest 1984;85:751–8.

[21] Wolkove N, Dajczman E, Colacone A, et al. The relationship between pulmonary function and dyspnea in obstructive lung disease. Chest 1989;96:1247–51.

[22] Nishimura K, Izumi T, Tsukino M, et al. Dyspnea is a better predictor of 5-year survival than airway obstruction in patients with COPD. Chest 2002;121: 1434–40.

[23] Celli BR, Cote CG, Marin JM, et al. The body mass index, airflow obstruction, dyspnea, and exercise capacity index in chronic obstructive pulmonary disease. N Engl J Med 2004;350:1005–12.

[24] Neff TA, Petty TL. Long-term continuous oxygen therapy in chronic airway obstruction. Ann Intern Med 1970;72:621–5.

[25] Medical Research Council Working Party. Long-term domiciliary oxygen therapy in chronic hypoxic cor pulmonale complicating chronic bronchitis and emphysema. Lancet 1981;1:681–6.

[26] Nocturnal Oxygen Therapy Trial Group. Continuous or nocturnal oxygen therapy in hypoxemic chronic obstructive lung disease. Ann Intern Med 1980;93:391–8.

[27] Burrows B, Earle RH. Prediction of survival in patients with chronic airway obstruction. Am Rev Respir Dis 1969;99:865–71.

[28] Boushy SF, Thompson HF, North LB, et al. Prognosis in chronic obstructive pulmonary disease. Am Rev Respir Dis 1973;108:1373–83.

[29] Postma DS, Burema J, Gimeno F, et al. Prognosis in severe chronic obstructive pulmonary disease. Am Rev Respir Dis 1979;119:357–67.

[30] Aida A, Miyamoto K, Nishimura M, et al, the Respiratory Failure Research Group in Japan. Prognostic value of hypercapnia in patients with chronic respiratory failure during long-term oxygen therapy. Am J Respir Crit Care Med 1998;158:188–93.

[31] Schols AM, Slangen J, Volovics L, et al. Weight loss is a reversible factor in the prognosis of chronic obstructive pulmonary disease. Am J Respir Crit Care Med 1998;157:1791–7.

[32] Casanova C, Cote C, de Torres JP, et al. Inspiratory-to-total lung capacity ratio predicts mortality in patients with chronic obstructive pulmonary disease. Am J Respir Crit Care Med 2005;171:591–7.

[33] Stevens D, Sharma K, Szidon P, et al. Severe pulmonary hypertension associated with COPD. Ann Transplant 2000;5:8–12.

[34] Scharf SM, Iqbal M, Keller C, et al. Hemodynamic characterization of patients with severe emphysema. Am Rev Respir Crit Care Med 2002;166:314–22.

[35] Chaouat A, Bugnet AS, Kadaoui N, et al. Severe pulmonary hypertension and chronic obstructive pulmonary disease. Am J Respir Crit Care Med 2005;172:189–94.

[36] Weitzenblum E, Sautegeau A, Ehrhart M, et al. Long-term oxygen therapy can reverse the progression of pulmonary hypertension in patients with chronic obstructive pulmonary disease. Am Rev Respir Dis 1985;131(4):493–8.

[37] Ashutosh K, Mead G, Dunsky M. Early effects of oxygen administration and prognosis in chronic obstructive pulmonary disease and cor pulmonale. Am Rev Respir Dis 1983;127(4):399–404.

[38] Kessler R, Faller M, Weitzenblum E, et al. Natural history of pulmonary hypertension in a series of 131 patients with chronic obstructive lung disease. Am J Respir Crit Care Med 2001;164(2):219–24.

[39] Engelen MP, Schols AM, Baken WC, et al. Nutritional depletion in relation to respiratory and peripheral skeletal muscle function in outpatients with COPD. Eur Respir J 1994;7:1793–7.

[40] Schols AM, Soeters PB, Dingemans AM, et al. Prevalence and characteristics of nutritional depletion in patients with stable COPD eligible for pulmonary rehabilitation. Am Rev Respir Dis 1993;147:1151–6.

[41] Wilson DO, Rogers RM, Wright EC, et al. Body weight in chronic obstructive pulmonary disease: the national institute of health intermittent positive-pressure breathing trial. Am Rev Respir Dis 1989;139:1435–8.

[42] Landbo C, Prescott E, Lange P, et al. Prognostic value of nutritional status in chronic obstructive pulmonary disease. Am J Respir Crit Care Med 1999; 160:1856–61.

[43] Gray-Donald K, Gibbons L, Shapiro SH, et al. Nutritional status and mortality in chronic obstructive pulmonary disease. Am J Respir Crit Care Med 1996;153:961–6.

[44] Marquis K, Debigare R, Lacasse Y, et al. Midthigh muscle cross-sectional area is a better predictor of mortality than body mass index in patients with chronic obstructive pulmonary disease. Am J Respir Crit Care Med 2002;166:809–13.

[45] Soler-cataluna JJ, Sanchez-Sanchez L, Martinez-Garcia MA, et al. Midarm muscle area is a better predictor of mortality than body mass index in COPD. Chest 2005;128(4):2108–15.

[46] Weisman I. Cardiopulmonary exercise testing in the preoperative assessment for lung resection surgery. Sem Thorac Cardiovasc Surg 2001;13:116–25.

[47] Bolliger C, Perruchoud A. Functional evaluation of lung resection candidates. Eur Respir J 1998;11: 198–212.

[48] Oga T, Nishimura K, Tsukino M, et al. Analysis of factors related to mortality in chronic obstructive pulmonary disease. Role of exercise capacity and health status. Am J Respir Crit Care Med 2002; 167:544–9.

[49] Epstein SK, Faling LJ, Daly BD, et al. Inability to perform bicycle ergometry predicts increased morbidity and mortality after lung resection. Chest 1995;107:311–6.

[50] Gerardi DA, Lovett L, Benoit-Connors ML, et al. Variables related to increased mortality following outpatient pulmonary rehabilitation. Eur Respir J 1996;9:431–5.

[51] Fishman A, Martinez F, Naunheim K, et al. A randomized trial comparing lung volume reduction surgery with medical therapy for severe emphysema. N Engl J Med 2003;348:2059–73.

[52] Szekely LA, Oelberg DA, Wright C, et al. Preoperative predictors of operative morbidity and mortality in COPD patients undergoing bilateral lung volume reduction surgery. Chest 1997;111:550–8.

[53] Pinto-Plata VM, Cote C, Cabral H, et al. The 6-min walk distance: change over time and value as a predictor of survival in severe COPD. Eur Respir J 2004;23:28–33.

[54] Engstrom CP, Persson LO, Larsson S, et al. Functional status and well being in chronic obstructive pulmonary disease with regard to clinical parameters and smoking: a descriptive and comparative study. Thorax 1996;51:825–30.

[55] Jones PW, Quirk FH, Baveystock CM, et al. A self-complete measure for chronic airflow limitation: the St. George's respiratory questionnaire. Am Rev Respir Dis 1992;142:1321–7.

[56] Domingo-Salvany A, Lamarca R, Ferrer M, et al. Health-related quality of life and mortality in male patients with chronic obstructive pulmonary disease. Am J Respir Crit Care Med 2002;166:680–5.

[57] Fan VS, Curtis JR, Tu SP, et al, from the Ambulatory Care Quality Improvement Project Investigators. Using quality of life to predict hospitalization

and mortality in patients with obstructive lung diseases. Chest 2005;122:429–36.

[58] Martinez FJ, Foster G, Curtis, et al, for the NETT research group. Predictors of mortality in patients with emphysema and severe airflow obstruction. Am J Respir Crit Care Med 2006;173:1326–34.

[59] John S, Hoerning S, Doehner W, et al. Anemia and inflammation in COPD. Chest 2005;127:825–9.

[60] Chambellan A, Chailleux E, Similoski T, the ANTADIR observatory group. Prognostic value of hematocrit in patients with severe chronic obstructive pulmonary disease receiving long-term oxygen therapy. Chest 2005;128:1201–8.

[61] Cote C, Zilberberg M, Mody S, et al. Hemoglobin level and its clinical impact in a cohort of patients with COPD. Eur Respir J 2007;29(3):535–40.

[62] Anto JM, Vermeire P, Vestbo J, et al. Epidemiology of chronic obstructive pulmonary disease. Eur Respir J 2001;17:982–94.

[63] Rahman I, Morrison D, Donaldson K, et al. Systemic oxidative stress in asthma, COPD, and smokers. Am J Respir Crit Care Med 1996;154:1055–60.

[64] Miller LG, Goldstein G, Murphy M, et al. Reversible alterations in immunoregulatory T cells in smoking. Analysis by monoclonal antibodies and flow cytometry. Chest 1982;82:526–9.

[65] Amadori A, Zamarchi R, De Silvestro G, et al. Genetic control of the CD4/CD8 T-cell ratio in humans. Nat Med 1995;1:1279–83.

[66] Sin DD, Anthonisen NR, Soriano JB, et al. Mortality in COPD: role of comorbidities. Eur Respir J 2006;28:1245–57.

[67] Soriano JB, Visick GT, Muellerova H, et al. Patterns of comorbidities of newly diagnosed COPD and asthma in the primary care. Chest 2005;128:2099–107.

[68] Almagro P, Calbo E, Ochoa de E, et al. Mortality after hospitalization for COPD. Chest 2002;121:1441–8.

[69] Charlson ME, Pompei P, Ales KL, et al. A new method of classifying prognostic comorbidity in longitudinal studies: development and validation. J Chronic Dis 1987;40:373–83.

[70] Scanlon PD, Connett JE, Waller LA, et al. Smoking cessation and lung function in mild-to-moderate chronic obstructive pulmonary disease. The Lung Health Study. Am J Respir Crit Care Med 2000; 161:381–90.

[71] Gaissert HA, Trulock EP, Cooper JD, et al. Comparison of early functional results after volume reduction or lung transplantation for chronic obstructive pulmonary disease. J Thorac Cardiovasc Surg 1996;111:296–306.

[72] Guell R, Casan P, Belda J, et al. Long-term effects of outpatient rehabilitation of COPD: a randomized trial. Chest 2000;117:976–83.

[73] O'Donnell DE, Voduc N, Fitzpatrick M, et al. Effect of salmeterol on the ventilatory response to exercise in chronic obstructive pulmonary disease. Eur Respir J 2004;24:86–94.

[74] Celli B, ZuWallack R, Wang S, et al. Improvement in resting inspiratory capacity and hyperinflation with tiotropium in COPD patients with increased static lung volumes. Chest 2003;124:1743–8.

[75] Ong KC, Earnest A, Lu SJ. A multidimensional grading system (BODE index) as predictor for hospitalization for COPD. Chest 2005;128:3810–6.

[76] Imfeld S, Bloch KE, Weder W, et al. The BODE index after lung volume reduction correlates with survival in COPD. Chest 2006;129:835–6.

[77] Cote CG, Celli BR. Pulmonary rehabilitation and the BODE index in COPD. Eur Respir J 2005;26: 630–6.

[78] Donaldson GC, Seemungal TAR, Bhowmik A, et al. Relationship between exacerbation frequency and lung function decline in chronic obstructive pulmonary disease. Thorax 2002;57:847–52.

[79] Cote CG, Dordelly LJ, Celli BR. Impact of exacerbations on patient-centered outcomes. Chest 2007; 131:696–704.

CLINICS
IN CHEST
MEDICINE

Clin Chest Med 28 (2007) 525–536

The Biology of a Chronic Obstructive Pulmonary Disease Exacerbation

John R. Hurst, PhD, Jadwiga A. Wedzicha, MD*

*Academic Unit of Respiratory Medicine, Royal Free and University College Medical School,
Royal Free Hospital, London, NW3 2PF, UK*

A defining characteristic of chronic obstructive pulmonary disease (COPD) is the relentless decline in lung function [1] that results in progressive symptoms and worsening exercise capacity. It also, however, long has been recognized that the course of COPD is punctuated by intermittent deteriorations in respiratory health termed exacerbations. The original and now classic study of Fletcher and Peto [2] describing the natural history of chronic airflow limitation suggested that exacerbations were no more than a troublesome increase in respiratory symptoms. This is now known not to be true, and it is apparent that exacerbations have profound implications for patients including accelerating the decline in lung function [3,4], impairing quality of life [5], and increasing mortality [6]. Exacerbations are therefore important outcome measures in COPD. With a greater understanding of the importance of exacerbations has come increasing research interest, and while there remain many unanswered questions, there is now a reasonable understanding of the biology of these events, the subject of this article.

What is an exacerbation?

The 2006 update to the World Health Organization (WHO)/US National Heart Lung and Blood Institute (NHLBI) Global initiative for chronic Obstructive Lung Disease (GOLD) document [1] included a definition of exacerbation for the first time. An exacerbation is defined as

"an event in the natural course of the disease characterized by a change in the patient's baseline dyspnoea, cough, and/or sputum that is beyond normal day-to-day variations, is acute in onset, and may warrant a change in regular medication in a patient with underlying COPD" [1].

It should be stated that establishing a universal definition of exacerbation has been controversial, and, indeed, there has been much debate about how exactly an exacerbation should be defined [7]. This is important when comparing results across research studies. Some previous definitions have included the necessity for an exacerbation to result in a change in treatment; yet it is apparent that many exacerbations remain unreported to health care professionals for treatment despite being no less severe than reported events [5]. As factors other than the underlying pathophysiology of exacerbation may affect the decision or ability of a patient to access treatment (consider, for example, differential global social and economic conditions), a definition such as that in the GOLD document [1], in which symptom changes may necessitate a change in treatment is now considered more appropriate.

A further complication to the definition of exacerbation, yet to be addressed in current criteria, although raised in a recent editorial [8], is that of comorbidities that may mimic or complicate exacerbation in a patient who has underlying COPD. Such conditions include, but are not restricted to pneumonia, pneumothorax, pulmonary embolism, and cardiac failure. The sections below discuss that exacerbations of COPD are associated with demonstrable changes in airway and systemic inflammation, and further impairment in lung function. The authors have suggested

---

* Corresponding author.
 E-mail address: j.a.wedzicha@medsch.ucl.ac.uk
(J.A. Wedzicha).

doi:10.1016/j.ccm.2007.05.003

that these comorbid conditions are primary diagnoses in their own right and do not exacerbate the airway inflammation that is characteristic of stable disease; therefore future definitions of exacerbation may evolve to include references to increased inflammation or specific physiological changes. As exacerbations are primarily defined by changes in symptoms, however, after discussing the epidemiology of exacerbation, it would seem appropriate to first examine what is known about symptom changes during exacerbations. The article then considers changes in lung function and inflammatory mediators, COPD being defined as a disease state associated with airflow limitation and an abnormal inflammatory response of the lung to noxious particles or gases [1].

Epidemiology of exacerbations in chronic obstructive pulmonary disease

COPD is a major global health problem, and one of the few diseases in which mortality rates continue to rise. This reflects an aging population and the relative greater effectiveness of therapies available for other common conditions such as cardiovascular disease and many cancers. Consequently, COPD is projected to be the third leading cause of death in the world by 2020 [9]. While many of these deaths are caused by exacerbations, especially in those with more severe underlying COPD, cardiovascular causes and lung cancer are also prominent, reflecting the shared etiology of these conditions.

In general, exacerbations become both more frequent and more severe as the severity of the underlying COPD increases [10]. The relationship between exacerbation frequency and disease severity is illustrated in Fig. 1. There remain large differences in annual exacerbation incidence rates between patients of similar COPD severity, however, and it now is recognized that the frequent exacerbator (usually defined as three or more exacerbations per year) is an important clinical phenotype. Frequent exacerbators have greater airway inflammation in the stable state [11], which may explain their more rapid decline in forced expiratory volume in 1 second (FEV_1) [4]. They also have a poorer quality of life [5] and greater mortality [6]. It should be noted that recent work demonstrating a relationship between exacerbation frequency and FEV_1 decline in COPD is not consistent with the original hypotheses of Fletcher and Peto [2].

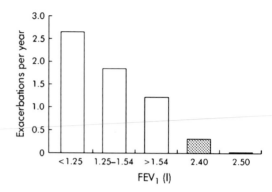

Fig. 1. Exacerbation frequency is related to the severity of the underlying chronic obstructive pulmonary disease: mean incidence of exacerbations per year in relation to forced expiratory volume in 1 second (FEV_1) in the placebo arms of three 3-year studies. From left to right, the first three bars are from the Inhaled Steroids in Obstructive Lung Disease in Europe (ISOLDE) study, in which exacerbations were defined as a worsening of respiratory symptoms that required treatment with oral corticosteroids or antibiotics. The next bar represents data from the Copenhagen City Lung Study, which defined exacerbations more broadly. The final bar shows data from the European Society Study on COPD, which used the same definition as the ISOLDE study. (*From* Burge S, Wedzicha JA. COPD exacerbations: definitions and classifications. Eur Respir J 2003;41:46; with permission.)

Given the importance of respiratory viruses in causing exacerbations, discussed further later in this article, it follows that exacerbation rates peak in the winter months, and indeed, they are around 50% more common at this time, when circulation of viruses within the community is greatest [12]. Exacerbations, therefore, contribute to seasonal peaks of health care use and hospital admission. In the United Kingdom, exacerbations of COPD account for around 1% of all admissions to hospital (approximately twice as many as for asthma), and with an average length of stay of 10 days, the associated health care costs are immense [12]. The in-hospital mortality for patients without respiratory failure is estimated at between 5% and 11%, and it is considerably higher for those in which respiratory failure is present. There is also a significant risk of mortality in the period after discharge [13], and the reasons for this remain poorly understood. In part, this on-going mortality risk may relate to clustering of exacerbations. This refers to the finding of symptom deterioration [14,15] or a second recurrent exacerbation in the period following a first exacerbation. The differential pathology and etiology of index and recurrent exacerbations remain to be explored, but the authors recently have shown that a heightened serum c-reactive protein in the recovery period predicts recurrence [16], suggesting that the mechanism may relate to non-resolution of the inflammatory response. Research in this area, and studies investigating factors underlying the frequent exacerbator phenotype, have the potential to impact on the particularly high burden of disease experienced by patients prone to frequent exacerbations.

Symptomatology: symptom changes during exacerbations of chronic obstructive pulmonary disease

The symptom changes and the timing of such changes that occur during exacerbation have been studied using diary card methodology in which patients are asked to record increases in symptoms above their usual daily severity. This approach has allowed practitioners to develop an understanding not only of the changes present at exacerbation onset, but also how symptoms develop in the prodromal period, and how symptoms resolve in response to therapy.

Seemungal and colleagues [17] studied 504 exacerbations in 101 patients who had severe COPD (mean FEV_1 41.9% predicted). After a short prodrome, and following exacerbation onset, the median time to symptom recovery was seven (interquartile range [IQR] 4 to 14) days. Fourteen percent of exacerbations still had not returned to baseline symptoms within 35 days, however, suggesting that the increases in symptoms observed in some exacerbations may never fully return to the baseline pre-exacerbation level. The symptoms present on the day of onset of exacerbation in the patients studied by Seemungal and colleagues [17] are described in Box 1. The same group subsequently demonstrated that these changes in symptoms are associated with a decrease in functional status, reflected in a greater proportion of patients remaining housebound during exacerbations than seen in stable disease [18]. The time course of changes in symptoms and functional status at exacerbation are illustrated in Fig. 2. In hospitalized patients who have more severe exacerbations, the recovery period also is associated with reduced physical activity that remains low and still is returning toward baseline even following discharge home [19].

Box 1. Symptoms present at the onset of 504 exacerbations in 101 patients

Increased dyspnoea (64%)
Increased sputum purulence (42%)
Increased sputum volume (26%)
Increased wheeze (35%)
Increased nasal symptoms (coryza) (35%)
Increased cough (20%)

Data from Seemungal TAR, Donaldson GC, Bhowmik A, et al. Time course and recovery of exacerbations in patients with chronic obstructive pulmonary disease. Am J Respir Crit Care Med 2000;161:1608–13.

Subsequently, it has been shown that exacerbations cause acute impairment to health status from which recovery also is prolonged and still continuing 1 month after exacerbation onset [20].

Assessing exacerbation severity

In the study by Seemungal and colleagues [17], just under half of exacerbations were reported directly to the clinical team, and the greater the number of increased symptoms present at

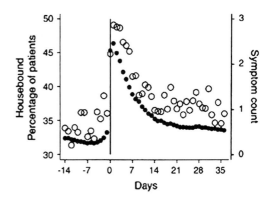

Fig. 2. Symptom time course of an exacerbation: evolution over a 51-day period of the time spent indoors (*open circles*) and the total number of new or worsening symptoms (symptom count, *solid circles*) from exacerbations in 136 patients with chronic obstructive pulmonary disease. (*Modified from* Donaldson GC, Wilkinson TM, Hurst JR, et al. Exacerbations and time spent outdoors in chronic obstructive pulmonary disease. Am J Respir Crit Care Med 2005;171:446–52; with permission.)

exacerbation onset, the longer it took for these symptoms to return to baseline. Assessing either the magnitude or duration of changes in exacerbation symptoms therefore provides an assessment of exacerbation severity. The same is true for the changes in lung function outlined in the following section. Both approaches, however, require the daily recording of data by patients, knowledge of the patient's individual baseline parameters and complex statistical techniques.

A simpler and more pragmatic assessment of exacerbation severity is to use the classification proposed by Anthonisen and colleagues [21] in a seminal paper on antibiotics at exacerbation of COPD. They considered the three cardinal symptoms of increased dyspnoea, increased sputum volume, and increased sputum purulence. A type 1 exacerbation was defined as having all three symptoms present, a type 2 exacerbation as having two symptoms present, and a type 3 exacerbation had just one of these three major symptoms in addition to other defined criteria that included upper respiratory infection, fever, increased wheeze, increased cough, tachycardia, or tachypnea. The proportion of exacerbations of each type will vary with the severity of the patient population and the definition of exacerbation employed.

Many researchers now use a third method of assessing exacerbation severity, based on the level of health care resources required, and in which exacerbation severity is graded as mild (the need for only an increased use of inhaled bronchodilators), moderate (the need for systemic corticosteroids), or severe (the need for hospital admission). Clearly this classification assesses factors other than those solely related to the underlying pathophysiological processes, and the search for a biomarker of exacerbation, physiological or biochemical, is ongoing [22] and discussed further in subsequent sections.

Physiology: lung function changes during exacerbations of chronic obstructive pulmonary disease

The relationships between symptoms and indices of lung function in COPD are complex, but it would be reasonable to assume that the increased symptoms present at exacerbation may be associated with evidence of additional impairment in pulmonary function, and this is indeed the case [23]. Complicating the assessment of changes in lung function is the fact that exacerbations of

COPD are extremely heterogenous events, ranging from no more than a transient worsening of symptoms in patients who have milder disease to the life-threatening episodes of respiratory failure observed in those who have more severe underlying lung function impairment.

In the study of exacerbation symptoms by Seemungal and colleagues [17] referred to previously, patients also were provided with peak-expiratory flow (PEF) meters and were instructed to record this measurement throughout the time course of the exacerbation. The results are illustrated in Fig. 3, which demonstrates numerous important points. First, PEF did not fall significantly during the prodromal period. Second, absolute changes in PEF are small with a median change of -8.6 (IQR 0 to -22.9) l/min [17]. Third, the median time to PEF recovery at 6 (1 to 14) days was similar to that for symptoms, and, likewise, some exacerbations have a prolonged recovery or may indeed never fully recover (around 25% and 7% of exacerbations still not returned to baseline PEF at 35 and 91 days respectively).

Therefore, while PEF provides a readily accessible method of assessing airflow, the changes observed are clearly too small to be useful in assessing individual patients. Furthermore, PEF is an assessment of larger airway obstruction and it is quite likely that much of the airflow obstruction in COPD is occurring in smaller airways, reflecting the major site of pathology in COPD [24].

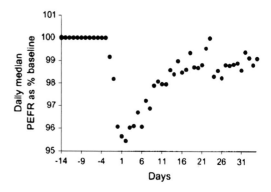

Fig. 3. Physiological time course of an exacerbation: median peak flow expressed as a percentage of baseline peak flow from 14 days prior, to 35 days following exacerbation onset in 504 exacerbations from 91 patients with chronic obstructive pulmonary disease. (*From* Seemungal TAR, Donaldson GC, Bhowmik A, et al. Time course and recovery of exacerbations in patients with chronic obstructive pulmonary disease. Am J Respir Crit Care Med 2000;161:1608–13; with permission.)

Moreover, the changes at exacerbation are likely to be much more complex than merely an increase in airflow obstruction.

Much of the more detailed work exploring physiological changes at exacerbation has been performed in severe exacerbations requiring mechanical ventilation, with the assumption made that the changes in milder exacerbations are quantitatively rather than qualitatively different [23]. The key physiological feature of COPD is expiratory flow limitation and various mechanisms may act to increase this at exacerbation, including greater mucus production, airway wall edema, and bronchoconstriction. The variable increase in end-expiratory lung volume that results is termed dynamic hyperinflation, the presence of which mechanically impairs the respiratory muscles, which are insulted further by systemic inflammation, hypoxia, acidosis, and oxidative stress. Mechanical disadvantage of the respiratory muscles may be affected further by tachypnea and result in an inability of the respiratory muscles to cope with the demands of central respiratory drive. This neuromechanical dissociation is thought to be a dominant mechanism for dyspnoea during exercise in COPD [25,26], and it is

likely also to be important during exacerbations [23]. The physiological changes associated with exacerbations, and their consequences, are summarized in Figs. 4 and 5. Although dynamic hyperinflation appears critical, it remains difficult to assess. One surrogate marker is inspiratory capacity, and Stevenson and colleagues [27] recently described improvements in inspiratory capacity with treatment of the exacerbation. The technique of forced oscillometry also has been used to detect improvements in airway resistance over the time course of an exacerbation [28].

Stable COPD can be associated with the presence of respiratory failure, and exacerbations may precipitate respiratory failure further, especially in patients who have more severe underlying disease. It is accepted that hypoxemia during exacerbation largely results from increased ventilation/perfusion (V/Q) mismatch [29], although increased peripheral oxygen utilization with a consequent reduction in mixed venous oxygen saturation also has been demonstrated. Hypercapnia also likely is caused by V/Q mismatch (rather than alveolar hypoventilation) and the mechanisms involved in worsening carbon dioxide retention seen in a proportion of patients exposed to

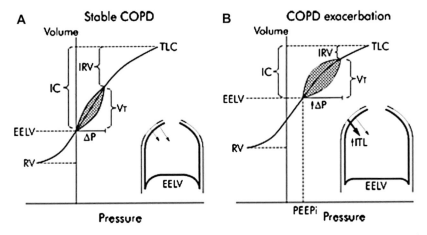

Fig. 4. Physiological changes at exacerbation of chronic obstructive pulmonary disease (COPD). Schematic of mechanical effects of COPD exacerbation. Representative pressure-volume plots during (A) stable COPD and (B) COPD exacerbation. During exacerbation, worsening expiratory flow limitation results in dynamic hyperinflation with increased end expiratory lung volume (EELV) and residual volume. Corresponding reductions occur in inspiratory capacity and inspiratory reserve volume. Total lung capacity (TLC) is unchanged. As a result, tidal breathing becomes shifted rightward on the pressure–volume curve, closer to TLC. Mechanically, increased pressures must be generated to maintain tidal volume. At EELV during exacerbation, intrapulmonary pressures do not return to zero, representing the development of intrinsic positive end expiratory pressure (PEEPi), which imposes increased inspiratory threshold loading on the inspiratory muscles (inset). During the subsequent respiratory cycle, PEEPi must first be overcome to generate inspiratory flow. (*From* O'Donnell DE, Parker CM. COPD exacerbations 3: pathophysiology. Thorax 2006;61:354–61; with permission.)

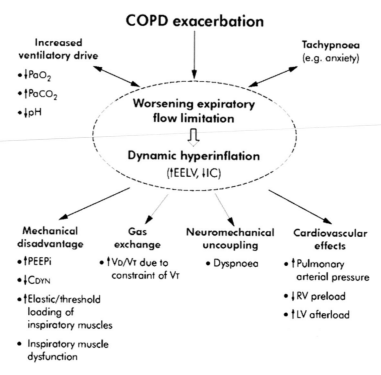

Fig. 5. Consequences of increased dynamic hyperinflation at exacerbation of chronic obstructive pulmonary disease. During exacerbation, dynamic hyperinflation develops as a consequence of worsening expiratory flow limitation. *Abbreviations*: LV, left ventricle; $PaCO_2$, partial pressure of arterial carbon dioxide; PaO_2, partial pressure of arterial oxygen; RV, right ventricle. (*From* O'Donnell DE, Parker CM. COPD exacerbations 3: pathophysiology. Thorax 2006;61:354–61; with permission.)

higher concentrations of inspired oxygen likely relate to both an impairment of central hypoxic drive [30,31] and a loss of hypoxic vasoconstriction with consequent worsening of V/Q relationships [32]. In contrast to the significance of changes in other physiological indices, the presence of acute hypercapnic respiratory failure is associated with poorer outcomes at exacerbation [33,34] and is therefore an important prognostic variable. Even following discharge, the outlook for patients whose exacerbation was associated with hypercapnic respiratory failure remains bleak. Around 80% will be admitted to hospital again within the following year, and the overall mortality in this period approaches 50% [35].

Inflammatory changes during exacerbations of chronic obstructive pulmonary disease

It is now well-established, indeed a defining characteristic [1], that COPD is associated with airway inflammation [36], and numerous individual studies (recently summarized in a meta-analysis) have demonstrated the presence of systemic inflammation in stable COPD [37]. Although highly variable, there is abundant evidence that exacerbations also are associated with increases in both pan-airway and systemic inflammatory markers [38]. The precise origins of systemic inflammation in COPD remain obscure, but the most plausible hypothesis is of spillover from the lungs. In contrast to stable disease, exacerbations appear to be associated with a direct correlation between the degree of airway inflammation and the magnitude of the systemic acute-phase response [38]. It is not known whether events that primarily result in increased systemic inflammation may secondarily trigger increases in airway inflammation and in turn COPD exacerbation.

A recent paper by Perera and colleagues [16] has, for the first time, described the time course of both airway and systemic inflammatory markers at exacerbation of COPD. Seventy-three patients were sampled in the baseline state, at exacerbation onset (before the initiation of therapy), and again at 7, 14, and 35 days later. Significant rises in both airway and systemic inflammatory markers were observed at exacerbation onset, and therapy (antibiotics and or corticosteroids) resulted in a return of concentrations to pre-exacerbation baseline levels, including an undershoot below the stable baseline value for serum interleukin (IL)-6. This is illustrated in Fig. 6.

Perera and colleagues [16] also demonstrated that nonrecovery of symptoms is related to a nonrecovery of inflammatory markers (Fig. 7) and that a raised CRP concentration 14 days after exacerbation onset may be predictive of recurrent exacerbation within the subsequent 50 days. The concept and significance of recurrence or clustering of exacerbations is discussed further in the subsequent sections, but these data do suggest that follow-up of patients 14 days following an exacerbation with assessment of systemic inflammatory markers may help to identify those most at risk of re-exacerbation and therefore those most likely to benefit from preventative therapies.

Etiology: causes of exacerbation in chronic obstructive pulmonary disease

The previous discussion, describing the biology of a COPD exacerbation, is summarized in Fig. 8,

which also illustrates that the causes of exacerbation are those insults that either increase airway inflammation or directly affect expiratory flow limitation.

Most literature focuses on micro-organisms as the causes of exacerbations. With molecular biological techniques, it is now possible to identify micro-organisms from airway secretions in most exacerbations, but there are numerous features of COPD that make the issue of causation more troublesome.

Numerous papers have investigated the role of respiratory viruses in stable COPD and at exacerbation [39–41]. Rohde and colleagues [41], for example, reported that respiratory viruses were detectable in either sputum or nasal lavage of 56% of patients during exacerbations, most commonly picornaviruses (36%), influenza A (25%), and respiratory syncytial virus (RSV, 22%). Viruses also were present in 19% of samples from stable patients, however, and the presence of an organism in a sample does not, of course, prove causation. More definitive evidence that these organisms are indeed causative had been absent until reports of a pilot study inducing mild exacerbations in COPD using experimental inoculation with rhinovirus 16 [42].

Experimental infection of patients has not been attempted with influenza or RSV, and this is not likely to be performed given the potential for

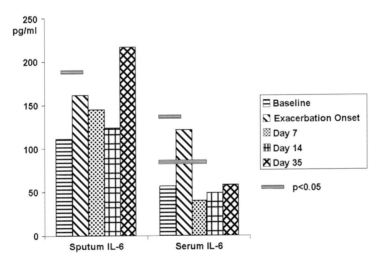

Fig. 6. Inflammatory time-course of an exacerbation: time course of airway (sputum) and systemic (serum) interleukin (IL)-6 in 73 patients at exacerbation of chronic obstructive pulmonary disease. Serum concentrations are expressed as 10 times those measured, and sputum concentrations are 10-fold dilutions by weight of the original sputum sample. (*Data from* Perera WR, Hurst JR, Wilkinson TMA, et al. Inflammatory changes, recovery, and recurrence at COPD exacerbation. Eur Respir J 2007;29:527–34.)

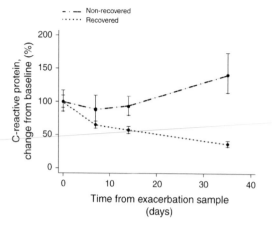

Fig. 7. Nonrecovery of symptoms at exacerbation is associated with nonrecovery of the systemic inflammatory response: difference in the time trend of serum C-reactive protein (CRP) concentration in patients whose symptoms had and had not recovered to baseline by day 35 following exacerbation onset, P = .03. (*Modified from* Perera WR, Hurst JR, Wilkinson TMA, et al. Inflammatory changes, recovery, and recurrence at COPD exacerbation. Eur Respir J 2007;29:527–34; with permission.)

catastrophic subsequent complications. RSV is particularly interesting, as some authors [43], but not others [44], have found significant RSV isolation in stable COPD, perhaps representing a chronic carrier state. This would be unusual for an RNA virus, but it may be important, given

an association between those patients who had more frequent isolation of RSV and a faster decline in lung function [43].

Establishing that bacteria cause exacerbation also is complicated by the frequent isolation of bacteria from lower airway samples of patients who have COPD in the stable state. This phenomenon, termed lower airway bacterial colonization, is not benign, as it is associated with increased frequency and severity of exacerbations [45] and a more rapid decline in FEV₁ [46]. Around 50% of patients whose FEV₁ is 50% or lower of that predicted have evidence of bacterial colonization. The most commonly isolated species include non-typeable *Haemophilus influenzae, Hs parainfluenzae, Streptococcus pneumoniae,* and *Moraxella catarrhalis.* This appears to coincide with the development of lymphoid follicles in the airway wall, and may suggest that bacterial antigens are driving an immune response [24]. Although the frequency at which bacterial species are isolated from lower airway samples is higher at exacerbation [38], as is the total bacterial load [38], this evidence still does not prove causation, but rather may represent a secondary phenomenon.

An alternative approach to the question of whether bacteria cause exacerbations of COPD has been to examine the benefit (or lack thereof) from antibiotics on exacerbation recovery. Meta-analysis has shown a small but statistically

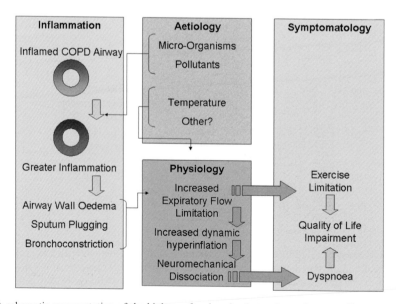

Fig. 8. A schematic representation of the biology of a chronic obstructive pulmonary disease exacerbation.

significant benefit in favor of antibiotics during these events [47]. The demonstration of strain-specific immune responses to colonizing bacterial species [48] provides further circumstantial evidence that the presence of bacterial species in the lower airways during exacerbations is not an epiphenomenon.

Work in this field has progressed recently with the development of molecular typing methods, allowing the detection of changes in bacterial strains, rather than species. Sethi and colleagues [49] prospectively studied 81 patients who had COPD and performed molecular typing on the most commonly isolated species. In 33% of visits at which a new strain was isolated, an exacerbation was present. This was statistically greater than the 14% of visits being exacerbations if no new strain had been identified. Clearly the situation is complex, however, as not all exacerbations were associated with strain change, and not all strain changes resulted in exacerbation.

Once again, an assumption is made that the presence of a micro-organism results in increased airway inflammation, and this precipitates the worsening expiratory flow limitation and symptoms that characterize exacerbations. There is considerable evidence that a higher total bacterial load is associated with both increased sputum [38] and broncho–alveolar lavage (BAL) [50] inflammation. The authors recently reported that the presence of a sputum bacterial species at exacerbation is associated with a greater systemic inflammatory response. It is important to remark, however, that associations observed between bacterial carriage and airway inflammation (which are also present in the stable state [51]) do not prove a causal relationship fully, and it is equally plausible that the increased airway inflammation may result in a greater susceptibility to bacterial carriage.

In health, the lower airways are sterile, and to reach the lung, a micro-organism must pass through the upper airway first. There is surprisingly little work investigating upper airway bacterial colonisation in COPD, and such studies are difficult to interpret, because many species that cause exacerbations are part of the normal upper respiratory tract flora. Additionally, the colonizing species of the upper airway vary greatly with the site of sampling. A recent study [38], however, has examined upper and lower airway bacterial carriage at COPD exacerbation, and in no patient was a potentially pathogenic micro-organism identified in nasal wash without there also being

an organism in sputum. This finding may lead to new preventative measures for exacerbation in COPD, using the analogy of topical antibiotics in the prevention of ventilator-associated pneumonia [52].

Whether atypical organisms such as *Chlamydia* and *Mycoplasma* species cause exacerbations remains unclear [53]. The question is complicated by the frequent isolation of atypical organisms in the stable state, and of copathogens in association with atypical organisms during exacerbations.

In summary, there is direct evidence that rhinovirus can induce airway inflammation and exacerbations, and considerable circumstantial evidence that exacerbations also may be caused by bacterial species. More recently, possible interactions between bacteria and viruses have been examined. Wilkinson and colleagues [54] reported a greater systemic inflammatory response in those exacerbations associated with both *H influenzae* and rhinovirus isolation. Additionally, if the isolation of *Haemophilus* was associated with new or worsening coryzal symptoms (a surrogate of viral infection), such infections were more severe as assessed by changes in symptoms and lung function at exacerbation onset. This has been confirmed in a further study demonstrating greater lung function impairment and longer hospitalizations in exacerbations associated with viral and bacterial coinfection [55].

In addition to micro-organisms, epidemiological studies have demonstrated a relationship between higher concentrations of atmospheric pollutants and increased admissions for COPD [56], suggesting that pollutants also may be capable of causing exacerbation. PM10 (particulate matter up to 10 μm in size), largely produced by diesel exhaust, appears to be particularly important, and inhalation of such particles is associated with a reduction in FEV_1 in patients who have COPD [57]. It is also recognized that changes in environmental temperature may provoke changes in airway caliber, and therefore may precipitate exacerbations of airways disease [58]. It seems likely, therefore, that exacerbations are induced either by agents such as micro-organisms or pollutants that increase airway inflammation, or by physiological stimuli that directly affect expiratory flow limitation. This is illustrated in Fig. 8, and may be one explanation for the reduction in exacerbation frequency seen with drugs such as the anticholinergic bronchodilator tiotropium bromide [59], which has dramatic effects on pulmonary physiology but is not thought to have anti-inflammatory properties.

Summary

Exacerbations are important events in the natural history of COPD and a tremendous burden both to the patient and to health care services. Exacerbations are associated with (and currently defined by) changes in symptoms, but there are characteristic underlying and demonstrable alterations in lung function parameters and both airway and systemic inflammation. Most exacerbations are caused by airway infection, and it is perhaps only by understanding the mechanisms of exacerbation that one may hope to improve the lives of the millions of people living with COPD in the 21st century.

References

[1] GOLD Executive committee. Global strategy for diagnosis, management, and prevention of COPD (Revised 2006). Available at: http://www.goldcopd.com/Guidelineitem.asp?l1=2&;l2=1&intId=989. Accessed 5th February 2007.

[2] Fletcher C, Peto R. The natural history of chronic airflow obstruction. BMJ 1977;6077:1645–8.

[3] Kanner RE, Anthonisen NR, Connett JE. Lower respiratory illnesses promote FEV_1 decline in current smokers but not ex-smokers with mild chronic obstructive pulmonary disease. Am J Respir Crit Care Med 2001;164:358–64.

[4] Donaldson GC, Seemungal TAR, Bhowmik A, et al. Relationship between exacerbation frequency and lung function decline in chronic obstructive pulmonary disease. Thorax 2002;57:847–52.

[5] Seemungal TA, Donaldson GC, Paul EA, et al. Effect of exacerbation on quality of life in patients with chronic obstructive pulmonary disease. Am J Respir Crit Care Med 1998;157:1418–22.

[6] Soler-Cataluna JJ, Martinez-Garcia MA, Roman Sanchez P, et al. Severe acute exacerbations and mortality in patients with chronic obstructive pulmonary disease. Thorax 2005;60:925–31.

[7] Rodriguez-Roisin R. Towards a consensus definition for COPD exacerbations. Chest 2000;117: 398s–401s.

[8] Hurst JR, Wedzicha JA. What is and is not an exacerbation of COPD? Thorax 2007;62:198–9.

[9] Murray CJ, Lopez AD. Alternative projections of mortality and disability by cause 1990–2020: global burden of disease study. Lancet 1997;349:1498–504.

[10] Donaldson GC, Seemungal TAR, Patel IS, et al. Longitudinal changes in the nature, severity, and frequency of COPD exacerbations. Eur Respir J 2003;22:931–6.

[11] Bhowmik A, Seemungal TAR, Sapsford RJ, et al. Relation of sputum inflammatory markers to symptoms and lung function changes in COPD exacerbations. Thorax 2000;55:114–20.

[12] Donaldson GC, Wedzicha JA. COPD exacerbations 1: epidemiology. Thorax 2006;61:164–8.

[13] Roberts CM, Lowe D, Bucknall CE, et al. Clinical audit indicators of outcome following admission to hospital with acute exacerbation of chronic obstructive pulmonary disease. Thorax 2002;57:137–41.

[14] Aaron SD, Vandemheen KL, Hebert P, et al. Outpatient oral prednisone after emergency treatment of chronic obstructive pulmonary disease. N Engl J Med 2003;348:2618–25.

[15] Hurst JR, Donaldson GC, Wedzicha JA. Prednisone for chronic obstructive pulmonary disease [letter]. N Engl J Med 2003;349:1288–90.

[16] Perera WR, Hurst JR, Wilkinson TMA, et al. Inflammatory changes, recovery, and recurrence at COPD exacerbation. Eur Respir J 2007;29:527–34.

[17] Seemungal TAR, Donaldson GC, Bhowmik A, et al. Time course and recovery of exacerbations in patients with chronic obstructive pulmonary disease. Am J Respir Crit Care Med 2000;161:1608–13.

[18] Donaldson GC, Wilkinson TM, Hurst JR, et al. Exacerbations and time spent outdoors in chronic obstructive pulmonary disease. Am J Respir Crit Care Med 2005;171:446–52.

[19] Pitta F, Troosters T, Probst VS, et al. Physical activity and hospitalization for exacerbation of COPD. Chest 2006;129:536–44.

[20] Spencer S, Jones PW. Time course of recovery of health status following an infective exacerbation of chronic bronchitis. Thorax 2003;58:589–93.

[21] Anthonisen NR, Manfreda J, Warren CP, et al. Antibiotic therapy in exacerbations of chronic obstructive pulmonary disease. Ann Intern Med 1987;106: 196–204.

[22] Hurst JR, Donaldson GC, Perera WR, et al. Use of plasma biomarkers at exacerbation of chronic obstructive pulmonary disease. Am J Respir Crit Care Med 2006;174:867–74.

[23] O'Donnell DE, Parker CM. COPD exacerbations 3: pathophysiology. Thorax 2006;61:354–61.

[24] Hogg JC, Chu F, Utokaparch S, et al. The nature of small airway obstruction in chronic obstructive pulmonary disease. N Engl J Med 2004;350: 2645–53.

[25] O'Donnell DE, Chau LKL, Bertley JC, et al. Qualitative aspects of exertional breathlessness in chronic airflow limitation: pathophysiologic mechanisms. Am J Respir Crit Care Med 1997;155:109–15.

[26] O'Donnell DE, Revill S, Webb KA. Dynamic hyperinflation and exercise intolerance in COPD. Am J Respir Crit Care Med 2001;164:770–7.

[27] Stevenson NJ, Walker PP, Costello RW, et al. Lung mechanics and dyspnea during exacerbations of chronic obstructive pulmonary disease. Am J Respir Crit Care Med 2005;172:1510–6.

[28] Johnson MK, Birch M, Carter R, et al. Measurement of physiological recovery from exacerbation of chronic obstructive pulmonary disease using within- breath forced oscillometry. Thorax 2007; 62:299–306.

[29] Barbera JA, Roca J, Ferrer A, et al. Mechanisms of worsening gas exchange during acute exacerbations of chronic obstructive pulmonary disease. Eur Respir J 1997;10:1285–91.

[30] Aubier M, Murciano D, Milic-Emili J, et al. Effects of the administration of O_2 on ventilation and blood gases in patients with chronic obstructive pulmonary disease during acute respiratory failure. Am Rev Respir Dis 1980;122:747–54.

[31] O'Donnell DE, D'Arsigny C, Fitzpatrick M, et al. Exercise hypercapnia in advanced chronic obstructive pulmonary disease. Am J Respir Crit Care Med 2002;166:663–8.

[32] Robinson TD, Freiberg DB, Regnis JA, et al. The role of hypoventilation and ventilation–perfusion redistribution in oxygen-induced hypercapnia during acute exacerbations of chronic obstructive pulmonary disease. Am J Respir Crit Care Med 2000; 161:1524–9.

[33] Seneff MG, Wagner DP, Wagner RP, et al. Hospital and 1-year survival of patients admitted to intensive care units with acute exacerbations of chronic obstructive pulmonary disease. JAMA 1995;274: 1852–7.

[34] Connors AF, Dawson NV, Thomas C, et al. Outcomes following acute exacerbations of severe chronic obstructive lung disease. Am J Respir Crit Care Med 1996;154:959–67.

[35] Chu CM, Chan VL, Lin AWN, et al. Readmission rates and life-threatening events in COPD survivors treated with noninvasive ventilation for acute hypercapnic respiratory failure. Thorax 2004;59: 1020–5.

[36] Di Stefano A, Caramori G, Ricciardolo FL, et al. Cellular and molecular mechanisms in chronic obstructive pulmonary disease: an overview. Clin Exp Allergy 2004;34:1156–67.

[37] Gan WQ, Man SF, Senthilselvan A, et al. Association between chronic obstructive pulmonary disease and systemic inflammation: a systematic review and a meta-analysis. Thorax 2004;59:574–80.

[38] Hurst JR, Perera WR, Wilkinson TMA, et al. Systemic and upper and lower airway inflammation at exacerbation of chronic obstructive pulmonary disease. Am J Respir Crit Care Med 2006;173:71–8.

[39] Greenberg SB, Allen M, Wilson J, et al. Respiratory viral infections in adults with and without chronic obstructive pulmonary disease. Am J Respir Crit Care Med 2000;162:167–73.

[40] Seemungal TAR, Harper-Owen R, Bhowmik A, et al. Respiratory viruses, symptoms, and inflammatory markers in acute exacerbations and stable chronic obstructive pulmonary disease. Am J Respir Crit Care Med 2001;164:1618–23.

[41] Rohde G, Wiethege A, Borg I, et al. Respiratory viruses in exacerbations of chronic obstructive pulmonary disease requiring hospitalisation: a case–control study. Thorax 2003;58:37–42.

[42] Mallia P, Message SD, Kebadze T, et al. An experimental model of rhinovirus-induced chronic pulmonary disease exacerbations: a pilot study. Respir Res 2006;7:116.

[43] Wilkinson TM, Donaldson GC, Johnston SL, et al. Respiratory syncytial virus, airway inflammation, and FEV_1 decline in patients with chronic obstructive pulmonary disease. Am J Respir Crit Care Med 2006;173:871–6.

[44] Falsey AR, Formica MA, Hennessey PA, et al. Detection of respiratory syncytial virus in adults with chronic obstructive pulmonary disease. Am J Respir Crit Care Med 2006;173:639–43.

[45] Patel IS, Seemungal TAR, Wilks M, et al. Relationships between bacterial colonisation and the frequency, character and severity of COPD exacerbations. Thorax 2002;57:759–64.

[46] Wilkinson TM, Patel IS, Wilks M, et al. Airway bacterial load and FEV_1 decline in patients with chronic obstructive pulmonary disease. Am J Respir Crit Care Med 2003;167:1090–5.

[47] Antibiotics for exacerbations of chronic obstructive pulmonary disease. Cochrane Database Syst Rev 2006;2:CD004403. doi:10.1002/14651858.CD004403. pub2.

[48] Yi K, Sethi S, Murphy TF. Human immune response to nontypeable Haemophilus influenzae in chronic bronchitis. J Infect Dis 1997;176:1247–52.

[49] Sethi S, Evans N, Grant BJ, et al. New strains of bacteria and exacerbations of chronic obstructive pulmonary disease. N Engl J Med 2002;347:465–71.

[50] Sethi S, Maloney J, Grove L, et al. Airway inflammation and bronchial bacterial colonization in chronic obstructive pulmonary disease. Am J Respir Crit Care Med 2006;173:991–8.

[51] Hill AT, Campbell EJ, Hill SL, et al. Association between airway bacterial load and markers of airway inflammation in patients with stable chronic bronchitis. Am J Med 2000;109:288–95.

[52] Bergmans DC, Bonten MJ, Gaillard CA, et al. Prevention of ventilator-associated pneumonia by oral decontamination: a prospective, randomized, double-blind, placebo-controlled study. Am J Respir Crit Care Med 2001;164:382–8.

[53] Wedzicha JA, Donaldson GC. Exacerbations of chronic obstructive pulmonary disease. Respir Care 2003;48:1204–15.

[54] Wilkinson TMA, Hurst JR, Perera WR, et al. Effect of interactions between lower airway bacterial and rhinoviral infection in exacerbation of COPD. Chest 2006;129:317–24.

[55] Papi A, Bellettato CM, Braccioni F, et al. Infections and airway inflammation in chronic obstructive pulmonary disease severe exacerbations. Am J Respir Crit Care Med 2006;173:1114–21.

[56] Anderson HR, Spix B, Medina S, et al. Air pollution and daily admissions for chronic obstructive pulmonary disease in 6 European cities: results from the APHEA project. Eur Respir J 1997;10:1064–71.

[57] Pope CA, Kanner RE. Acute effects of PM10 pollution on pulmonary function of smokers with mild to moderate chronic obstructive pulmonary disease. Am Rev Respir Dis 1993;137:1336–40.

[58] Eccles R. An explanation for the seasonality of acute upper respiratory tract viral infections. Acta Otolaryngol 2002;122:183–91.

[59] Niewoehner DE, Rice K, Cote C, et al. Prevention of exacerbations of chronic obstructive pulmonary disease with tiotropium, a once-daily inhaled anticholinergic bronchodilator: a randomized trial. Ann Intern Med 2005;143:317–26.

ELSEVIER
SAUNDERS

Clin Chest Med 28 (2007) 537–552

Systemic Inflammation and Skeletal Muscle Dysfunction in Chronic Obstructive Pulmonary Disease: State of the Art and Novel Insights in Regulation of Muscle Plasticity

Alexander H. Remels, MSc, Harry R. Gosker, PhD,
Jos van der Velden, BSc, Ramon C. Langen, PhD,
Annemie M. Schols, PhD*

*Department of Respiratory Medicine, Nutrition and Toxicology Research Institute, University of Maastricht,
P.O. Box 5800, 6202 AZ Maastricht, The Netherlands*

Chronic obstructive pulmonary disease (COPD) is a chronic lung disease characterized by at least partially irreversible airway obstruction and an abnormal chronic inflammatory response of the airways. Dominant symptoms are dyspnea and impaired exercise capacity. These symptoms lead to progressive disability and poor health status but correlate poorly with severity of local impairment in the lungs. Surprisingly, even in the most recent international guidelines for diagnosis of COPD, staging is still based on severity of airways obstruction only. There is increasing evidence in the literature that COPD should not be considered a localized pulmonary disorder but a systemic disease that involves pathology in several extrapulmonary tissues. Well-characterized systemic features include chronic low-grade systemic inflammation and altered regulation of protein metabolism, which result initially in muscle atrophy only (commonly referred to as sarcopenia) but in later stages also result in cachexia [1,2].

Muscle atrophy is associated with increased mortality risk independent of disease staging based on severity of airflow obstruction [3]. Besides muscle atrophy, it is well established that intrinsic abnormalities in muscle structure and metabolism are present in moderate to severe cases of COPD and that both processes contribute to reduced strength and endurance of the muscle. In turn, skeletal muscle dysfunction adversely affects clinical outcome in COPD, because it is an independent determinant of exercise limitation [4,5]. In this article we present a state-of-the-art update on skeletal muscle dysfunction and systemic inflammation in patients who have COPD and discuss the therapeutic potential of novel insights from experimental research in the regulation of muscle plasticity.

Characterization and causes of skeletal muscle dysfunction in chronic obstructive pulmonary disease

Skeletal muscle dysfunction in COPD is characterized by a reduction in strength and endurance of the muscle. Skeletal muscle strength is largely determined by muscle mass. Data clearly indicate that atrophy of skeletal muscles is apparent in COPD and that the disease selectively affects the predominant glycolytic type IIA/IIX fibers [6,7]. Loss of muscle mass is a complex process that involves changes in the control of substrate and protein metabolism and changes in muscle cell turnover. Impaired protein metabolism may result in muscle atrophy when protein degradation exceeds protein synthesis. To date, a limited number of studies have addressed protein metabolism in patients who have COPD. Using stable isotope techniques, two studies have

---

* Corresponding author.
E-mail address: schols@pul.unimaas.nl (A.M. Schols).

investigated muscle protein turnover in patients who have COPD. Morrison and colleagues [8] demonstrated a decreased muscle protein synthesis in underweight patients with emphysema. More recently, Rutten and colleagues [9] showed an elevated myofibrillar protein breakdown in cachectic patients who had COPD, whereas no difference was seen between noncachectic patients who had COPD and healthy controls. At the cellular level, increased apoptosis of muscle cells has been demonstrated in skeletal muscle of severely underweight patients who have COPD [10], although this observation was not confirmed in weight-stable patients who have COPD and are suffering from muscle wasting [11]. This finding could implicate different mechanisms in loss of muscle mass in the absence or presence of weight loss (ie, sarcopenia versus cachexia).

Reduced muscle endurance, on the other hand, is not associated with muscle wasting but may be secondary to either intrinsic muscle alterations (mitochondrial abnormalities and loss of contractile proteins) or alterations in the external milieu in which the muscle works (hypoxia, hypercapnia, and acidosis) that result from the abnormalities of pulmonary gas exchange that exist in COPD. Gosker and colleagues [12] showed that in COPD there is a shift in muscle fiber type from type I (slow twitch, oxidative fibers) to type II (fast twitch glycolytic) fibers. Type I fibers are resistant to fatigue, whereas type II fibers are more fatigable. A decrease in the percentage of type I fibers in the vastus lateralis of patients who have COPD compared with age-matched controls was reported together with a corresponding increase in type IIx fibers [12]. Research has shown consistently that peripheral muscles of patients who have COPD are characterized by reduced activities of enzymes involved in muscle oxidative metabolism as citrate synthase and β-hydroxyacylCoA dehydrogenase [12,13]. Conversely, activities of glycolytic enzymes were found to be increased in lower limb muscle of patients who have COPD by some studies [13]. Because these enzyme activities depend largely on fiber type [14], it is likely that this shift in activities is related to the shift in fiber distribution mentioned previously. Whether enzyme activities adapt to the fiber type or the other way around remains unclear.

Further indication of an impaired energy metabolism in patients who have COPD is derived from studies that measured substrate and cofactor concentrations in peripheral skeletal muscle of patients who have COPD. Most striking was the observation of reduced concentrations of high-energy phosphates at rest, as indicated by elevated levels of inosine monophosphate [15]. Muscle glycogen content in COPD also tends to be lower, whereas lactate concentrations are higher than in healthy persons [16,17]. These data indicate that anaerobic energy metabolism is enhanced in COPD. Because this process yields far less ATP than complete oxidative degradation of glucose, a reduced energy state in COPD could not only limit exercise endurance but also contribute to a decreased work efficiency that has been reported during cycle exercise [18] and elevated energy expenditure in some patients [19]. We hypothesized that uncoupling protein 3 (UCP-3), which uncouples oxidative phosphorylation from ATP production, is implicated in the elevated energy expenditure in COPD. Gosker and colleagues [20], however, demonstrated that instead of the expected increase in skeletal muscle UCP-3 content, UCP-3 protein levels were decreased in skeletal muscle of patients who have COPD. UCP-3 also has been postulated as an important factor in the defense against lipid-induced oxidative muscle damage [21]. Markers of oxidative stress are elevated in skeletal muscle of patients who have COPD at rest and during exercise [22]. Consequently, impaired skeletal muscle antioxidant defenses also have been reported [23].

Characterization and sources of systemic inflammation in chronic obstructive pulmonary disease

By definition, COPD is a disorder characterized by reduced maximum expiratory flow and slow forced emptying of the lungs caused by varying combinations of diseases of the airways and emphysema. Progression of the disease is associated with an intense chronic inflammation of the lungs, and the critical role of this local inflammatory process in the pathogenesis and progression of COPD is generally recognized and accepted. In addition to airway inflammation, there is increasing evidence of low-grade systemic inflammation in COPD. In contrast to extensive knowledge of the inflammatory process in the airways of patients who have COPD, surprisingly less is known about systemic inflammation in this disorder. Although the exact relationship between inflammation in the lung and in the systemic compartment remains to be established, an inverse relationship has been shown between the presence of systemic inflammation and the mean forced expiratory volume in 1 second in patients, which highlights the importance of systemic inflammation in disease progression [24].

According to a recent meta-analysis, several clinical studies have reported persistent systemic inflammation in COPD, as evidenced by elevated levels of the proinflammatory cytokines tumor necrosis factor-alpha (TNF-α), interleukin-6 (IL-6), IL-8, and the soluble TNF-α receptors (sTNFR-55 and sTNFR-75) [25,26]. Proinflammatory cytokines such as IL-6 and TNF-α have been shown to induce the formation of acute phase reactants. One of the major acute phase proteins, C-reactive protein, is increased in the circulation of patients who have COPD compared to healthy controls [27]. High C-reactive protein levels in the circulation of patients who have COPD have been associated with reduced quadriceps strength, lower maximal and submaximal exercise capacity, and increased mortality [28,29].

The origin of the systemic inflammation in patients who have COPD remains poorly understood; several (independent) pathways may be involved. Although a relationship between lung and systemic inflammation has been suggested, evidence from available cross-sectional studies indicates no clear correlation between the presence of inflammation in the pulmonary and systemic compartments [30]. This finding suggests that the systemic inflammatory response is not caused by an overflow of inflammatory mediators from the pulmonary compartment but is regulated differently. Potential nonpulmonary sources of systemic inflammatory mediators include inflammatory cells in the circulation, because several studies have shown increased levels of various circulating inflammatory cells, including neutrophils and lymphocytes, in peripheral blood of patients who have COPD. The activation of peripheral blood lymphocytes, which results in potentiation of cytotoxic and migratory responses, also has been shown [31].

A second pathway involved in the process of systemic inflammation could be hypoxia, which is often present in patients who have severe COPD. Several in vitro studies have shown that hypoxia results in enhanced cytokine production by macrophages, which could contribute to activation of the TNF-α system in COPD. Takabatake and colleagues [32] showed a significant inverse relationship between arterial oxygen pressure and circulating levels of TNF-α and soluble TNF-R in patients who have COPD. Alternatively, increased levels of inflammatory mediators in the blood of patients who have COPD may originate from

muscle cells or yet-unexplored extrapulmonary cells, including endothelium and fat tissue. Skeletal muscle itself is capable of constitutive and inducible production of proinflammatory cytokines, such as TNF-α and IL-6 [33,34]. Data on the contribution of extrapulmonary cells to the ongoing inflammatory process in COPD is, to date, lacking.

Several studies have shown that systemic inflammatory cytokines, such as TNF-α and IL-6, are proximal markers of cachexia and selectively target myosin protein content in skeletal muscle. High levels of IL-6 have been associated with reduced quadriceps strength and diminished exercise capacity [29], and TNF-α has been shown to be inversely related to muscle mass [35]. These cytokines may cause skeletal muscle weakness without causing muscle wasting by directly compromising contractile properties of the skeletal musculature. De Oca and colleagues [36] showed that TNF-α protein levels in skeletal muscle of patients who have COPD were markedly higher compared to healthy control subjects. A study by Agusti and colleagues [37] also suggested that patients who have severe COPD and are suffering from weight loss are characterized by increased activation of the transcription factor nuclear factor kappa B (NF-κB), a major signaling pathway that conveys inflammatory signals, in skeletal muscle.

These studies indicated that the systemic inflammatory process in COPD also involves the skeletal musculature itself. Although recent studies showed a clear association between C-reactive protein and impaired muscle function and exercise capacity, even after adjustment for mean forced expiratory volume in 1 second, it is unclear if this association is linked to effects on muscle mass or caused by direct effects on muscle contractility [38]. In summary, a large body of evidence suggests that systemic inflammation is present in patients who have COPD, and several lines of evidence indicate a significant role of inflammatory mediators in disturbed regulation of muscle mass and muscle functional capacity. Because most data in this context originated from studies with a cross-sectional design, longitudinal studies are needed to unravel the exact role of systemic inflammation in the progression of COPD and the impairment of skeletal muscle function.

Novel insights in the regulation of muscle mass during muscle wasting

Abundant evidence from in vitro research and experimental models indicates that inflammatory stimuli trigger weight loss and muscle atrophy [35,39–41]. Muscle loss has been documented in animals treated with exogenous TNF-α, in animals that express a TNF transgene, and in diseases that elevate endogenous TNF-α (ie, experimental sepsis or tumor implantation) [41]. Several studies also point to the importance of IL-6 in the regulation of muscle wasting [35,42]. Little information is available, however, on how elevated and circulatory levels of inflammatory mediators, such as TNF-α and IL-6, convey signaling cues that cause skeletal muscle to atrophy. Upon binding to their cognate receptors at the myofiber surface, proinflammatory cytokines, such as TNF-α and IL-1β, cause activation of the transcription factor NF-κB. Under basal conditions, NF-κB is present within the cytoplasm in an inactive state, bound to its inhibitory protein IκBα. Upon stimulation with an inflammatory stimulus (eg, TNF-α) an intracellular signaling cascade is initiated, which results in the phosphorylation of IκBα by IκB kinase and subsequent degradation of IκBα. Once liberated from its inhibitory protein, NF-κB translocates into the nucleus, where it regulates transcription of various inflammatory genes [43]. Although the intracellular signaling initiated by inflammatory stimuli is certainly not limited to NF-κB activation in skeletal muscle, recent work suggests that this pathway is involved in muscle atrophy signaling.

The exact intracellular mechanisms responsible for inflammation-induced wasting of skeletal muscle remain to be elucidated. At the protein level, an imbalance between protein synthesis and protein degradation may favor muscle catabolism. At the cellular level, a disturbed balance between the loss and gain of nuclei in muscle fibers through apoptosis and myonuclear accretion, respectively, may contribute to loss of skeletal muscle mass. These processes are discussed in further detail later in this article. Importantly, these processes are not mutually exclusive but are likely to occur in parallel during muscle wasting, as has been shown for their involvement in muscle plasticity in response to physiologic stimuli.

Effects of inflammation on regulation of muscle protein turnover

Protein degradation

Work using cultured murine myotubes (eg, the in vitro equivalents of muscle fibers) demonstrated that TNF-α directly stimulates a time- and concentration-dependent decrement in total muscle protein content and loss of muscle-specific proteins, including fast-type myosin heavy chain (MyHC). MyHC losses were not accompanied by a change in synthesis rate, which suggests that TNF-α stimulated degradation of myofibrillar proteins rather than inhibited their synthesis [41,44]. Research also has demonstrated that infusion with TNF-α increased muscle proteolysis in rats [45]. Several proteolytic systems could contribute to enhanced protein degradation in chronic inflammatory disorders, including the lysosomal pathway, the Ca^{2+}-dependent pathway, caspases, and the ATP-dependent ubiquitin proteasome pathway (UPP). Recent in vitro and animal model–derived evidence postulates the UPP as the predominant pathway involved in skeletal muscle atrophy. In this pathway, proteins to be degraded are tagged by at least four moieties of the polypeptide ubiquitin (Ub), which are covalently bound at the lysine 48 residue. This process, named K48-Ub conjugation, requires the sequential activity of a series of specific enzymes: E1, or Ub-activation enzyme; E2, or Ub-conjugating enzyme; and E3, or Ub-ligase. K48-polyubiquitinated proteins are recognized and degraded by the 26S-proteasome complex into short peptides that are further rapidly degraded to free amino acids in the cytosol [46].

Elevated Ub gene expression and Ub conjugation were reported in skeletal muscle after the administration of TNF-α in vitro [47]. MyHC depletion in response to TNF-α also occurred via an upregulation of certain components of the Ub-proteasome pathway [48]. Several in vivo models confirm the involvement of TNF-α and the UPP in wasting of skeletal muscle mass. Increased expression of muscular Ub and Ub conjugation were observed in rats after injection of TNF-α [49]. Two muscle-specific Ub (E3) ligases, atrogin-1/MAFbx and MuRF1, also are rate limiting for muscle protein loss in various catabolic conditions. Expression of these two Ub ligases is upregulated in the muscle of various animal models of inflammation-associated muscle atrophy, including cancer, diabetes, and sepsis, whereas the muscle mass of MAFbx-/- and MuRF1-/- gene knockout animals is spared in several of these atrophy models [50–52].

Muscle proteins targeted for degradation by the UPP in response to inflammatory cytokines include MyHC and MyoD [53,54]. MyHC is a myofibrillar protein involved in muscle contraction, whereas MyoD is a muscle regulatory factor essential for muscle-specific gene expression and muscle growth implicating a mechanism by which the UPP contributes to muscle atrophy, not only through degradation of specific muscle proteins but also via the selective degradation of regulatory proteins. Several studies have postulated an important role for NF-κB in this regulation of protein degradation through the UPP during muscle atrophy. For instance, loss of MyHC protein in response to TNF-α corresponded with NF-κB activation in cultured myotubes, and inhibition of NF-κB activity blocked cytokine-mediated decreases in muscle-specific proteins [48]. TNF-α increases Ub-conjugating activity in skeletal muscle cells in vitro in an NF-κB–dependent manner [47]. It was recently established that through muscle-specific transgenic expression of activated IκB kinase 2, constitutive activation of NF-κB in skeletal muscle was sufficient to induce profound muscle atrophy. Muscle loss in this model was caused by accelerated protein breakdown through Ub-dependent proteolysis, because expression of the E3 ligase MuRF1, a mediator of muscle atrophy, was increased and muscle atrophy was ameliorated in MuRF1-deficient mice [55]. Conversely, skeletal muscle-specific inhibition of NF-κB activation preserved muscle tissue in various experimental models of muscle atrophy [56], which indicated that muscular NF-κB activation may be required for the loss of muscle mass in certain (pathologic) conditions.

Protein synthesis

In addition to increased proteolysis, systemic inflammation is also associated with decreased protein synthesis. Protein synthesis is impaired in muscles of animals subjected to experimental sepsis [57], and this response seems to involve systemic inflammation, because TNF-α and IL-1β antagonists have been reported to improve muscle protein balance in septic rats by preventing decreased synthesis rates [58,59]. Conversely, administration of TNF-α or IL-1β reduced synthesis of the major muscle proteins in rats [59,60]. Muscle protein synthesis is under positive control of insulin-like growth factor-1 (IGF-1) signaling. Decreased circulating IGF-1 levels have been reported in response to sepsis and IGF-1 resistance of skeletal muscle exposed to inflammatory cytokines [61]. Skeletal muscle production of IGF-1, which stimulates protein synthesis and suppresses degradation in an autocrine fashion, is reduced by inflammatory mediators [61].

Binding of IGF-1 to its receptor initiates a signal transduction cascade that promotes mRNA translation and consequently increases protein synthesis [62]. Incubation of skeletal muscle cells with inflammatory cytokines, including TNF-α and IL-1β, induces IGF-1 resistance, which is characterized by decreased protein synthesis as a result of impaired signaling proximal to receptor activation [63]. The exact molecular mechanism of inflammation-induced IGF-1 resistance in skeletal muscle remains to be elucidated but may involve ceramide as an intermediate, because inhibition of de novo synthesis of this second messenger prevented impaired IGF-1–induced protein synthesis by TNF-α or IL-1β [64].

Effects of inflammation on regulation of myonuclear turnover

Because of its multinucleated nature, the cytoplasm (sarcoplasm) of a myofiber is shared by multiple nuclei, each of which is thought to regulate protein expression for a defined volume of the sarcoplasm (eg, the myonuclear domain). Experimental evidence indicates that the dimensions of the myonuclear domain are relatively constant, implying flexibility of the myonuclear number to accommodate muscle plasticity, which is accomplished by the addition (myonuclear accretion) or loss (by apoptosis) of myonuclei during muscle (fiber) growth and atrophy, respectively [65]. In addition to an inequity in muscle protein synthesis and degradation, an imbalanced myonuclear turnover may contribute to muscle atrophy in patients with disorders associated with chronic inflammation. The effects of inflammatory mediators on cellular mechanisms that regulate apoptosis and myonuclear accretion are described herein.

Apoptosis

Apoptosis, or programmed cell death, is an important process in multicellular organisms during development but also in postnatal tissue homeostasis. Apoptosis can be initiated by ligand binding to so-called "death receptors" (which include Fas and members of the TNF receptor family) or by the release of apoptosis-inducing factors from mitochondria [66]. Subsequently, protein-cleaving enzymes (caspases) and endonucleases are activated, which results in the degradation of regulatory proteins and DNA fragmentation, respectively. In mononuclear cells, this process ultimately culminates in the formation of apoptotic bodies that are cleared by macrophages. Because of the multinucleated nature of myofibers, however, the elimination of one myonucleus by apoptosis is not necessarily followed by the destruction of the entire myofiber, and this process is referred to as apoptotic nuclear death. As a consequence, the mechanisms involved in apoptosis signaling in skeletal muscle are likely distinct from mononucleated cells.

DNA fragmentation that suggests apoptosis has been reported in skeletal muscle of septic rats, which was prevented by administration of a TNF-α antagonist, which suggests that TNF-α may trigger apoptotic events in skeletal muscle during inflammatory conditions [67]. This notion is further supported by experiments in cultured myoblasts and myotubes, which revealed DNA fragmentation after chronic exposure to TNF-α [68], although differentiated myofibers seem to be more resistant to TNF-α–induced apoptosis than undifferentiated myoblasts [41]. Myoblasts exposed to TNF-α show procaspase-8 cleavage [69], whereas TNF-α–induced apoptosis in skeletal muscle of patients who have COPD may be mediated by upregulation of inducible nitric oxide synthase in myofibers [37]. Caspase-3 activation was reported to contribute to myofibrillar protein degradation in catabolic conditions [70] and was associated with muscle weakness in sepsis [71]. In chronic heart failure, circulatory levels of TNF-α are increased, which is paralleled by a rise in the number of apoptotic nuclei in the soleus and tibialis anterior muscles [72]. Despite these recent studies suggesting a role of TNF-α and other inducers and mediators of apoptotic signaling in skeletal muscle atrophy, the relevance of these pathways in myofibers remains to be established because of their multinucleated nature and potential cell death–unrelated consequences.

Myonuclear accretion and muscle regeneration

During conditions such as muscle growth, recovery from atrophy, and muscle regeneration after damage, myonuclear accretion is increased, which requires activation of local muscle precursor cells, called satellite cells [65,73]. Upon activation, these cells proliferate to form a pool of myoblasts, which differentiate to fuse with existing myofibers or form new myofibers, processes that are essential for efficient muscle growth, regrowth, and regeneration [74]. Several groups have demonstrated that TNF-α [40,75] and the related ligand TWEAK [76] as well as IL-1β inhibit

muscle differentiation and myoblast fusion [75,77]. Inhibition of myogenesis by TNF-α requires activation of NF-κB and involves repression of MyoD synthesis and protein stability [78]. MyoD is a master regulator of myogenesis, which explains the inability of myoblasts to express muscle-specific gene transcripts or form multinucleated myotubes in the presence of these proinflammatory cytokines. Recent evidence also showed that TNF-α could inhibit myogenesis through the activation of caspases [79]. In a model of chronic pulmonary (and systemic) inflammation, impaired muscle differentiation and regeneration was observed during muscle regrowth after atrophy [35]. These data indicated that inflammatory signaling may impair muscle differentiation and myonuclear accretion, thereby compromising the ability of the muscle to recover after injury or atrophy and contributing to the loss of muscle mass observed in several inflammatory conditions.

To conclude, the effects of inflammation on the regulation of muscle mass may favor muscle atrophy as a result of imbalances in protein turnover and myonuclear turnover and likely involve enhanced myofibrillar protein degradation and/or reduced protein synthesis and activation of apoptotic mechanisms and/or impaired myonuclear accretion. These processes are summarized in Fig. 1.

Novel insights in the regulation of fiber type and muscle oxidative phenotype

One of the most prominent features of skeletal muscle is its high level of plasticity. Physical activity level, nutritional status, and the presence and/or absence of disease are important factors determining muscle mass, fiber type composition, and oxidative capacity. The muscle senses these factors as mechanical, metabolic, neuronal, or hormonal stimuli that lead to intracellular signaling cascades that switch on or off specific gene expression profiles (Fig. 2). In the following section, some of the major key regulators of muscle fiber type and oxidative phenotype are discussed. A shift in muscle fiber type from type I (slow twitch, oxidative, fatigue resistant) to type II (fast twitch, glycolytic, fatigue prone) fibers has been noted in muscle of patients who have COPD [20].

Peroxisome proliferator-activated receptors

In the past decade, peroxisome proliferator-activated receptors (PPARs) have emerged as

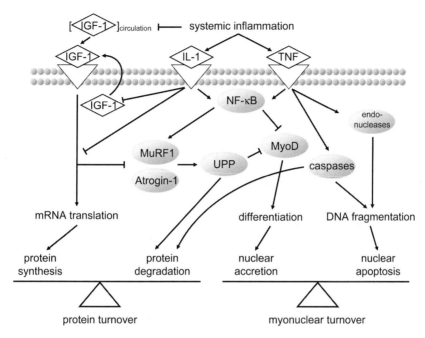

Fig. 1. Schematic overview of the effects of inflammation on regulation of skeletal muscle mass by protein- and myonuclear turnover. Growth factors and cytokines that exert receptor-mediated effects (*inverted triangles*) are shown as diamonds, intracellular mediators/signaling proteins are displayed as ovals, and intracellular processes are in plain text. Arrows indicate activation, whereas blunted arrows indicate inhibition. IGF-1, insulin growth factor 1; IL-1, interleukin 1; MuRF1, muscle ring finger-1; NF-κB, nuclear factor kappa B; TNF, tumor necrosis factor; UPP, ubiquitin proteasome pathway.

positive regulators of skeletal muscle oxidative phenotype [80,81]. There are three PPAR isotypes: PPAR-α, PPAR-δ, and PPAR-γ, with the latter having a low expression in skeletal muscle and being implicated in storage of fatty acids. On the other hand, the PPAR-α and PPAR-δ isotypes are highly expressed in skeletal muscle and play a role in the transcriptional control of genes that encode mitochondrial fatty acid β-oxidation enzymes [80,81]. Many muscle genes that promote selective use of lipid substrates are upregulated by in vivo administration of PPAR-α activators. It has been shown that skeletal muscle PPAR-α protein content is increased by exercise training and is induced during myocyte differentiation, coincident with an increased oxidative capacity [82,83]. PPAR-α also regulates fatty acid use and expression of several genes involved in fatty acid β-oxidation [84]. Based on these results, one would expect that PPAR-α deficiency results in low rates of β-oxidation in skeletal muscle [85].

Inconsistent with this hypothesis, however, skeletal muscles from PPAR-α knock-out mice exhibited only minor changes in fatty acid homeostasis, and neither constitutive nor inducible expression of known PPAR-α target genes was negatively affected by its absence. Skeletal muscle also expresses high levels of PPAR-δ. Activation of the PPAR-δ subtype increases fatty acid β-oxidation and mRNA levels of several classical PPAR-α target genes in rodent and human skeletal muscle cells, and PPAR-δ protein, like PPAR-α protein, is induced in skeletal muscle after exercise [86]. These results indicate that in addition to PPAR-α, PPAR-δ also plays an important role in mediating lipid-induced regulation of oxidative pathways in skeletal muscle. Because PPAR-δ is the predominant subtype in skeletal muscle and because isolated rat muscle is more sensitive to a PPAR-δ– than a PPAR-α–specific agonist, a more prominent role for PPAR-δ in regulating skeletal muscle oxidative capacity has been suggested [87]. Targeted overexpression of PPAR-δ or a constitutively active form of PPAR-δ in mouse skeletal muscle results in a greater number of type I oxidative fibers in various muscles. This remodeling was caused by hyperplasia or conversion of fibers to a more oxidative phenotype, similar to what is observed in endurance training [88].

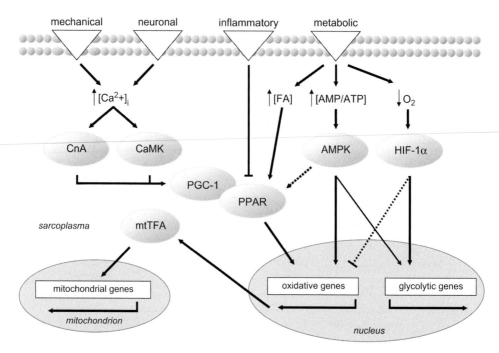

Fig. 2. Schematic overview of muscle oxidative phenotype regulation. Depending on the nature of the stimuli, specific transcriptional pathways are switched on. Arrows indicate activation, whereas blunted arrows indicate inhibition. Dashed arrows indicate less established relationships. FA, fatty acids; CnA, calcineurin; CaMK, calcium/calmodulin-dependent kinases; AMPK, AMP-activated protein kinase; HIF-1α, hypoxia-inducible factor-1α; PPAR, peroxisome proliferator-activated receptor; PGC-1, PPAR-γ coactivator-1; mtTFA, mitochondrial transcriptional factor A.

These histologic observations were confirmed by the finding that muscle-specific PPAR-δ over-expression led to an increase of oxidative enzymes, such as citrate synthase and β-hydroxyacylCoA dehydrogenase. Conversely, activities of glycolytic enzymes remained unchanged [88]. These observations were accompanied by the finding that trans-genic mice with a constitutively activated form of PPAR-δ in skeletal muscle were capable of running nearly twice as long as their wild-type littermates without any physical training, which gave func-tional meaning to these observations. Together, these data strongly support a key role of PPAR-α and PPAR-δ in the regulation of fatty acid oxida-tion in skeletal muscle and in the adaptive response of this tissue to lipid catabolism [89].

Peroxisome proliferator-activated receptor-γ coactivator-1α

Probably the master regulator of oxidative phenotype is the peroxisome proliferator-acti-vated receptor-γ coactivator-1 (PGC-1α). Its name is misleading in two ways: it is not just some coactivator secondary to the PPARs, and it is not only a coactivator of PPAR-γ. PGC-1α is described most in the context of mitochondrial biogenesis, but it is likely that PGC1-β is also somehow involved in the regulation of mitochon-drial function [90]. PGC-1 overexpressing muscle cells showed increased mitochondrial respiration, upregulation of genes involved in oxidative phos-phorylation, and increased mitochondrial DNA content, all of which indicated enhanced mito-chondrial biogenesis [91]. Two key transcription factors in the regulation of mitochondrial func-tion—the nuclear respiratory factor-1 and the mitochondrial transcription factor A—were tran-scriptionally upregulated by PGC-1. Nuclear re-spiratory factor-1 coordinates the transcription of genes involved in the electron transport chain and that of mitochondrial transcription factor A, which migrates to the mitochondria and initiates transcription of mitochondrial-encoded genes [92]. In transgenic mice that overexpress PGC-1α in the skeletal muscles, a clear fiber type II → I (fast-to-slow) shift was observed, associated with increased mitochondrial gene expression [93].

Calcineurin

An illustrative study for a role of calcineurin in muscle phenotype is that of Talmadge and colleagues [94], which showed that in transgenic mice with muscle-specific overexpression of an active form of calcineurin, the result was a fast-to-slow fiber type shift. Similar results were observed in cultured skeletal myotubes, in which transcription of the slow fiber-specific genes troponin I slow and myoglobin was stimulated by overexpression of active calcineurin. Conversely, administration of cyclosporin A, a calcineurin antagonist, induced a slow-to-fast fiber type shift in rat muscles [95]. Calcium (Ca^{2+}) plays an important role in the excitation-relaxation of muscle fibers upon neural activation but also in the regulation of gene expression. The calcineurin-calmodulin complex is activated by binding to Ca^{2+} and activates the nuclear factor of activated T cells, which then translocates to the nucleus and switches on slow fiber-specific promoters. It is possible that this is mediated through PGC-1α [96]. This process preferentially occurs with low frequency or tonic motor nerve activity (typical for slow fibers), which is associated with a sarcolemmal Ca^{2+}-influx ($[Ca2+]_i$) of low concentration but of sufficient duration. In contrast, the calcineurin-nuclear factor of activated T cells pathway is insensitive to shorter high-amplitude $[Ca2+]_i$ evoked by high frequency motor nerve activity (typical for fast fibers). It is postulated that calcineurin plays an important role in the translation of motor nerve activity patterns into the expression profiles of muscle fiber type–specific genes [95].

Calcium/calmodulin-dependent kinases

Other pathways by which Ca^{2+} influences muscle oxidative phenotype are that of the calcium/calmodulin-dependent kinases (CaMKs): CaMKII and CaMKIV [97]. CaMKIV, when bound to calmodulin-Ca^{2+}, is phosphorylated by CaMK kinase and becomes transcriptionally active. Transgenic mice that overexpress CaMKIV in skeletal muscles showed increased proportions of slow fibers and enhanced mitochondrial biogenesis [98]. In these mice, the increase in mitochondrial content was associated with PGC-1, which suggested that CaMKIV regulates oxidative phenotype through PGC-1. Cultured myocytes that overexpress CaMKIV showed enhanced PGC-1 reporter gene expression [96]. CaMKII also has been suggested to be involved in the regulation of mitochondrial biogenesis [97]. It consists of 12 subunits that become sequentially autophosphorylated the longer CaMKII is bound to calmodulin-Ca^{2+}, subsequently associated with an increasing transcriptional activity of CaMKII. Like calcineurin, CaMKII seems to be able to decode stimulation frequencies [97].

AMP-activated protein kinase

AMP-activated protein kinase (AMPK) plays a critical role in regulating energy metabolism in situations of critical energy demands (eg, as a consequence of exercise) [99,100]. Contraction-induced AMPK activity is highest in red muscles, which are largely composed of slow (type I) fibers, compared to white muscle, which contains mostly fast (type II) fibers [101]. Acutely, low-energy status (ie, increased AMP/ATP ratio) activates AMPK, which in turn inhibits ATP-consuming processes and activates substrate metabolism to restore ATP levels. AMPK is also involved in chronic adaptations through regulation of gene expression. However, a broad range of genes involved in energy metabolism have been shown to be controlled by AMPK, most of which are involved in oxidative metabolism, such as components of the Krebs cycle and fatty acid oxidation [99]. It has been demonstrated that chronic energy deprivation enhances AMPK-dependent mitochondrial biogenesis associated with increased protein levels of CaMKIV and PGC-1α [102], which play an important role in muscle oxidative phenotype.

Hypoxia-inducible factor-1α

Hypoxia-inducible factor-1α (HIF-1α) mediates numerous adaptations of tissue to hypoxia. Intramuscular partial pressure of oxygen drops during exercise, and increased HIF-1α protein levels have been reported in muscle from healthy humans after exercise [103]. Likewise, it is possible that this also occurs as a consequence of reduced oxygen supply in diseases such as COPD and chronic heart failure. During normoxia, HIF-1α is hydroxylated at two proline residues by prolyl-hydroxylases, which promote binding of von Hippel-Lindau protein and target HIF-1α to degradation by the ubiquitin-proteasome pathway. When oxygen is limited, the prolyl-hydroxylases are inhibited, and HIF-1α becomes stabilized, migrates to the nucleus, dimerizes with HIF-1β, and induces transcription of its target genes [104]. With respect to metabolic profiles, these target genes are mainly genes involved in glycolytic metabolism, and HIF-1α should be regarded as a negative mediator of oxidative capacity [105]. Exposure to hypoxia often induces a shift toward glycolytic metabolism away from oxidative metabolism [106]. Whether HIF-1α directly downregulates enzymes involved in oxidative metabolism is less obvious, although data from muscle-specific HIF-1α knock-out mice do support this notion. Recent data also show that the expression of PPARs is inhibited by HIF-1α [107]. HIF-1α directly controls muscle oxidative phenotype through regulation of the glycolytic genes and possibly indirectly influences oxidative phenotype via PPAR-dependent pathways.

It is plausible that all of these regulators are to some degree involved in the loss of muscle oxidative phenotype in COPD. Systemic inflammation, a hallmark of COPD, may affect muscle oxidative phenotype by downregulation of the PPARs. It has been shown that a bidirectional antagonism between the PPAR and NF-kB signaling pathway exists. Several studies independently reported that TNF-α and other proinflammatory cytokines under transcriptional control of NF-kB (eg, IL-6)—in vitro and in vivo—exert a downregulating effect on the expression of PPAR mRNAs and have an inhibitory effect on the transcriptional activity of PPAR proteins [108–110]. Remels and colleagues [111] recently demonstrated reduced PPAR levels that correlated negatively with TNF-α levels in the circulation in skeletal muscle of patients who have COPD. The reduced daily physical activity patterns of these patients imply reduced muscular activity, especially endurance related, which could attenuate the expression of oxidative genes through the Ca^{2+}-dependent calcineurin and CaMK pathways or via downregulation of the PPARs [86]. In patients who have COPD, particularly persons who suffer from severe hypoxemia, local hypoxia could cause a shift away from oxidative metabolism through stabilization of HIF-1α. Further investigation is needed to understand more fully the spectrum of processes that regulate fiber type shift and loss of muscle oxidative capacity in skeletal muscle of patients who have COPD.

Therapeutic implications

Modulation of muscle atrophy

Several studies have investigated the effects of exercise training and pharmacologic anabolic stimuli to promote protein synthesis in patients who have COPD. Resistance exercise [112] and a combined strength and endurance exercise approach [113] resulted in gain of muscle mass. Anabolic steroids, testosterone, growth hormone, and growth hormone–releasing factor also showed a variable but overall positive response on muscle mass [114–116]. These studies illustrated that stimulation of protein synthesis is a feasible therapeutic strategy. No data are available yet regarding the effects of these interventions on muscle IGF-1, mechano growth factor-1 levels, and downstream markers of IGF-1 signaling in COPD. The therapeutic potential of IGF-1 has been reflected mainly by experimental studies in cultured cells and animals, in which stimulation of muscle growth and prevention of aging- or disease-associated muscle loss have been well documented. Recent insights reveal that two distinct cellular processes are involved in postnatal muscle (re)growth: myofiber hypertrophy and muscle regeneration. As a result, the effect of IGF-1 depends on which of these processes participates in the growth response, because IGF-1 signaling differs between muscle cells involved in myofiber hypertrophy and muscle regeneration. Basal IGF-1/insulin signaling is also required for the maintenance of muscle mass by suppression of muscle degradation pathways. It is essential to dissect IGF-1 signal transduction in maintenance of muscle mass and muscle growth responses involving myofiber hypertrophy and regeneration (during the stable clinical state and recovery from acute exacerbations) to identify regulatory molecules as putative candidates for specific pharmacologic modulation of muscle growth and atrophy.

Another yet relatively unexplored possibility for inducing or enhancing muscle weight gain is by nutritional modulation of protein synthesis. Optimizing protein intake may stimulate protein synthesis per se but also may enhance efficacy of anabolic drugs and physiologic stimuli, such as resistance exercise. It has been shown in underweight patients who have COPD that exercise training without nutritional rehabilitation is insufficient to increase weight loss and muscle mass [117]. Amino acids are the building blocks of protein, and several studies have to date reported an abnormal plasma amino acid pattern in COPD. Of interest are the consistently reduced plasma levels of branched chain amino acids in underweight patients who have COPD and in patients with low muscle mass [9]. In particular, leucine is an interesting nutritional substrate because it not only serves as precursor but also activates signaling pathways that enhance activity and synthesis of proteins involved in mRNA translocation to upregulate protein synthesis in skeletal muscle [118].

The anabolic response after tailored rehabilitation and pharmacologic stimulation is, however, soon reversed when the anabolic stimulus is terminated. Some patients who have COPD do not respond at all [119]. Muscle wasting in COPD may be the result of a perpetuating systemic inflammatory response, because studies in experimental models have demonstrated cachexia-inducing effects of proinflammatory cytokines, such as TNF-α, IL-1, and IL-6. Cross-sectional studies provide evidence for inflammation as a trigger of muscle atrophy, and systemic inflammation seemed to discriminate patients with a poor therapeutic response to a standardized and controlled clinical rehabilitation program from so-called "responders" [120]. Because increased levels of multiple inflammatory mediators have been reported in COPD, further work is needed to determine which of these mediators should be targeted to prevent muscle atrophy in patients who have COPD.

From a therapeutic perspective, it would theoretically be more effective to modulate muscle metabolism at a level at which many of these stimuli converge (ie, activation of NF-κB in skeletal muscle itself). Evidence to support such a strategy is provided by several recent studies that revealed that NF-κB activation in skeletal muscle is required for the induction of muscle loss by several atrophy stimuli [55,56,121], and induction of NF-κB specifically in skeletal muscle is sufficient to induce atrophy [55]. Importantly, inactivation of muscular NF-κB was also documented to stimulate muscle differentiation [55,75,122], promote muscle regeneration, and increase muscle strength [121]. Alternatively, strategies to increase local IGF-1 also may exert inflammatory signaling-suppressive effects [123]. This strategy would positively modulate muscle mass by overcoming the suppressive effects of inflammation on muscle regeneration and stimulation of muscle growth via IGF-1 signaling.

Regulation of muscle metabolism

Positive effects of pulmonary rehabilitation (particularly endurance exercise training) on oxidative enzymes and exercise capacity illustrate that decreased muscle oxidative capacity in COPD is at least partly reversible [124]. Exercise training also seemed to restore UCP-3 content in limb muscles, especially in patients who showed no increase in hydroxyacylCoA dehydrogenase activity, whereas lipid peroxidation levels were unaltered [125]. The nature of this response complies with the hypothesis that UCP-3 may protect against lipotoxicity (possibly induced or aggravated by oxidative stress) and that antioxidant modulation or fatty acid modulation may positively affect these processes. This may be useful in pulmonary and systemic circumstances that limit high-intensity exercise, such as severe respiratory impairment or cachexia.

A recent report provided evidence for electron transport chain dysfunction of mitochondria in cachectic patients who have COPD and were otherwise characterized by low UCP-3 mRNA expression and abnormal adaptations of skeletal muscle redox status after exercise training [22,126]. A recent randomized clinical trial of patients who have COPD participating in a pulmonary rehabilitation program showed that polyunsaturated fatty acids markedly enhanced exercise capacity compared to placebo [127]. These positive effects also could be explained by modulating effects on PPAR content and activity in skeletal muscle, because polyunsaturated fatty acids are natural ligands of the PPARs. Importantly, there is experimental evidence that PPARs also can exert anti-inflammatory effects in airways and muscle cells, thereby not limiting their promising beneficial effects on the pathogenesis of COPD to the extrapulmonary manifestations of the disease but expanding them to the level of the primary organ dysfunction [128,129].

Summary

Efficacy of known interventions to modulate skeletal muscle function, together with novel insights in the regulation of muscle mass and muscle metabolism as summarized in this article, provides increasing evidence of the need for therapeutic strategies to improve skeletal muscle oxidative capacity and muscle protein synthesis and regulate systemic inflammation and oxidative stress, which are strongly associated with skeletal muscle atrophy and dysfunction in COPD and other chronic disorders.

References

[1] Agusti AG. Systemic effects of chronic obstructive pulmonary disease. Proc Am Thorac Soc 2005;2: 367–70 [discussion: 71–2].

[2] Balasubramanian VP, Varkey B. Chronic obstructive pulmonary disease: effects beyond the lungs. Curr Opin Pulm Med 2006;12:106–12.

[3] Mador MJ. Muscle mass, not body weight, predicts outcome in patients with chronic obstructive pulmonary disease. Am J Respir Crit Care Med 2002;166:787–9.

[4] Gosker HR, Wouters EF, van der Vusse GJ, et al. Skeletal muscle dysfunction in chronic obstructive pulmonary disease and chronic heart failure: underlying mechanisms and therapy perspectives. Am J Clin Nutr 2000;71:1033–47.

[5] Satta A, Migliori GB, Spanevello A, et al. Fibre types in skeletal muscles of chronic obstructive pulmonary disease patients related to respiratory function and exercise tolerance. Eur Respir J 1997;10:2853–60.

[6] Gosker HR, Engelen MP, van Mameren H, et al. Muscle fiber type IIX atrophy is involved in the loss of fat-free mass in chronic obstructive pulmonary disease. Am J Clin Nutr 2002;76:113–9.

[7] Jagoe RT, Engelen MP. Muscle wasting and changes in muscle protein metabolism in chronic obstructive pulmonary disease. Eur Respir J 2003; 46(Suppl):52s–63s.

[8] Morrison WL, Gibson JN, Scrimgeour C, et al. Muscle wasting in emphysema. Clin Sci (Lond) 1988;75:415–20.

[9] Rutten EP, Franssen FM, Engelen MP, et al. Greater whole-body myofibrillar protein breakdown in cachectic patients with chronic obstructive pulmonary disease. Am J Clin Nutr 2006;83:829–34.

[10] Agusti AG, Sauleda J, Miralles C, et al. Skeletal muscle apoptosis and weight loss in chronic obstructive pulmonary disease. Am J Respir Crit Care Med 2002;166:485–9.

[11] Gosker HR, Kubat B, Schaart G, et al. Myopathological features in skeletal muscle of patients with chronic obstructive pulmonary disease. Eur Respir J 2003;22:280–5.

[12] Gosker HR, van Mameren H, van Dijk PJ, et al. Skeletal muscle fibre-type shifting and metabolic profile in patients with chronic obstructive pulmonary disease. Eur Respir J 2002;19:617–25.

[13] Jakobsson P, Jorfeldt L, Henriksson J. Metabolic enzyme activity in the quadriceps femoris muscle in patients with severe chronic obstructive pulmonary disease. Am J Respir Crit Care Med 1995; 151:374–7.

[14] Essen-Gustavsson B, Henriksson J. Enzyme levels in pools of microdissected human muscle fibres of identified type: adaptive response to exercise. Acta Physiol Scand 1984;120:505–15.

[15] Pouw EM, Schols AM, van der Vusse GJ, et al. Elevated inosine monophosphate levels in resting muscle of patients with stable chronic obstructive pulmonary disease. Am J Respir Crit Care Med 1998;157:453–7.

[16] Kutsuzawa T, Shioya S, Kurita D, et al. Muscle energy metabolism and nutritional status in patients with chronic obstructive pulmonary disease: a 31P magnetic resonance study. Am J Respir Crit Care Med 1995;152:647–52.

[17] Maltais F, Simard AA, Simard C, et al. Oxidative capacity of the skeletal muscle and lactic acid kinetics during exercise in normal subjects and in patients with COPD. Am J Respir Crit Care Med 1996;153:288–93.

[18] Franssen FM, Broekhuizen R, Janssen PP, et al. Limb muscle dysfunction in COPD: effects of muscle wasting and exercise training. Med Sci Sports Exerc 2005;37:2–9.

[19] Baarends EM, Schols AM, Akkermans MA, et al. Decreased mechanical efficiency in clinically stable patients with COPD. Thorax 1997;52:981–6.

[20] Gosker HR, Schrauwen P, Hesselink MK, et al. Uncoupling protein-3 content is decreased in peripheral skeletal muscle of patients with COPD. Eur Respir J 2003;22:88–93.

[21] Bezaire V, Seifert EL, Harper ME. Uncoupling protein-3: clues in an ongoing mitochondrial mystery. FASEB J 2007;21:312–24.

[22] Rabinovich RA, Ardite E, Troosters T, et al. Reduced muscle redox capacity after endurance training in patients with chronic obstructive pulmonary disease. Am J Respir Crit Care Med 2001;164:1114–8.

[23] Couillard A, Maltais F, Saey D, et al. Exercise-induced quadriceps oxidative stress and peripheral muscle dysfunction in patients with chronic obstructive pulmonary disease. Am J Respir Crit Care Med 2003;167:1664–9.

[24] Donaldson GC, Seemungal TA, Patel IS, et al. Airway and systemic inflammation and decline in lung function in patients with COPD. Chest 2005;128:1995–2004.

[25] Wouters EF, Creutzberg EC, Schols AM. Systemic effects in COPD. Chest 2002;121:127S–30S.

[26] Yanbaeva DG, Dentener MA, Creutzberg EC, et al. Systemic inflammation in COPD: is genetic susceptibility a key factor? COPD 2006;3:51–61.

[27] Pinto-Plata VM, Mullerova H, Toso JF, et al. C-reactive protein in patients with COPD, control smokers and non-smokers. Thorax 2006;61:23–8.

[28] Broekhuizen R, Wouters EF, Creutzberg EC, et al. Raised CRP levels mark metabolic and functional impairment in advanced COPD. Thorax 2006;61:17–22.

[29] Yende S, Waterer GW, Tolley EA, et al. Inflammatory markers are associated with ventilatory limitation and muscle dysfunction in obstructive lung disease in well functioning elderly subjects. Thorax 2006;61:10–6.

[30] Vernooy JH, Kucukaycan M, Jacobs JA, et al. Local and systemic inflammation in patients with chronic obstructive pulmonary disease: soluble tumor necrosis factor receptors are increased in

sputum. Am J Respir Crit Care Med 2002;166: 1218–24.

[31] Noguera A, Busquets X, Sauleda J, et al. Expression of adhesion molecules and G proteins in circulating neutrophils in chronic obstructive pulmonary disease. Am J Respir Crit Care Med 1998;158:1664–8.

[32] Takabatake N, Nakamura H, Abe S, et al. The relationship between chronic hypoxemia and activation of the tumor necrosis factor-alpha system in patients with chronic obstructive pulmonary disease. Am J Respir Crit Care Med 2000;161: 1179–84.

[33] Bartoccioni E, Michaelis D, Hohlfeld R. Constitutive and cytokine-induced production of interleukin-6 by human myoblasts. Immunol Lett 1994; 42:135–8.

[34] Tews DS, Goebel HH. Expression of cell adhesion molecules in inflammatory myopathies. J Neuroimmunol 1995;59:185–94.

[35] Langen RC, Schols AM, Kelders MC, et al. Muscle wasting and impaired muscle regeneration in a murine model of chronic pulmonary inflammation. Am J Respir Cell Mol Biol 2006;35:689–96.

[36] Montes de Oca M, Torres SH, De Sanctis J, et al. Skeletal muscle inflammation and nitric oxide in patients with COPD. Eur Respir J 2005;26:390–7.

[37] Agusti A, Morla M, Sauleda J, et al. NF-kappaB activation and iNOS upregulation in skeletal muscle of patients with COPD and low body weight. Thorax 2004;59:483–7.

[38] Broekhuizen R, Grimble RF, Howell WM, et al. Pulmonary cachexia, systemic inflammatory profile, and the interleukin 1beta -511 single nucleotide polymorphism. Am J Clin Nutr 2005;82: 1059–64.

[39] Buck M, Chojkier M. Muscle wasting and dedifferentiation induced by oxidative stress in a murine model of cachexia is prevented by inhibitors of nitric oxide synthesis and antioxidants. EMBO J 1996;15:1753–65.

[40] Guttridge DC, Mayo MW, Madrid LV, et al. NF-kappaB-induced loss of MyoD messenger RNA: possible role in muscle decay and cachexia. Science 2000;289:2363–6.

[41] Li YP, Schwartz RJ, Waddell ID, et al. Skeletal muscle myocytes undergo protein loss and reactive oxygen-mediated NF-kappaB activation in response to tumor necrosis factor alpha. FASEB J 1998;12:871–80.

[42] Smith BK, Conn CA, Kluger MJ. Experimental cachexia: effects of MCA sarcoma in the Fischer rat. Am J Physiol 1993;265:R376–84.

[43] Pahl HL. Signal transduction from the endoplasmic reticulum to the cell nucleus. Physiol Rev 1999;79:683–701.

[44] Reid MB, Li YP. Tumor necrosis factor-alpha and muscle wasting: a cellular perspective. Respir Res 2001;2:269–72.

[45] Ling PR, Schwartz JH, Bistrian BR. Mechanisms of host wasting induced by administration of cytokines in rats. Am J Physiol 1997;272:E333–9.

[46] Ventadour S, Attaix D. Mechanisms of skeletal muscle atrophy. Curr Opin Rheumatol 2006;18: 631–5.

[47] Li YP, Lecker SH, Chen Y, et al. TNF-alpha increases ubiquitin-conjugating activity in skeletal muscle by up-regulating UbcH2/E220k. FASEB J 2003;17:1048–57.

[48] Ladner KJ, Caligiuri MA, Guttridge DC. Tumor necrosis factor-regulated biphasic activation of NF-kappa B is required for cytokine-induced loss of skeletal muscle gene products. J Biol Chem 2003;278:2294–303.

[49] Garcia-Martinez C, Llovera M, Agell N, et al. Ubiquitin gene expression in skeletal muscle is increased by tumour necrosis factor-alpha. Biochem Biophys Res Commun 1994;201:682–6.

[50] Gomes MD, Lecker SH, Jagoe RT, et al. Atrogin-1, a muscle-specific F-box protein highly expressed during muscle atrophy. Proc Natl Acad Sci U S A 2001;98:14440–5.

[51] Lecker SH, Jagoe RT, Gilbert A, et al. Multiple types of skeletal muscle atrophy involve a common program of changes in gene expression. FASEB J 2004;18:39–51.

[52] Wray CJ, Mammen JM, Hershko DD, et al. Sepsis upregulates the gene expression of multiple ubiquitin ligases in skeletal muscle. Int J Biochem Cell Biol 2003;35:698–705.

[53] Drexler H, Riede U, Munzel T, et al. Alterations of skeletal muscle in chronic heart failure. Circulation 1992;85:1751–9.

[54] Inoue I, Katayama S. The possible therapeutic actions of peroxisome proliferator-activated receptor alpha (PPAR alpha) agonists, PPAR gamma agonists, 3-hydroxy-3-methylglutaryl coenzyme A (HMG-CoA) reductase inhibitors, angiotensin converting enzyme (ACE) inhibitors and calcium (Ca)-antagonists on vascular endothelial cells. Curr Drug Targets Cardiovasc Haematol Disord 2004;4:35–52.

[55] Cai D, Frantz JD, Tawa NE Jr, et al. IKKbeta/ NF-kappaB activation causes severe muscle wasting in mice. Cell 2004;119:285–98.

[56] Hunter RB, Kandarian SC. Disruption of either the Nfkb1 or the Bcl3 gene inhibits skeletal muscle atrophy. J Clin Invest 2004;114:1504–11.

[57] Lang CH, Frost RA. Sepsis-induced suppression of skeletal muscle translation initiation mediated by tumor necrosis factor alpha. Metabolism 2007;56: 49–57.

[58] Garcia-Martinez C, Lopez-Soriano FJ, Argiles JM. Acute treatment with tumour necrosis factor-alpha induces changes in protein metabolism in rat skeletal muscle. Mol Cell Biochem 1993;125:11–8.

[59] Lang CH, Frost RA, Nairn AC, et al. TNF-alpha impairs heart and skeletal muscle protein synthesis

by altering translation initiation. Am J Physiol Endocrinol Metab 2002;282:E336–47.

[60] Cooney RN, Maish GO 3rd, Gilpin T, et al. Mechanism of IL-1 induced inhibition of protein synthesis in skeletal muscle. Shock 1999;11: 235–41.

[61] Thissen JP. How proinflammatory cytokines may impair growth and cause muscle wasting. Horm Res 2007;67(Suppl 1):64–70.

[62] Glass DJ. Skeletal muscle hypertrophy and atrophy signaling pathways. Int J Biochem Cell Biol 2005; 37:1974–84.

[63] Broussard SR, McCusker RH, Novakofski JE, et al. Cytokine-hormone interactions: tumor necrosis factor alpha impairs biologic activity and downstream activation signals of the insulin-like growth factor I receptor in myoblasts. Endocrinology 2003;144:2988–96.

[64] Strle K, Broussard SR, McCusker RH, et al. Proinflammatory cytokine impairment of insulin-like growth factor I-induced protein synthesis in skeletal muscle myoblasts requires ceramide. Endocrinology 2004;145:4592–602.

[65] Allen DL, Roy RR, Edgerton VR. Myonuclear domains in muscle adaptation and disease. Muscle Nerve 1999;22:1350–60.

[66] Danial NN, Korsmeyer SJ. Cell death: critical control points. Cell 2004;116:205–19.

[67] Almendro V, Carbo N, Busquets S, et al. Sepsis induces DNA fragmentation in rat skeletal muscle. Eur Cytokine Netw 2003;14:256–9.

[68] Phillips T, Leeuwenburgh C. Muscle fiber specific apoptosis and TNF-alpha signaling in sarcopenia are attenuated by life-long calorie restriction. FASEB J 2005;19:668–70.

[69] Stewart CE, Newcomb PV, Holly JM. Multifaceted roles of TNF-alpha in myoblast destruction: a multitude of signal transduction pathways. J Cell Physiol 2004;198:237–47.

[70] Mitch WE, Du J. Cellular mechanisms causing loss of muscle mass in kidney disease. Semin Nephrol 2004;24:484–7.

[71] Callahan LA, Supinski GS. Diaphragm and cardiac mitochondrial creatine kinases are impaired in sepsis. J Appl Physiol 2007;102:44–53.

[72] Setsuta K, Seino Y, Ogawa T, et al. Ongoing myocardial damage in chronic heart failure is related to activated tumor necrosis factor and Fas/Fas ligand system. Circ J 2004;68:747–50.

[73] van der Velden J, Langen R, Kelders M, et al. Myogenic differentiation during regrowth of atrophied skeletal muscle is associated with inactivation of GSK-3{beta}. Am J Physiol Cell Physiol 2007; 292(5):C1636–44.

[74] Hawke TJ, Garry DJ. Myogenic satellite cells: physiology to molecular biology. J Appl Physiol 2001;91:534–51.

[75] Langen RC, Schols AM, Kelders MC, et al. Inflammatory cytokines inhibit myogenic differentiation

through activation of nuclear factor-kappaB. FASEB J 2001;15:1169–80.

[76] Dogra C, Changotra H, Wedhas N, et al. TNF-related weak inducer of apoptosis (TWEAK) is a potent skeletal muscle-wasting cytokine. FASEB J 2007;21(8):1857–69.

[77] Broussard SR, McCusker RH, Novakofski JE, et al. IL-1beta impairs insulin-like growth factor i-induced differentiation and downstream activation signals of the insulin-like growth factor i receptor in myoblasts. J Immunol 2004;172:7713–20.

[78] Langen RC, Van Der Velden JL, Schols AM, et al. Tumor necrosis factor-alpha inhibits myogenic differentiation through MyoD protein destabilization. FASEB J 2004;18:227–37.

[79] Tolosa L, Morla M, Iglesias A, et al. IFN-gamma prevents TNF-alpha-induced apoptosis in C2C12 myotubes through down-regulation of TNF-R2 and increased NF-kappaB activity. Cell Signal 2005;17:1333–42.

[80] Fredenrich A, Grimaldi PA. Roles of peroxisome proliferator-activated receptor delta in skeletal muscle function and adaptation. Curr Opin Clin Nutr Metab Care 2004;7:377–81.

[81] Lefebvre P, Chinetti G, Fruchart JC, et al. Sorting out the roles of PPAR alpha in energy metabolism and vascular homeostasis. J Clin Invest 2006;116: 571–80.

[82] Cresci S, Wright LD, Spratt JA, et al. Activation of a novel metabolic gene regulatory pathway by chronic stimulation of skeletal muscle. Am J Physiol 1996;270:C1413–20.

[83] Horowitz JF, Leone TC, Feng W, et al. Effect of endurance training on lipid metabolism in women: a potential role for PPARalpha in the metabolic response to training. Am J Physiol Endocrinol Metab 2000;279:E348–55.

[84] Minnich A, Tian N, Byan L, et al. A potent PPAR-alpha agonist stimulates mitochondrial fatty acid beta-oxidation in liver and skeletal muscle. Am J Physiol Endocrinol Metab 2001;280:E270–9.

[85] Muoio DM, MacLean PS, Lang DB, et al. Fatty acid homeostasis and induction of lipid regulatory genes in skeletal muscles of peroxisome proliferator-activated receptor (PPAR) alpha knock-out mice: evidence for compensatory regulation by PPAR delta. J Biol Chem 2002;277:26089–97.

[86] Fritz T, Kramer DK, Karlsson HK, et al. Low-intensity exercise increases skeletal muscle protein expression of PPARdelta and UCP3 in type 2 diabetic patients. Diabetes Metab Res Rev 2006;22:492–8.

[87] Brunmair B, Staniek K, Dorig J, et al. Activation of PPAR-delta in isolated rat skeletal muscle switches fuel preference from glucose to fatty acids. Diabetologia 2006;49:2713–22.

[88] Luquet S, Lopez-Soriano J, Holst D, et al. Peroxisome proliferator-activated receptor delta controls muscle development and oxidative capability. FASEB J 2003;17:2299–301.

[89] Furnsinn C, Willson TM, Brunmair B. Peroxisome proliferator-activated receptor-delta, a regulator of oxidative capacity, fuel switching and cholesterol transport. Diabetologia 2007;50:8–17.

[90] St-Pierre J, Lin J, Krauss S, et al. Bioenergetic analysis of peroxisome proliferator-activated receptor gamma coactivators 1alpha and 1beta (PGC-1-alpha and PGC-1beta) in muscle cells. J Biol Chem 2003;278:26597–603.

[91] Wu Z, Puigserver P, Andersson U, et al. Mechanisms controlling mitochondrial biogenesis and respiration through the thermogenic coactivator PGC-1. Cell 1999;98:115–24.

[92] Scarpulla RC. Nuclear activators and coactivators in mammalian mitochondrial biogenesis. Biochim Biophys Acta 2002;1576:1–14.

[93] Lin J, Wu H, Tarr PT, et al. Transcriptional coactivator PGC-1 alpha drives the formation of slow-twitch muscle fibres. Nature 2002;418:797–801.

[94] Talmadge RJ, Otis JS, Rittler MR, et al. Calcineurin activation influences muscle phenotype in a muscle-specific fashion. BMC Cell Biol 2004;5:28.

[95] Chin ER, Olson EN, Richardson JA, et al. A calcineurin-dependent transcriptional pathway controls skeletal muscle fiber type. Genes Dev 1998;12:2499–509.

[96] Handschin C, Rhee J, Lin J, et al. An autoregulatory loop controls peroxisome proliferator-activated receptor gamma coactivator 1alpha expression in muscle. Proc Natl Acad Sci U S A 2003;100:7111–6.

[97] Chin ER. Role of Ca2+/calmodulin-dependent kinases in skeletal muscle plasticity. J Appl Physiol 2005;99:414–23.

[98] Wu H, Kanatous SB, Thurmond FA, et al. Regulation of mitochondrial biogenesis in skeletal muscle by CaMK. Science 2002;296:349–52.

[99] Aschenbach WG, Sakamoto K, Goodyear LJ. 5′ adenosine monophosphate-activated protein kinase, metabolism and exercise. Sports Med 2004;34:91–103.

[100] Reznick RM, Shulman GI. The role of AMP-activated protein kinase in mitochondrial biogenesis. J Physiol 2006;574:33–9.

[101] Ai H, Ihlemann J, Hellsten Y, et al. Effect of fiber type and nutritional state on AICAR- and contraction-stimulated glucose transport in rat muscle. Am J Physiol Endocrinol Metab 2002;282:E1291–300.

[102] Zong H, Ren JM, Young LH, et al. AMP kinase is required for mitochondrial biogenesis in skeletal muscle in response to chronic energy deprivation. Proc Natl Acad Sci U S A 2002;99:15983–7.

[103] Ameln H, Gustafsson T, Sundberg CJ, et al. Physiological activation of hypoxia inducible factor-1 in human skeletal muscle. FASEB J 2005;19:1009–11.

[104] Semenza GL. HIF-1, O(2), and the 3 PHDs: how animal cells signal hypoxia to the nucleus. Cell 2001;107:1–3.

[105] Semenza GL. HIF-1: mediator of physiological and pathophysiological responses to hypoxia. J Appl Physiol 2000;88:1474–80.

[106] Hoppeler H, Vogt M. Muscle tissue adaptations to hypoxia. J Exp Biol 2001;204:3133–9.

[107] Narravula S, Colgan SP. Hypoxia-inducible factor 1-mediated inhibition of peroxisome proliferator-activated receptor alpha expression during hypoxia. J Immunol 2001;166:7543–8.

[108] Delerive P, De Bosscher K, Besnard S, et al. Peroxisome proliferator-activated receptor alpha negatively regulates the vascular inflammatory gene response by negative cross-talk with transcription factors NF-kappaB and AP-1. J Biol Chem 1999;274:32048–54.

[109] Sung CK, She H, Xiong S, et al. Tumor necrosis factor-alpha inhibits peroxisome proliferator-activated receptor gamma activity at a posttranslational level in hepatic stellate cells. Am J Physiol Gastrointest Liver Physiol 2004;286:G722–9.

[110] Tham DM, Martin-McNulty B, Wang YX, et al. Angiotensin II is associated with activation of NF-kappaB-mediated genes and downregulation of PPARs. Physiol Genomics 2002;11:21–30.

[111] Remels AH, Schrauwen P, Broekhuizen R, et al. Expression and contents of PPARs is reduced in skeletal muscles of COPD patients. Eur Respir J 2007;30(2).

[112] Bernard S, Whittom F, Leblanc P, et al. Aerobic and strength training in patients with chronic obstructive pulmonary disease. Am J Respir Crit Care Med 1999;159:896–901.

[113] Franssen FM, Broekhuizen R, Janssen PP, et al. Effects of whole-body exercise training on body composition and functional capacity in normal-weight patients with COPD. Chest 2004;125:2021–8.

[114] Casaburi R. Anabolic therapies in chronic obstructive pulmonary disease. Monaldi Arch Chest Dis 1998;53:454–9.

[115] Creutzberg EC, Casaburi R. Endocrinological disturbances in chronic obstructive pulmonary disease. Eur Respir J 2003;46(Suppl):76s–80s.

[116] Ferreira I, Brooks D, Lacasse Y, et al. Nutritional intervention in COPD: a systematic overview. Chest 2001;119:353–63.

[117] Schols AM, Soeters PB, Mostert R, et al. Physiologic effects of nutritional support and anabolic steroids in patients with chronic obstructive pulmonary disease: a placebo-controlled randomized trial. Am J Respir Crit Care Med 1995;152:1268–74.

[118] Anthony JC, Anthony TG, Kimball SR, et al. Signaling pathways involved in translational control of protein synthesis in skeletal muscle by leucine. J Nutr 2001;131:856S–60S.

[119] Bolton CE, Broekhuizen R, Ionescu AA, et al. Cellular protein breakdown and systemic

inflammation are unaffected by pulmonary rehabilitation in COPD. Thorax 2007;62:109–14.

[120] Creutzberg EC, Schols AM, Weling-Scheepers CA, et al. Characterization of nonresponse to high caloric oral nutritional therapy in depleted patients with chronic obstructive pulmonary disease. Am J Respir Crit Care Med 2000;161:745–52.

[121] Mourkioti F, Kratsios P, Luedde T, et al. Targeted ablation of IKK2 improves skeletal muscle strength, maintains mass, and promotes regeneration. J Clin Invest 2006;116:2945–54.

[122] Guttridge DC, Albanese C, Reuther JY, et al. NF-kappaB controls cell growth and differentiation through transcriptional regulation of cyclin D1. Mol Cell Biol 1999;19:5785–99.

[123] Pelosi L, Giacinti C, Nardis C, et al. Local expression of IGF-1 accelerates muscle regeneration by rapidly modulating inflammatory cytokines and chemokines. FASEB J 2007;21(7): 1393–402.

[124] Puente-Maestu L, Tena T, Trascasa C, et al. Training improves muscle oxidative capacity and oxygenation recovery kinetics in patients with chronic obstructive pulmonary disease. Eur J Appl Physiol 2003;88:580–7.

[125] Gosker HR, Schrauwen P, Broekhuizen R, et al. Exercise training restores uncoupling protein-3 content in limb muscles of patients with chronic obstructive pulmonary disease. Am J Physiol Endocrinol Metab 2006;290(5):E976–81.

[126] Rabinovich RA, Bastos R, Ardite E, et al. Mitochondrial dysfunction in COPD patients with low body mass index. Eur Respir J 2007;29:643–50.

[127] Broekhuizen R, Wouters EF, Creutzberg EC, et al. Polyunsaturated fatty acids improve exercise capacity in chronic obstructive pulmonary disease. Thorax 2005;60:376–82.

[128] Birrell MA, Patel HJ, McCluskie K, et al. PPAR-gamma agonists as therapy for diseases involving airway neutrophilia. Eur Respir J 2004;24:18–23.

[129] Patel HJ, Belvisi MG, Bishop-Bailey D, et al. Activation of peroxisome proliferator-activated receptors in human airway smooth muscle cells has a superior anti-inflammatory profile to corticosteroids: relevance for chronic obstructive pulmonary disease therapy. J Immunol 2003;170:2663–9.

ELSEVIER
SAUNDERS

Clin Chest Med 28 (2007) 553–557

CLINICS
IN CHEST
MEDICINE

Other Systemic Manifestations of Chronic Obstructive Pulmonary Disease

Andrew C. Stone, MD, MPH[a], Linda Nici, MD[b,c],*

[a]Providence, RI, USA
[b]Brown University School of Medicine, Providence, RI, USA
[c]Pulmonary and Critical Care Section, Providence Veterans Administration Medical Center,
830 Chalkstone Avenue, Providence, RI 02908, USA

Clinically relevant systemic effects of chronic obstructive pulmonary disease (COPD) include skeletal muscle, cardiovascular, neurologic, psychiatric, and endocrine system dysfunction. Systemic inflammation and skeletal muscle dysfunction in COPD are discussed in detail in the article by Remels and colleagues elsewhere in this issue. This article focuses on other systemic manifestations of COPD. Recognition and understanding of these extrapulmonary effects of COPD will point to additional areas for intervention, which should lead to improved functional status, performance, and enhanced quality of life for these patients.

Inflammatory markers

A large body of evidence now suggests the presence of systemic inflammation in COPD. There are many studies and reviews in the literature evaluating increased levels of inflammatory cytokines, acute phase proteins, and markers of oxidant stress in patients who have COPD [1–5]. Increases in inflammatory cytokines are documented in sputum, exhaled breath condensate, bronchoalveolar lavage (BAL) fluid, and plasma in patients who have COPD. They include tumor necrosis factor α (TNF-α), transforming growth factor-beta, interferon-γ, and interleukins (ILs) 6 and 8 [1]. Many of these inflammatory markers are elevated in patients who have clinically stable

COPD and increase further with exacerbations [2]. Increased inflammatory cytokines and C-reactive protein (CRP) also are associated with skeletal muscle dysfunction, heart disease, and atherosclerosis in patients who have COPD [1,2].

There is increased oxidant stress in the lungs of patients who have COPD as compared with healthy nonsmokers. This is demonstrated by measuring hydrogen peroxide and nitric oxide levels in BAL fluid and exhaled breath condensate [3]. These increases in oxidative burden are hypothesized as responsible for many of the systemic effects of COPD, including changes in fibrinolysis [6], which may contribute to atherosclerosis. Acute phase proteins, such as CRP and fibrinogen, are elevated in smokers [6], and increased plasma fibrinogen levels in smokers are associated with decreased lung function and increased risk for COPD [7]. Fibrinogen and IL-6 are elevated in patients who have stable COPD and rise with exacerbations [8]. Because CRP and fibrinogen are implicated in heart disease and atherosclerosis, it is postulated that reducing the number of COPD exacerbations might decrease these acute phase protein levels and, thus, reduce the risk for coronary artery disease. The association between COPD and cardiovascular disease is discussed later.

Cardiovascular disease

The previous section introduced the concept that systemic inflammation occurs in COPD and may play a role in its pathogenesis. These inflammatory processes also may lead to cardiovascular pathology and dysfunction. Additionally,

* Corresponding author. Pulmonary and Critical Care Section, Providence Veterans Administration Medical Center, 830 Chalkstone Avenue, Providence, RI 02908.
  E-mail address: linda_nici@brown.edu (L. Nici).

structural changes in the chest wall and lungs may affect cardiac performance independent of the systemic inflammatory response. In this section, cardiovascular dysfunction and pathology are discussed in relation to COPD.

The cardiovascular system is affected by COPD in several ways, the most important being an increase in right ventricular afterload due to elevated pulmonary vascular resistance from direct vascular injury or destruction of the vascular bed [9,10], hypoxic vasoconstriction [11], or increases in effective pulmonary vascular resistance resulting from erythrocytosis [12]. The overloaded right ventricle in turn leads to right ventricular hypertrophy, which, if severe or left untreated, may result in right ventricular failure [13]. Left ventricular (LV) filling also may be compromised through septal shifts. This, in turn, can reduce the heart's ability to meet exercise demands [14]. Air trapping, with resultant hyperinflation, and the consequent rise in right atrial pressure may compromise cardiac function further [15].

Although pulmonary hypertension is known to be associated with the factors discussed previously, structural changes in pulmonary arteries also are seen early in COPD, before the onset of hypoxemia [16,17]. These findings suggest that hypoxemia may not be the sole cause of structural alterations in the vascular bed or increased pulmonary artery pressure. In one cross-sectional study of patients who had COPD and pulmonary hypertension (most neither were hypoxemic nor on supplemental oxygen), blood levels of TNF-α and CRP were independent predictors of systolic pulmonary artery pressure [18]. These investigators suggest a pathogenic role of systemic inflammation in pulmonary hypertension associated with COPD.

Right ventricular dysfunction also is noted in patients who have COPD and who have normal oxygenation or mild hypoxemia and normal pulmonary artery pressures. Vonk-Noordegraaf and colleagues [19] noted concentric right ventricular hypertrophy in patients who had COPD compared with controls. The investigators concluded that changes in the right ventricle happen early in COPD and may be the result of nocturnal hypoxemia or increased pulmonary arterial pressures during exercise. Another possible mechanism for these findings could be cardiac structural changes secondary to inflammatory mediators, but this has not been studied to date.

The progression of pulmonary hypertension is believed to lead to the clinical syndrome of right heart failure [20]. This hypothesis may prove too simplistic, however. Some controversy exists as to whether or not high pulmonary artery pressures result in lower extremity edema, as some patients who have lower extremity edema have normal resting right atrial pressures. Naejie [20] suggests that pulmonary vascular resistance with exercise or possibly nocturnal desaturation can explain this apparent paradox. Further work is needed to understand the pathogenesis of right heart failure in patients who have COPD.

In epidemiologic studies, atherosclerosis and coronary artery disease are associated with decline in forced expiratory volume in 1 second (FEV_1) even when corrected for smoking and other established cardiovascular risk factors. Decreased FEV_1 also is shown to be an independent predictor of cardiac death in patients who have COPD. In a careful review of the topic, Sin and Man concluded the increased risk for cardiovascular death was 75% greater for patients who had an FEV_1 in the lowest quintile as compared with the highest [21]. They did note heterogeneity in many of these population-based studies despite controlling for established risk factors, such as cigarette smoking, cholesterol level, and hypertension. There are at least four additional studies that have looked at this association and all corrected for smoking status and other risk factors [22–25]. In the Lung Health Study [26], Anthonisen and coworkers noted that for every decrease in FEV_1 by 10%, cardiovascular death increased by 28% and hospitalizations for cardiovascular causes increased by 42%. Hospitalizations for lower respiratory tract infection were one third those of cardiac admissions. Thus, there seems to be a relationship between loss of lung function and risk for cardiac death. The mechanisms underlying this association are as yet unknown.

Thrombosis may be influenced by inflammatory and coagulation cascade interactions [6,27]. This may be an explanation for the increased incidence of myocardial infarction in patients who have COPD and the increased incidence of venous thromboembolic disease [6,27].

LV diastolic dysfunction increasingly is recognized as having as poor a prognosis as systolic dysfunction in patients who have clinical congestive heart failure [28,29]. Population studies show equally poor survival regardless of ejection fraction. COPD is seen more commonly in patients who have diastolic dysfunction than in patients who have systolic dysfunction, despite similar risk factors. The association of COPD with LV diastolic dysfunction is ascribed to the concept of ventricular dependency and pericardial constraint. As right-sided pressures increase, left-sided filling is impeded [20], resulting in decreased LV end-diastolic volumes. As stroke volume and cardiac output decreases, the clinical syndrome of left heart failure ensues. It remains to be seen whether or not this finding is simply a manifestation of COPD severity or another pathogenic association, such as systemic inflammation.

Hyperinflation and alterations in intrathoracic pressures also may impede LV filling by way of either increasing pulmonary vascular resistance and right-sided pressures or by increasing LV afterload causing decreases in left-sided cardiac output [30]. Hyperinflated lungs also compress the heart and may decrease LV filling, causing diastolic dysfunction by way of decreasing end-diastolic LV stroke volume. It is unknown if therapies designed to improve hyperinflation also can improve LV performance.

Improvement of clinical outcomes among patients who have COPD may depend on the results of future studies that focus on this interaction between the cardiovascular system and COPD. Optimization of programs that improve exercise tolerance and quality of life for COPD patients will require increased understanding and awareness of the overlap between limitations in pulmonary function and limitations in cardiac performance.

Neurocognitive and psychiatric effects

Disordered sleep, anxiety, depression, and cognitive decline all are associated with COPD [31–43]. In turn, these problems are associated with decreased quality of life [31], increased hospitalizations [32], and earlier mortality [33]. The prevailing theory suggests hypoxia as the central feature in these complications of COPD [31,36]. There is one small study suggesting cognitive decline can occur in the absence of hypoxemia or with mild disease [34]; however, a larger earlier study found the opposite to be true [35]. A study of 10 patients who had COPD given long-term oxygen therapy showed improvements in neurocognitive function; however, the results did not reach statistical significance [36]. Further studies are needed to characterize the pathogenesis of cognitive decline in COPD better.

Depression and anxiety are seen more commonly in patients who have COPD than in healthy age-matched controls and in patients who have other chronic diseases [44]. Theories of increased prevalence of depression and anxiety in COPD suggest earlier onset of smoking in depressed adolescents, hypoxia-induced neuronal damage, and repeated reactive depression from losses associated with exacerbations, such as loss of functional status/independence and decreased self-perception [37]. Depression and anxiety in adolescents are linked with increased amount and earlier onset of smoking [44]. Smoking initiation at a young age is associated with more difficulty in quitting later in life and earlier onset of smoking-related lung disease.

Pharmacologic antidepressant therapy is not shown clearly beneficial in this patient population [38]. Some improvement of symptoms and quality of life scores occurs, however, with behavioral therapy [39]. Large well-designed studies are needed to develop treatment modalities that further address depression in patients who have COPD.

Disordered sleep is common in COPD. Mechanisms underlying nonapneic oxygen desaturation during sleep include decreased functional residual capacity, diminished ventilatory responses to hypoxia and hypercapnia, and impaired respiratory mechanical effectiveness. Additionally, diminished arousal responses, respiratory muscle fatigue, diminished nonchemical respiratory drive, and increased upper airway resistance also may play a role in sleep interruption [40].

In addition to poor sleep from hypoxemia, obstructive sleep apnea (OSA) is seen in association with COPD and is termed "overlap syndrome." It is estimated that 10% to 15% of patients who have COPD also have OSA [41]. The combination of OSA and COPD is shown to have an even more profound affect on patients' oxygenation, gas exchange, and breathing patterns than either disease alone. Identification of patients who have overlap syndrome is important because their 5-year survival is lower than that of patients who have OSA alone and there may be an increased risk for pulmonary hypertension and right heart failure in these patients [41,42].

Insomnia in COPD also has been reviewed. It is believed that more than 50% of COPD patients have sleep complaints characterized by longer latency falling asleep, more frequent awakenings, or generalized insomnia. Sleep disturbances tend to be more severe with advancing disease and contribute to decreased quality of life [43].

Osteoporosis

Although osteoporosis is a well-known consequence of oral glucocorticoid therapy [45], it also is seen in patients taking inhaled steroids and may be more prevalent in those who have had minimal steroid exposure [46]. Compression fractures of the vertebrae and hip fractures are common manifestations of osteoporosis. Thoracic vertebral compression fractures may lead to more compromised lung function as kyphosis and resultant restriction ensues. Pain related to thoracic vertebral compression fractures also may alter breathing pattern and worsen gas exchange disturbances.

In a cross-sectional study, osteopenia and osteoporosis were seen in 68% of patients who had COPD (predominantly females). The investigators concluded that steroid use alone was insufficient to explain the high prevalence [46]. Bolton and coworkers [47], in 2004, reported finding osteoporosis/osteopenia in 69% of patients who had COPD with FEV_1 greater than 50% and in 89% of patients who had FEV_1 less than 50% compared with 45% of controls. In a Veterans Administration study, McEvoy and colleagues reported vertebral compression fractures in 63% of patients who had COPD on oral steroids, 57% of patients who had COPD and were on inhaled steroids, and 49% of patients who had COPD who had never received steroids [48].

Despite the prevalence of osteoporosis in patients who have COPD, there are no studies to date on therapeutic approaches for these patients. Clearly, smoking cessation and increased physical activity is recommended for all patients suspected of having osteopenia. When to start calcium and vitamin D supplementation or bisphosphonate therapy in COPD is an area in need of future research.

Summary

COPD has broad-reaching consequences in multiple organ systems in addition to the lungs, either from systemic inflammation, hypoxemia, decreased function, or mechanical effects of hyperinflation. The involvement of these other organ systems provides ample opportunity for interdisciplinary collaborative research, which may lead to improved outcomes in these chronic disease states, which currently exact a heavy toll on patients, families, and society.

References

[1] Wouters EF. Local and systemic inflammation in chronic obstructive pulmonary disease. Proc Am Thorac Soc 2005;2(1):26–33.

[2] van Eeden SF, Yeung A, Quinlam K, et al. Systemic response to ambient particulate matter: relevance to chronic obstructive pulmonary disease. Proc Am Thorac Soc 2005;2(1):61–7.

[3] MacNee W. Pulmonary and systemic oxidant/antioxidant imbalance in chronic obstructive pulmonary disease. Proc Am Thorac Soc 2005;2(1):50–60.

[4] Agusti AG, Noguera A, Sauleda J, et al. Systemic effects of chronic obstructive pulmonary disease. Eur Respir J 2003;21(2):347–60.

[5] Oudijk EJ, Lammers JW, Koenderman L. Systemic inflammation in chronic obstructive pulmonary disease. Eur Respir J Suppl 2003;46:5s–13s.

[6] MacCallum PK. Markers of hemostasis and systemic inflammation in heart disease and atherosclerosis in smokers. Proc Am Thorac Soc 2005;2(1):34–43.

[7] Dahl M, Tybjaerg-Hansen A, Vestbo J, et al. Elevated plasma fibrinogen associated with reduced pulmonary function and increased risk of chronic obstructive pulmonary disease. Am J Respir Crit Care Med 2001;164(6):1008–11.

[8] Wedzicha JA, Seemungal TA, MacCallum PK, et al. Acute exacerbations of chronic obstructive pulmonary disease are accompanied by elevations of plasma fibrinogen and serum IL-6 levels. Thromb Haemost 2000;84(2):210–5.

[9] World Health Organization. Definition of chronic cor pulmonale. Circulation 1963;27:594–615.

[10] Santos S, Peinado VI, Ramirez J, et al. Characterization of pulmonary vascular remodelling in smokers and patients with mild COPD. Eur Respir J 2002; 19:632–8.

[11] Voelkel NF, Tuder RM. Hypoxia-induced pulmonary vascular remodeling: a model for what human disease? J Clin Invest 2000;106:733–8.

[12] Chetty KG, Brown SE, Light RW. Improved exercise tolerance of the polycythemic lung patient following phlebotomy. Am J Med 1983;74: 415–20.

[13] Sietsema K. Cardiovascular limitations in chronic pulmonary disease. Med Sci Sports Exerc 2001;33: S656–61.

[14] MacNee W. Pathophysiology of cor pulmonale in chronic obstructive pulmonary disease. Part One. Am J Respir Crit Care Med 1994;150:833–52.

[15] Butler J, Schrijen F, Henriquez A, et al. Cause of the raised wedge pressure on exercise in chronic obstructive pulmonary disease. Am Rev Respir Dis 1988; 138:350–4.

[16] Wright JL, Levy RD, Churg A. Pulmonary hypertension in chronic obstructive pulmonary disease: current theories of pathogenesis and their implications for treatment. Thorax 2005;60: 605–9.

[17] Peinado VI, Barbera JA, Abate P, et al. Inflammatory reaction in pulmonary muscular arteries of patients with mild chronic obstructive pulmonary disease. Am J Respir Crit Care Med 1999;159: 1605–11.

[18] Joppa P, Petrasova D, Stancak B, et al. Systemic in-flammation in patients with COPD and pulmonary hypertension. Chest 2006;130(2):326–33.

[19] Vonk-Noordegraaf A, Marcus JT, Holverda S, et al. Early changes of cardiac structure and function in COPD patients with mild hypoxemia. Chest 2005; 127(6):1898–903.

[20] Naeije R. Pulmonary hypertension and right heart failure in chronic obstructive pulmonary disease. Proc Am Thorac Soc 2005;2(1):20–2.

[21] Sin DD, Man SF. Chronic obstructive pulmonary disease as a risk factor for cardiovascular morbidity and mortality. Proc Am Thorac Soc 2005;2(1):8–11.

[22] Hole DJ, Watt G, Davey-Smith G, et al. Impaired lung function and mortality risk in men and women: findings from the Renfrew and Paisley prospective population study. BMJ 1996;313:711–5.

[23] Schunemann HJ, Dorn J, Grant BJ, et al. Pulmonary function is a long-term predictor of mortality in the general population: 29-year follow-up of the Buffalo Health Study. Chest 2000;118(3): 656–64.

[24] Hospers JJ, Postma DS, Rijcken B, et al. Histamine airway hyper-responsiveness and mortality from chronic obstructive pulmonary disease: a cohort study. Lancet 2000;356:1313–7.

[25] Knuiman MW, James AL, Divitini ML, et al. Lung function, respiratory symptoms, and mortality: results from the Busselton Health Study. Ann Epidemiol 1999;9(5):297–306.

[26] Anthonisen NR, Connett JE, Enright PL, et al. Lung Health Study Research Group. Hospitalizations and mortality in the Lung Health Study. Am J Respir Crit Care Med 2002;166(3):333–9.

[27] Tapson VF. The role of smoking in coagulation and thromboembolism in chronic obstructive pulmonary disease. Proc Am Thorac Soc 2005;2(1):71–7.

[28] Bursi F, Bursi F, Weston SA, et al. Systolic and diastolic heart failure in the community. JAMA 2006;296(18):2209–16.

[29] Bhatia RS, Tu JV, Lee DS, et al. Outcome of heart failure with preserved ejection fraction in a population-based study. N Engl J Med 2006;355:260–9.

[30] Pinsky MR. Cardiovascular issues in respiratory care. Chest 2005;128:592s–7s.

[31] Norwood R, Balkissoon R. Current perspectives on management of co-morbid depression in COPD. COPD 2005;2(1):185–93.

[32] Gudmundsson G, Gislason T, Janson C, et al. Risk factors for rehospitalisation in COPD: role of health status, anxiety and depression. Eur Respir J 2005; 26(3):414–9.

[33] Raffaele AI, Andrea C, Claudio P, et al. Drawing impairment predicts mortality in severe COPD. Chest 2006;130(6):1687–94.

[34] Liesker JJ, Postma DS, Beukema RJ, et al. Cognitive performance in patients with COPD. Respir Med 2004;98(4):351–6.

[35] Incalzil RA, Bellia V, Maggi S, et al. Mild to moderate chronic airways disease does not carry an excess risk of cognitive dysfunction. Aging Clin Exp Res 2002;14(5):395–401.

[36] Hjalmarsen A, Waterloo K, Dahl A, et al. Effect of long-term oxygen therapy on cognitive and neurological dysfunction in chronic obstructive pulmonary disease. Eur Neurol 1999;42(1):27–35.

[37] Norwood R. Prevalence and impact of depression in chronic obstructive pulmonary disease patients. Curr Opin Pulm Med 2006;12:113–7.

[38] Eiser N, Harte R, Karvounis S, et al. Effect of treating depression on quality-of life and exercise tolerance in severe COPD. COPD 2005;2:233–41.

[39] Eiser NM, Evans S, Jeffers A, et al. Effects of psychotherapy on dyspnoea in moderately severe COPD: a pilot study. Eur Respir J 1997;10:1581–4.

[40] Mohsenin V. Sleep in chronic obstructive pulmonary disease. Semin Respir Crit Care Med 2005;26(1): 109–16.

[41] Bhullar S, Phillips B. Sleep in COPD patients. COPD 2005;2(3):355–61.

[42] Kutty K. Sleep and chronic obstructive pulmonary disease. Curr Opin Pulm Med 2004;10:104–12.

[43] George CF, Bayliff CD. Management of insomnia in patients with chronic obstructive pulmonary disease. Drugs 2003;63(4):379–87.

[44] Ferguson DM. Comorbidity between depressive disorders and nicotine dependence in a cohort of 16 year olds. Arch Gen Psychiatry 1996;53:1043–7.

[45] Gluck O, Colice G. Recognizing and treating glucocorticoid-induced osteoporosis in patients with pulmonary diseases. Chest 2004;125(5):1859–76.

[46] Jorgensen NR, Schwarz P, Holme I, et al. The prevalence of osteoporosis in patients with chronic obstructive pulmonary disease-A cross sectional study. Respir Med 2007;101(1):177–85.

[47] Bolton CE, Ionescu AA, Shiels KM, et al. Associated loss of fat-free mass and bone mineral density in chronic obstructive pulmonary disease. Am J Respir Crit Care Med 2004;170(12):1286–93.

[48] McEvoy CE, Ensrud KE, Bender E, et al. Association between corticosteroid use and vertebral fractures in older men with chronic obstructive pulmonary disease. Am J Respir Crit Care Med 157 (3 Pt 1):704–9.

ELSEVIER
SAUNDERS

Clin Chest Med 28 (2007) 559–573

CLINICS
IN CHEST
MEDICINE

Environmental Tobacco Smoke: Respiratory and Other Health Effects

Jane Z. Reardon, MSN, RN

Departments of Medicine and Nursing, Hartford Hospital, 80 Seymour Street, Hartford, CT 06102, USA

In general, people are better informed about the risks of active smoking than the dangers of environmental tobacco smoke (ETS). As more information is gathered, however, it has become clear that the dangers of ETS are undeniable. There is no safe level of exposure to ETS. In the 2006 Surgeon General's report on secondhand smoke, Dr. Richard H. Carmona declared, "the debate is over." The data reported since the landmark 1986 Surgeon General's report on the health hazards of secondhand smoke documents beyond any doubt that second hand smoke harms people's health. Millions of Americans still are exposed to ETS in their homes and workplaces despite the considerable progress in tobacco control. Written by 22 scientists, the 2006 Surgeon General's report was reviewed by at least 40 peer reviewers and 30 independent investigators [1]. The damaging effects of ETS reach far beyond the lungs. As discussed in this article, multiple body systems are harmed. The recognized adverse health effects of ETS exposure include chronic obstructive pulmonary disease (COPD); asthma; upper and lower respiratory tract infections; cardiovascular disease; lung, breast, and cervical cancer; and childhood illnesses, such as middle ear disease and sudden infant death syndrome (SIDS). It is reported that ETS exposure is the third leading cause of preventable death in the United States, resulting in more than 50,000 deaths per year [2]. The United States Environmental Protection Agency classifies ETS as a group A carcinogen, given the large number of known or suspected carcinogens in tobacco smoke [3].

Although there is a large body of evidence on the health effects of chronic exposure to ETS, there also is growing evidence regarding its short-term or immediate effects. For example, it has been shown that even very brief exposures to ETS can trigger intense bronchopulmonary responses that could be life threatening for infants, children, or adults who have asthma or highly sensitive respiratory systems. Some scientists, however, warn that the data on acute risks should be disseminated with caution so that media coverage does not distort the evidence and convince the public prematurely that brief, transient exposure is enough to cause chronic health problems [4].

ETS has been targeted as a public health priority for disease prevention. Although legislation has become increasingly effective in reducing ETS in public places, a significant amount of ETS exposure still occurs in the home, affecting particularly vulnerable groups, such as children and the elderly. Although it is impossible to legislate a ban on smoking in the home, educational efforts must be strengthened, and barriers to adopting ETS risk-reducing behaviors must be explored. ETS now is considered an unacceptable and entirely preventable public health hazard.

Definitions

The term, ETS, has been defined as the sum of sidestream smoke (SS) released from the burning tip of a cigarette and mainstream smoke (MS), which is exhaled by smokers. Each type of smoke is comprised of a particulate and a vapor phase. The physical and chemical characteristics of ETS are dynamic and differ significantly between MS and fresh SS. MS contributes 15% of total ETS whereas SS, a product of incomplete combustion,

E-mail address: jreardo@harthosp.org

doi:10.1016/j.ccm.2007.06.006

constitutes 85% [5]. Particles present in SS have one tenth the particle diameter of MS and, as such, have the potential to reach the most distal alveoli from where they cannot be expelled easily [6].

ETS also is referred to commonly as passive cigarette smoking, involuntary smoking, and secondhand smoking. ETS can be a major component of air pollution in indoor environments.

Composition of environmental tobacco smoke

More than 4000 compounds have been identified in tobacco smoke and of these, at least 60 are known or suspected carcinogens [7,8]. These chemicals comprise approximately 95% of MS weight. This complex mixture of chemical substances also has unique proinflammatory and cytotoxic effects [9]. Inorganic compounds, such as nickel, chromium, cadmium, arsenic, and hydrazine, are related to lung cancer whereas ammonia, nitrogen dioxide, sulfur dioxide, hydrogen cyanide, and acrolein are among the many irritant gases that can contribute to development of airways disease, such as COPD and asthma. In addition, other cancers can be caused by compounds, such as benzene, urethane, vinyl chloride, and aniline [6]. The tobacco-related carcinogens also are associated with a decreased capacity for DNA repair, which is associated with an increased risk for non–small cell lung cancer [10]. Yields per cigarette of some carcinogens have been reported to be greater in SS than with MS. For example, the release of volatile N-nitrosamines and aromatic amines is higher in SS than in MS. A major reason that undiluted SS and MS have different concentrations of toxic and carcinogenic agents is that peak temperatures in the burning cone of a cigarette reach 800°C to 900°C during puffing but only 600°C between puffs, resulting in less complete combustion of tobacco during generation of SS [11]. Table 1 lists many of the toxic and carcinogenic agents identified in SS and MS. Individual chemicals remain relatively constant in different commercial brands, including filter and nonfilter brands of cigarettes [12].

Assessing exposure to environmental tobacco smoke

Overall, the extent of adverse health effects resulting from ETS exposure is related to two major factors: the duration and intensity of exposure and individual susceptibility, believed to be genetically controlled [13].

The determination of an individual's exposure to ETS is a complex task, given the multiple variables involved. The number of cigarettes smoked by people in an environment, the length of time over which smoking occurs, the ventilation properties of a building, and the absorptive qualities of a structure, furniture, carpets, and curtains all contribute to the final exposure assessment [14]. Two approaches can be used to estimate ETS exposure. In the first, data on the smoking habits of the people in an environment in which individuals spend time are collected by questionnaire. This may be data from home, workplace, or other environments in which individuals spend time. Questionnaires can be informative in determining exposure to ETS; however, the lack of standardized, validated tools and the misclassification of exposure (inaccurate recall or inability to estimate accurately) must be considered. The second approach involves quantification of ETS components or their metabolites, either in the environmental air or in individual serum, saliva, urine, or hair. Various biomarkers of ETS (nicotine and its metabolite cotinine) have been developed that can be used to validate questionnaire responses and are useful in assessing recent exposure. Although nicotine has a short half-life (less than 2 hours) cotinine has a 3 to 4 day half-life and can be measured in urine, saliva, blood, and hair [15].

Exposure prevalence

Several studies have estimated the prevalence of ETS exposure [13,16]. Reported prevalence rates of exposure vary between 30% and 80% [17] for adults, with many studies showing the workplace as a major source of exposure. Increased regulation on smoking in the workplace and in most public places in recent years has made the home the leading unregulated source of ETS. This has significant potential impact on preschool-aged children who spend proportionately more time in the home [16]. One source estimates that approximately 43% of children in the United States live with a smoker, whereas in the United Kingdom, 40% to 60% of children are exposed to ETS in the home [18]. Studies of the potential effects of ETS on fetal and child health have multiplied over the past 20 years and an increased risk for multiple disease states has been demonstrated clearly (detailed later). Other areas needing further regulation include several

Table 1
Toxic and carcinogenic agents in undiluted cigarette sidestream smoke

Compound	Type of toxicity	Amount in sidestream smoke (per cigarette)	Ratio of sidestream smoke/mainstream smoke
Vapor phase			
Carbon monoxide	T	26.8–61 mg	2.5–14.9
Carbonyl sulfide	T	2–3 mg	0.03–0.13
Benzene	C	400–500 µg	8–10
Formaldehyde	C	1,500 µg	50
3-Vinylpyridine	SC	300–450 µg	24–34
Hydrogen cyanide	T	14–110 g	0.06–0.4
Hydrazine	C	90 ng	3
Nitrogen oxides	T	500–2000 µg	3.7–12.8
N-nitrosodimethylamine	C	200–1040 ng	20–130
N-nitrosopyrrolidine	C	30–390 ng	6–120
Particulate phase			
Tar	C	14–30 mg	1.1–15.7
Nicotine	T	2.1–46 mg	1.3–21
Phenol	TP	70–250 µg	1.3–3.0
Catechol	CoC	58–290 µg	0.67–12.8
o-Toluidine	C	3 µg	18.7
2-Naphthylamine	C	70 ng	39
4-Aminobiphenyl	C	140 ng	3.1
Benz(a)anthracene	C	40–200 ng	2–4
Benzo(a)pyrene	C	40–70 ng	2.5–20
Quinoline	C	15–20 µg	8–11
N-nitrosonomicotine	C	0.15–1.7 µg	0.5–5.0
NNK	C	0.2–1.4 µg	1.0–22
N-nitrosodiethanolamine	C	43 ng	1.2
Cadmium	C	0.72 µg	7.2
Nickel	C	0.2–2.5 µg	13–30
Polonium-210	C	0.5–1.6 pCi	1.06–3.7

Abbreviations: C, carcinogenic; CoC, cocarcinogenic; SC, suspected carcinogen; T, toxic; TP, tumor promoter.

Data from National Institute of Occupational Safety and Health. Reducing the health consequences of smoking: 25 years of progress. A report of the Surgeon General. Rockville (MD): US Department of Health and Human Services, DHHS publication no. (CDC) 89-8411; and Hoffman D, Hecht SS. Advances in tobacco carcinogens. In: Grover P, editor. Handbook of experimental pharmacology 1988. New York: Springer Verlag. Available at: http://www.cdc.gov/niosh/91108_54.html. Accessed April 9, 2007.

service-type workplace establishments, namely the five Bs: *b*ars, *b*owling alleys, *b*illiard halls, *b*etting establishments (casinos), and *b*ingo parlors [19]. Three overlapping waves of clean indoor air policy have addressed public buildings and workspace, but office settings and restaurants were the primary focal points until recently. Because of this pattern of policy adoption, workers in the five Bs have not had the same level of protection from ETS as the general public. A major reason why the five Bs have remained largely exempt is the relationship that exists between these establishments and the tobacco industry and the support the tobacco industry has provided them to help oppose smoking regulations [20,21]. In the United States, there are more than 800,000 workers in bars, bowling alleys, and casinos alone [22]. Workers in these areas have the highest occupational levels of exposure to secondhand smoke, with unacceptable levels of excess mortality risk [19].

Health problems and environmental tobacco smoke exposure

The increased risk for a wide range of adverse health effects associated with ETS is well established from experimental animal data and human studies in children and adults. The multitude of health risks linked to ETS is shown in Box 1. The following sections review the literature on these health effects in more detail.

Box 1. Environmental tobacco smoke–related health risks

Respiratory illnesses
- COPD
- Asthma in children and adults
- Exacerbation of cystic fibrosis
- Allergies
- Bronchitis
- Pneumonia
- Bronchiolitis
- Croup

Adverse effects on fertility
Miscarriage
Low birth weight
SIDS
Middle ear infections
Periodontal disease
Ulcerative colitis
Neurocognitive decrements
Cardiovascular disease
- Ischemic heart disease
- Acute stroke

Malignancies
- Lung
- Head and neck
- Breast
- Bladder
- Cervix

Children's health, fertility, and environmental tobacco smoke

Almost 60% of United States children aged 3 to 11 years—or almost 22 million children—are exposed to ETS [1]. The reproductive health effects of cigarette smoke exposure for women are far reaching [23]. Children's exposure to ETS during fetal development and during childhood likely is the most pervasive and hazardous of children's environmental exposures [24]. The first report detailing the adverse effects of ETS on children's health was published in 1967 [25]. Several comprehensive reviews have been published on fetal and child health, systematically reviewing the evidence for different diseases [26–29]. The endpoints of such studies include fetal, perinatal, and postnatal effects.

Fetal and perinatal effects

Review of the literature on ETS and adverse reproductive outcomes shows that ETS consistently is associated with increased risks for low birth weight and slower intrauterine growth rate [18,30]. The reduction in birth weight attributed to ETS varies from 25 to 125 grams, with a smaller range in studies adjusting for gestational age [31].

Neal and colleagues recently conducted a retrospective study of 225 female patients, reviewing the effects of ETS on in vitro fertilization in women exposed to SS versus active smokers versus their nonexposed counterparts (NS) [32]. Despite similar embryo quality, there was a striking difference in implantation and pregnancy rates of active smokers and SS smokers compared with nonsmokers (NS) (AS = 12%, SS = 12.6%, and NS = 25%). Their data demonstrated clearly that the effects of SS on fertility are equally as damaging as active smoking. The mechanisms underlying the reduced fertility success in women exposed to cigarette smoke are unknown. Toxicants can impair reproduction by acting in men, women, or both [33]. Sofikitis and colleagues [34] reported that cotinine concentrations similar to those seen in heavy smokers (>400 ng/mL) reduced hamster sperm performance with respect to in vitro tests but did not affect fertilization of hamster ova when intracytoplasmic sperm injection (ICSI) was used. One explanation regarding the higher rate of early pregnancy loss in women exposed to smoke is that the inhibition of granulose-luteal cell function (due to toxins from cigarette smoke) may lead to corpus luteal deficiency [35]. It seems that the reproductive consequences of ETS may be as great as those observed in active smokers. Fortunately for women who seek medical attention, a recent randomized controlled trial found that a simple explanation of the reproductive consequences of smoking and ETS was as effective as a structured intervention in achieving compliance with smoking cessation [36].

Postnatal effects and timeframes of critical exposure

Studies of the relationship between ETS and postnatal health are difficult to conduct because of the need to distinguish between prenatal and postnatal ETS exposure and the extent of exposure and the truthfulness of parent reporting. Fetal development represents a critical time of pulmonary vulnerability. Investigations of lung function in infants of mothers who smoked during pregnancy show that in utero exposure to maternal smoking is associated with reduced lung function in the perinatal period [37]. Also, women who smoke during pregnancy are likely to continue smoking after delivery [7]. This fact makes it difficult to isolate the effect of in utero exposure to maternal smoking from that of postnatal ETS exposure [7]. Gilliland and colleagues [38] studied lifetime tobacco smoke exposure histories and parental reports of wheezing and physician-diagnosed asthma in nearly 6000 school-aged children from 12 different communities in Southern California. Their findings concluded that children exposed to in utero tobacco smoke were 1.8 times more likely to develop asthma and a lifetime history of wheezing than those who did not have in utero ETS exposure. Nestled within that Children's Health Study, these investigators conducted a smaller case-controlled study, which examined the association of maternal and grand-maternal smoking before, during, and after pregnancy with childhood asthma [39]. Detailed information on maternal and household smoking histories and other asthma risk factors were obtained by telephone interview. In utero exposure to maternal smoking was associated with increased risk for asthma diagnosed in the first 5 years of life (odds ratio [OR] 1.5; 95% CI, 1.0–2.3) and for persistent asthma (OR 1.5; 95% CI, 1.0–2.3). Children of mothers who quit smoking before pregnancy showed no increased risk (OR 0.9; 95% CI, 0.5–1.5). Grandmaternal smoking during the mother's fetal period also was associated with increased asthma risk in the grand-children (OR 2.1; 95% CI, 1.4–3.2). In another 10-year longitudinal study of school children's respiratory health, investigators suggest that perinatal deficits in lung function are persistent and actually may increase during adolescence [40]. A more recent large Norwegian cohort study by Skorge and colleagues [41] gave further strength to this hypothesis. They examined the incidence of respiratory symptoms and asthma among adults associated with passive smoking in utero or in childhood, after adjustment for several important confounders. The adjusted attributable fractions of the adult incidence of asthma were 17.3% (95% CI, 5.2–27.9) caused by maternal smoking and 9.3% (95% CI, −23.2–33.2) caused by smoking by household members. Several other investigators reported similar results [42–44]. Other studies have examined further the increased risk for asthma in relation to a cumulative ETS exposure over a lifetime [45,46].

The association between active maternal smoking and SIDS also is well established. It is the major suspected risk factor for SIDS now that public health campaigns successfully have advised parents to place sleeping infants on their back. Epidemiologic evidence also points to a causal relationship between SIDS and postnatal exposure to ETS [28]. The distinction between prenatal versus postnatal exposure and the risk for SIDS warrants additional investigation.

Childhood respiratory illnesses

According to the World Health Organization, approximately 1 billion adults smoke worldwide and at least 700 million children (nearly 50% of the world's children) breathe the air polluted by tobacco smoke at home [47]. In addition to the effects of ETS on asthma, it is estimated that each year 150,000 to 300,000 respiratory tract infections are caused in part by ETS, resulting in 7500 to 15,000 hospitalizations in infants and children less than 18 months of age [48]. Exposure of children to ETS increases the incidence of middle ear disease, asthma, wheeze, cough, mucus production, bronchitis, bronchiolitis, pneumonia, and impaired pulmonary function [24]. It also is associated with snoring [49], adenoid hypertrophy [50], tonsillitis, and sore throats [51]. Frequent respiratory infections in childhood are associated significantly with increased risk for developing COPD later in life [52,53].

Childhood asthma

Pediatric asthma, in particular, constitutes a significant public health problem. Asthma mortality rates nearly doubled from 1980 to 1993 among children aged 5 to 15 years old, and African American children were 6 times more likely than white children to die from asthma [54]. The link between ETS and asthma is well established. Minority children from the inner city have disproportionately higher rates of morbidity and mortality caused by asthma, and this disparity is linked closely to socioeconomic status, poverty, and environmental exposures, especially ETS [55,56]. ETS exposure during childhood aggravates asthma, often leading to emergency room visits and hospitalizations [55]. The influence of smoking in the household on asthma is especially formidable until the age of 6. Thereafter, the association becomes less strong, at least partially because of reduced ETS exposure as children grow up and spend more time away from home [47,57]. Even light cigarette smoking (ie, 10 cigarettes/day) by adults corresponded to the level of environmental irritants at which children who had asthma experienced nocturnal symptoms [48]. If exposed to higher levels of ETS, these children were 3 times as likely to be in the mild persistent disease category and twice as likely to be in the moderate to severe disease category compared with those who had lower levels of ETS exposure [48]. Asthmatic children exposed to multiple household smokers face a 4.5-fold increased risk for respiratory illness–related absences from school, having an adverse impact on the children's education and family functioning [58]. Childhood asthma, if poorly controlled, poses a potential risk for developing fixed airflow obstruction (COPD) as an adult [52].

Finally, atopy is a significant risk factor for childhood asthma, with more than 80% of the children who develop asthma having an antigen-specific IgE. A large body of evidence supports the theory that ETS increases development of atopy in susceptible individuals [59]. Several mechanisms are believed to enhance atopy in those exposed to ETS, including increased airway mucosal permeability or direct effects on immune function [59].

Multiple genetic and environmental factors also contribute to asthma. A multicenter collaborative study supported by the National Heart, Lung, and Blood Institute (NHLBI) [60] found genetic loci that contribute to the development of asthma and asthma-related phenotypes. In this study, regions were found that showed a nominally significant increased lod score when accounting for exposure to ETS. A lod score is a statistical estimate of whether or not two genetic loci are likely to lie near each other on a chromosome and, therefore, likely to be inherited together. A lod score of 3 or more generally is taken to indicate that the two loci are close [61]. The NHLBI study's results indicated that a gene-environment interaction might exist between ETS and unobserved susceptibility genes in several regions. Although more research is needed in this area, the studies indicate that the genetic predisposition for the development of an IgE-mediated response to common allergens (such as ETS) is the strongest identifiable predisposing factor in developing asthma.

Behavior and cognitive functioning

The literature on the impact of prenatal and postnatal exposure to tobacco smoke on human behavior and neurologic development (some dating back more than 2 decades) strongly suggests that such exposures lead to negative behavioral and neurocognitive effects in children. Olds [62] reported that 10 of 11 human studies reviewed found increased rates of child behavior problems

and attention-deficit hyperactivity disorder– type behaviors in children exposed to ETS even after controlling for many potential confounders. Exposure to maternal smoking also is shown to affect children's performance adversely on intelligence and achievement tests and performance in school [24], although findings in this area are not as consistent as those for increased rates of behavior problems. Butler and Goldstein [63] demonstrated that children whose mothers smoked 10 or more cigarettes per day were between 3 and 5 months delayed in reading, mathematics, and general ability. Several studies found similar effects [64,65], whereas others found effects significantly minimized after controlling for confounders [66,67]. When mothers smoked during some pregnancies but not during others, children who were exposed performed worse on intelligence tests than their unexposed siblings [61]. More recent evidence confirming the negative effects of ETS on behavior and cognitive functioning also is available [68–70].

Environmental tobacco smoke and adult health

Evaluating ETS exposure in adults is more complex than in children. Adults are exposed to ETS in multiple venues other than the home, including the workplace and many other public arenas. Because active smoking is a well-established cause of chronic respiratory disease and lung function decline, more information regarding the relationship of ETS with these health effects has been sought over the past several decades. As discussed in the section that follows, a causal relationship between acute and chronic respiratory symptoms of the nose, eyes, throat, and lower airways and exposure to ETS is established clearly.

Allergies, asthma, and environmental tobacco smoke

There is wide agreement that the prevalence of allergic airway disease has risen dramatically over the past few decades [71]. The causes of this increase are the source of much controversy and discussion. Epidemiologic studies have been helpful in establishing associations between allergy or asthma and diet, childhood infections, allergen levels, and indoor and outdoor pollutants [72,73]. Until now, mostly observational studies postulated that the ETS influence on development of asthma was primarily mechanical (ie, a direct irritant causing a gross inflammatory process that led to airway damage). A recent study by Diaz-Sanchez and colleagues [74], however, demonstrated that ETS can interact with allergen to modulate immune responses in the upper airway. Subjects who have allergy who were exposed to ragweed allergen and short-term ETS showed an enhanced allergic response (as opposed to those not exposed to ETS) characterized by IgE antibody production against the inhaled protein allergen. The ETS/allergen subjects also showed a local formation of a T_H2-type cytokine milieu, characteristic of active allergic inflammation. Moreover, nasal histamine levels were 3.3-fold greater after a combination ETS/ragweed challenge than after clean air/ragweed challenge. Thus, in this study [74], it is shown that in addition to direct irritant effects, ETS can work through another mechanism of adjuvancy: the interaction with allergen, to alter the immune system and enhance allergic responses.

ETS is associated with the induction and the exacerbation of adult asthma. In a study comparing 231 never-smoking cases of newly diagnosed asthma with 487 never-smoking referents, the risk related to ETS exposure in the previous year was significant for exposure in the workplace (OR 2.15, 95% CI, 1.26–3.72) and for the home (OR 4.77, 95% CI, 1.29–17.7) [45].

Chronic obstructive pulmonary disease in nonsmokers and environmental tobacco smoke

Although the majority of COPD is seen in active or former smokers, the disease also occurs among persons who have never smoked. Proposed risk factors for COPD include ETS, genetic predisposition, air pollution, *Helicobacter pylori* infection, and autoimmune thyroid disease [75]. Acute smoke exposure activates cells, such as neutrophils and macrophages in the airways, has a suppressive effect on the numbers of eosinophils and may result in tissue damage [76]. Repeated smoke exposure may promote a chronic inflammatory process resulting in thicker, inflamed, deformed, and narrow airways with emphysematous changes around them [77].

Eisner and colleagues [78] evaluated the longitudinal impact of ETS exposure on validated measures of COPD severity, physical health status, quality of life (QOL), and dyspnea measures at 1-year follow-up in 77 nonsmokers. Monitoring was based on urine cotinine and a personal badge that measured nicotine. In longitudinal analysis, the highest level of baseline cotinine was associated with worse COPD severity (mean score

increment 4.7 points; CI, 0.1–9.4), disease-specific QOL (2.9 points; CI, −0.16–5.9; $P = .063$), and dyspnea (0.9 points; 95% CI, 0.2–1.6 points; $P < .05$). According to an epidemiologic study in nonsmokers [79], the prevalence of COPD is greater among women than men until age 60, at which time prevalence no longer differs by gender. In that study, neither urban residence nor occupation was associated with COPD in nonsmokers. In a more recent study [80] (the Third National Health and Nutrition Examination Survey [NHANES]: 1988–1994), Behrendt reported that among nearly 14,000 people examined, 48.7 ± 0.9% were nonsmokers (never smokers and former smokers with < 5 pack-year smoking history), 8.8 ± 0.3% had mild COPD, and 4.1 ± 0.3% had moderate to severe COPD. Spirometry was done in addition to medical history and assessment of medication use and risk behaviors. One fourth of those who had COPD were nonsmokers. Among nonsmokers, physician-diagnosed asthma increased the risk for mild and especially of moderate to severe COPD. The risk for moderate to severe disease in nonsmokers was associated markedly with male gender, peaked at middle age, and was related inversely to nonwhite ethnicity. COPD risks did not vary by minimal smoking history, longest-held occupation, urban residence, income, allergies, thyroid disease, or *H pylori* antibody. In this study, people who had mild COPD tended to avoid exposure to smoking in the home and at work, whereas those who had moderate to severe COPD did not. Nonsmokers who did and did not have COPD are described in Table 2. Behrendt concludes that among nonsmokers, mild and moderate to -severe COPD is associated with asthma but otherwise they have distinct demographic profiles. The investigator suggests that moderate to severe disease is not simply a progression of mild COPD.

Most of the longitudinal studies of COPD span only 5 to 10 years. Therefore, knowledge of the rate of development and progression of COPD stems from extrapolated results from individuals followed for relatively short periods. Little information is reported on the influence of ETS and other exposures. As a part of the Copenhagen City Heart Study, more than 8000 men and women from the general population aged 30 to 60 years who had normal lung function at baseline were followed for 25 years. Lokke and colleagues [81] reported on the absolute risk for developing COPD in this population and related this risk to changes in tobacco consumption. They concluded

Table 2

Characteristics, respiratory symptoms, and physician diagnoses among nonsmokers aged 18 to 80 years, by level of chronic obstructive pulmonary disease

Characteristics	No chronic obstructive pulmonary disease	Mild chronic obstructive pulmonary disease	Moderate to severe chronic obstructive pulmonary disease
Subjects, no.	7031	403	92
Population represented, millions	70.923	3.587	1.437
Mean age, year	39.1 ± 0.4	60.9 ± 1.3[a]	39.3 ± 1.3
Female gender	63.2 ± 0.9	82.5 ± 2.3[a]	11.9 ± 4.2[a]
Ever smoked	12.1 ± 0.6	15.3 ± 2.8	9.1 ± 4.4
Now exposed to smoking at home	15.2 ± 1.0	6.2 ± 1.4[a]	16.9 ± 5.5
Now exposed to smoking at work	9.7 ± 0.7	1.3 ± 0.7[a]	23.1 ± 8.3
Thyroid disease	10.1 ± 0.7	22.6 ± 3.3[b]	12.8 ± 8.3
H pylori antibody positive	27.1 ± 1.9	41.9 ± 4.6[b]	35.9 ± 15.8
Education < 12 years	16.7 ± 1.0	30.3 ± 2.4[a]	10.6 ± 3.2
White race	79.5 ± 1.2	87.1 ± 1.6[a]	88.8 ± 2.1[b]
Respiratory symptoms in past year			
Chronic cough	3.9 ± 0.3	12.3 ± 2.7[b]	8.3 ± 3.5
Chronic phlegm	4.1 ± 0.4	7.0 ± 1.2[b]	7.3 ± 2.6
Wheezing	10.0 ± 0.6	21.6 ± 3.1[b]	43.0 ± 10.2[b]
Dyspnea on exertion	15.0 ± 0.9	26.9 ± 2.8[a]	23.4 ± 6.2
Any of the above symptoms	25.5 ± 1.0	41.1 ± 2.8[a]	52.0 ± 9.7[c]
Physician diagnosis, ever			
Asthma	5.7 ± 0.4	16.6 ± 2.6[a]	45.1 ± 8.3[a]
Chronic bronchitis	3.2 ± 0.3	12.7 ± 2.6[b]	6.8 ± 3.3
Emphysema	0.2 ± 0.1	2.7 ± 1.2	1.6 ± 1.1
Any of the above diagnoses	8.1 ± 0.5	24.3 ± 3.2[a]	45.8 ± 8.3[a]

Data are presented as percentages (± SE) unless otherwise indicated.

[a] $P < .001$ versus nonsmokers who did not have COPD.

[b] $P < .01$ versus nonsmokers who did not have COPD.

[c] $P < .05$ versus nonsmokers who did not have COPD.

From Behrendt CE. Mild and moderate-to-severe COPD in nonsmokers. Chest 2005;128:1239–44; with permission.

that among continuous smokers, the risk was at least 25%, much higher than studies spanning a shorter period of time [82]. The report did not include information of the exposure to ETS among the never smokers who developed COPD (9%), although it would be expected to have been a significant risk factor. Investigators from one recent study [83] examined the association between lifetime ETS exposure and the risk for developing COPD. Using structured telephone interview, more than 2000 adults aged 55 to 75 years were recruited from 48 contiguous United States states. Higher cumulative lifetime home and work exposure to ETS was associated with a greater risk for COPD. The highest quartile of lifetime home ETS exposure was associated with a greater risk for COPD, controlling for age, sex, race, personal smoking history, education,

marital status, and occupational exposures (OR 1.55; 95% CI, 1.09–2.21). The population attributable fraction was 11% for the highest quartile of home ETS exposure and 7% for work exposure. Of considerable significance, Skogstad and colleagues [84] reported a larger cross shift decrease in lung function of employees in bars and restaurants in Norway before compared with after the implementation of a smoking ban in these establishments. ETS exposure may be an important cause of COPD.

Cardiovascular effects of environmental tobacco smoke

ETS has been estimated to cause up to 70,000 deaths per year from heart disease in nonsmokers (never smokers and former smokers < 5 pack years) [85]. Nonsmokers who are exposed to ETS at home or at work increase their risk for developing heart disease by 25% to 30% [1]. A substantial number of meta-analyses and studies [86–91] have been conducted to investigate the relationship between ETS exposure and fatal and nonfatal coronary heart disease (CHD). Most of the studies adjusted for demographic variables and other factors, such as obesity, lipid levels, blood pressure, and diet. In general, most individual studies have shown that among nonsmokers, increased risk for CHD is associated with living with a smoker. This holds true despite the differences in study design, date performed, years of follow-up, method of ascertaining the adverse health endpoint, and degree of adjustment for other risk factors. One of the suggested causal mechanisms for CHD is evidence of reduced exercise tolerance in healthy individuals exposed to ETS. Exposure to ETS in the short-term causes an increase in resting heart rate, blood pressure, and blood levels of carbon monoxide (CO) and carboxyhemoglobin, the compound formed when inhaled CO combines with hemoglobin in the blood. It also increases myocardial oxygen demand and causes an increase in platelet aggregation and endothelial cell damage [2,92]. Other evidence suggests that ETS can contribute to atherosclerotic plaque formation and atherosclerosis [2]. Results from meta-analyses vary slightly, but pooled results are of the same order of magnitude. Law and colleagues [88], for example, found a summary relative risk [RR] of 1.30 (95% CI, 1.22–1.38) for CHD among never smokers whose spouses were active smokers relative to those whose spouses never smoked. To give further strength to the association between CHD and ETS, several studies looked at the dose-response relationship between level of ETS exposure and CHD death [93,94]. There is a pattern of increasing the RR of fatal CHD with increasing levels of ETS. The combined risk associated with being exposed to more than 20 cigarettes per day is 1.18 (1.04–1.33) [93].

Lung cancer

More than 50 investigations, mostly case-controlled studies, have shown that involuntary smoking (ETS) is associated with an increased risk for lung cancer [95,96]. Lung cancer is the leading cause of death in the United States and in the world [1]. In women, there has been a 600% increase in death rates from lung cancer since 1950, surpassing breast cancer as the leading cause

of cancer death in women in 1997 [97]. More than 125,000 Americans die from smoking-attributable lung cancers each year. Of these, approximately 3000 are believed caused by passive smoking [98,99]. Three population-based studies [100–102] and several meta-analyses [95,103,104] have provided further evidence for a direct association between ETS and lung cancer among people who have never smoked. Because the cumulative amount of tobacco smoke exposure may be underestimated significantly if only personal smoking history is obtained, de Andrade and colleagues [105] conducted a descriptive study of 810 women who had newly diagnosed primary lung cancer from 1997 to 2001. These women were interviewed to obtain data, including the source, intensity, and duration of ETS exposure. Relationships between smoking history, ETS exposure, and lung cancer histologic subtypes were analyzed. More than 95% of these women reported active smoking, ETS exposure, or both. Among those who never smoked but had a history of ETS exposure, the mean years of exposure were 27 from a smoking spouse, 19 from parents, and 15 from coworkers. For each major subtype of lung cancer (adenocarcinoma, squamous cell, unclassified non–small cell lung cancer, small cell, or carcinoids) among never smokers, 75% to 100% of patients had ETS exposure. Compared with women who had been active smokers, never smokers (divided into ETS and non-ETS exposed) had relatively more adenocarcinoma (68.1% versus 48.1%) and carcinoid tumor cells (15.9% versus 5.1%), fewer squamous (5.8% versus 20.1%) and small cell carcinomas (2.4% versus 13.1%), and no large cell carcinomas (0% versus 3.8%). This is interesting when considering the small particle size of the SS that is likely to reach alveoli. Never smokers who did not have ETS exposure and who developed lung cancer had a higher proportion of adenocarcinoma (76%) compared with never smokers who had ETS exposure (66%), former smokers (53%), and current smokers (41%), whereas the opposite trend was observed for squamous and small cell carcinoma. These results were consistent with a multicenter case-controlled study of ETS exposure in Europe, which observed a statistically significant trend of increased risk for squamous cell ($P = .03$) and a suggestive trend for small cell ($P = .08$) carcinoma with increasing duration of ETS exposure from the spouse and workplace compared with those not exposed to ETS from these sources [106]. In contrast, a meta-analysis of case-controlled studies, which included never-smoking Chinese women [107], reported no statistically significant relationship between the amount or duration of ETS exposure and lung cancer risk. The results of this study, however, must be extrapolated to the United States population with caution, as lung cancer risk factors differ markedly between Chinese and American women.

Accurate measurements of ETS are important for establishing accurate dose-response relationships between levels of tobacco smoke exposure and risk for lung cancer. Identifying the amount and source of ETS for never smokers provides critical evidence supporting the association between ETS and tobacco-related health consequences. In a large European prospective nested case-controlled study, the European Prospective Investigation into Cancer and Nutrition, Vineis and colleagues investigated the association between ETS, measuring plasma cotinine concentration and lung cancer in more than 1500 healthy volunteers who had never actively smoked or who had stopped smoking for at least 10 years [108]. They confirmed that ETS is a risk factor for lung cancer and other respiratory diseases, particularly in exsmokers. The greater risk among former smokers could indicate greater susceptibility due to already existing cell mutations. Over 7 years of follow-up, 97 people had newly diagnosed lung cancer, 20 had upper respiratory cancers, and 14 died from COPD. The advantage of this cohort design is the lack of recall bias (as information about exposure was collected before onset of disease).

Clinicians are just beginning to understand how genes have an impact on lung cancer susceptibility. ETS exposure can be linked to gene mutations, especially the p53 and GSTM1, both of which are linked to an increased risk for developing lung cancer [108]. Future studies, especially those involving genetic-environmental interactions, would benefit from defining patient phenotype more accurately by validating ETS exposure with personal nicotine monitors or biomarkers.

Cervical cancer and environmental tobacco smoke

Many studies have reported an increased risk for cervical cancer in smokers, which remains significant after adjustment for age, the number of sexual partners, and infection with the human papilloma virus [16]. The presence of cotinine in cervical mucus of nonsmoking women who are exposed to ETS makes it reasonable to postulate that passive smoking can contribute to carcinogenesis through the same potential pathways as active

smoking, including genotoxic and immunomodulatory effects [109,110]. In a large prospective cohort study with multivariate analysis [111], the investigators interviewed 623 women referred to a colposcopy clinic for evaluation of abnormal Papanicolaou's smears (showing either repeated inflammatory changes, low-grade squamous intraepithelial lesion, or high-grade squamous intraepithelial lesion [HSIL]). In this study, it was reported that the risk for HSIL increased by 4.6% for every cigarette smoked in a patient's presence. Eight studies relating to ETS exposure to risk for cervical cancer were reviewed by Lee [112]. Only one of these studies found a decreased risk, whereas the others all found a statistically significant increase. A meta-analysis based on the seven studies gave a RR for developing cervical cancer of 1.27 (95% CI, 1.03–1.56) after exposure to ETS.

Breast cancer and environmental tobacco smoke

Most studies have found either no association or only a weak association between active smoking and breast cancer risk. In a review of 13 studies investigating the role of ETS in breast cancer, no significant association was found in four prospective studies, but significantly raised risks were evident in four case-controlled studies, giving a pooled weak RR of 1.29 (95% CI, 1.3–1.46) [112]. No study showed a strong dose-response relation with ETS exposure. One possible reason that associations have not been found is that incomplete measures of ETS exposure have been obtained. Morabia [113] suggested that the model for carcinogenesis might be different for the lung, which is exposed to smoke directly, whereas the mammary gland is exposed only to its metabolites. Gammon and colleagues analyzed data from a large population-based case-controlled study that included a detailed assessment of passive smoking [114]. Subjects who had available ETS information assessed by questionnaire and in-person interviews included 1356 newly diagnosed cases of breast cancer and 1383 controls. Although no dose response was evident, an increased OR was noted among nonsmokers who lived with a smoking spouse for more than 27 years (2.10; 95% CI, 1.47–3.02). Also, among women who had hormone-receptor-positive tumors only, the OR for active and passive smoking was increased (1.42; 95% CI, 1.00–2.00). Despite the inconsistent results across epidemiologic studies in this area, research continues to be sustained and propelled by the known mammary carcinogenicity of some tobacco smoke constituents (such as polycyclic aromatic hydrocarbons) in laboratory animals [115]. Further work is needed to clarify whether or not exposure to ETS increases risk for breast cancer and to identify subgroups of patients who may be at greatest risk.

Reducing exposure to environmental tobacco smoke

As a result of the wide body of research presented in this article, ETS now is considered a serious public health hazard. The demonstration that ETS can augment allergic airway responses makes it a public health issue of extreme importance. Workers in the 5 Bs have the highest occupational levels of exposure to ETS and many children remain in situations at home or in cars with adults who smoke. Intervention studies on domestic ETS exposure have focused primarily on children and on achieving parental smoking cessation. Interventions have varied from minimal contact to intensive counseling but many show only short-lived effects. Home-based interventions with more contact were more effective than physician-based interventions [116].

Involuntary exposure to ETS is a common, serious public health hazard that is entirely preventable by adopting and enforcing appropriate regulatory policies. Healthy People 2010 objectives address this issue and seek optimal protection of nonsmokers through policies, regulations, and laws requiring smoke-free environments in all schools, work sites, and public places [98].

The dangers from ETS and the need for legislation to protect children also is receiving much public support. In Connecticut, House Bill 5204 would prohibit motorists from smoking when driving if there is a child in the car under 7 years old or weighing less than 60 pounds, which is the same standard applied for existing seatbelt violations. Other states (Arkansas and Louisiana) already have passed similar measures and nine other states are considering doing so.

It is time for a new wave of clean indoor air policy promotion in which public health advocates insist that all people be protected from the ill effects of ETS.

Summary

In general, people have been less well informed of the risks of ETS than the risks of active smoking. ETS exposure, however, has been determined to be the third leading cause of preventable death in this country, resulting in more than 50,000 deaths each year [93].

As discussed in this review, ETS can lead to a broad spectrum of adverse health consequences affecting the respiratory tract, the cardiovascular and central nervous systems, systemic metabolic and immunologic functions, and fetal development. The elimination of smoking in children's homes, in all forms of transportation used by children, and in multiple settings not yet included in indoor air legislation must be promoted aggressively. Future research should investigate effective means of lowering ETS exposure, preventing smoking initiation, and facilitating smoking cessation. Better data are needed on the effects of maternal smoking cessation and alterations in asthma, neurocognitive functioning, and behavior problems. Independent of active smoking, ETS exposure is a modifiable risk factor for COPD, and clinicians should assess ETS exposure in their patients and counsel its avoidance. Finally, Celli and colleagues [117] recommend that lung health screening programs should be considered not only for smokers but also for never smokers who have possible ETS to better identify and enable early treatment intervention for persons who have ETS-associated respiratory disease.

References

[1] U.S. Department of Health and Human Services. The health consequences of involuntary exposure to tobacco smoke: a report of the surgeon general. U.S. Department of Health and Human Services, Centers for Disease Control and Prevention, National Center for Chronic Disease Prevention and Health Promotion, Office on Smoking and Health, 2006; Available at: http://www.surgeongeneral.gov/library/secondhandsmoke/factsheets. Accessed February 3, 2007.

[2] Glantz SA, Parmley WW. Passive smoking and heart disease: epidemiology, physiology and biochemistry. Circulation 1991;83:1.

[3] Environmental Health Information Service. 9th. Report on Carcinogens. U.S. Department of Health and Human Services, Public Health Service, National Toxicology Program. 2000.

[4] Kuehn BM. Report reviews secondhand smoke risks—some scientists question risk level. JAMA 2006;296(8):922–3.

[5] Manuel J. Double exposure. Environ Health Perspect 1999;107(4):A197–201.

[6] Chan-Yeung M, Dimich-Ward H. Respiratory health effects of exposure to environmental tobacco smoke. Respirology 2003;8:131–9.

[7] Dhala A, Pinsker K, Prezant DJ. Respiratory health consequences of environmental tobacco smoke. Med Clin North Am 2004;88:1535–52.

[8] Law MR, Hackshaw AK. Environmental tobacco smoke. Br Med Bull 1996;52:22–34.

[9] Rustemeier K, Stabbert R, Haussman HJ, et al. Evaluation of the potential effects of ingredients added to cigarettes. Part 2: chemical composition of mainstream smoke. Food Chem Toxicol 2002; 40:93–104.

[10] Shen H, Spitz MR, Qiao Y, et al. Smoking, DNA repair and risk of non-small cell lung cancer. Int J Cancer 2003;107:84–8.

[11] DHHS (NIOSH) Publication No. 91–108. Environmental smoke in the workplace. Lung Cancer and other health effects; June 1991.

[12] Guerin MR, Jenkins RA. The chemistry of environmental tobacco smoke: composition and measurement. Second edition. Boca Raton (FL): CRC Press; 2000.

[13] National Cancer Institute. Health effects of exposure to environmental tobacco smoke: the report of the California environmental protection agency. Smoking and Tobacco Control Monograph No. 10. Bethesda, Maryland, USA: U.S. Department of Health and Human Services, National Institutes of Health, NCI; 1999.

[14] Kamholz SL. Health consequences of tobacco smoking. In: Hurst JW, editor. Medicine for the practicing physician. 4th edition. Stamford (CT): Appleton & Lange; 1996. p. 936–8.

[15] Benowitz NL. Cotinine as a biomarker of environmental tobacco smoke exposure. Epidemiol Rev 1996;18:188–204.

[16] Rushton L, Courage C, Green E. Estimation of the impact on children's health of environmental tobacco smoke in England and Wales. J R Soc Health 2003;123:175–80.

[17] Boffetta P. Involuntary smoking and lung cancer. Scand J Work Environ Health 2002;28(Suppl 2):30–40.

[18] Rushton L. Health impact of environmental tobacco smoke in the home. Rev Environ Health 2004;19(3):291–309.

[19] Siegel M, Skeer M. Exposure to secondhand smoke and excess lung cancer mortality risk among workers in the "5 B's": bars, bowling alleys, billiard halls, betting establishments, and bingo parlours. Tob Control 2003;12:333–8.

[20] Ritch WA, Begay ME. Strange bedfellows: the history of collaboration between the Massachusettes Restaurant Association and the tobacco industry. Am J Public Health 2001;91:598–603.

[21] Dearlove JV, Bialous SA, Glantz SA. Tobacco industry manipulation of the hospitality industry to maintain smoking in public places. Tob Control 2002;11:94–104.

[22] US Census Bureau. No. 593. Employed civilians by occupation, sex, race and Hispanic origin: 1983 and 2000. US Census Bureau, Statistical abstract of the United States, 2001. Available at: www.census.gov/prod/2002pubs/01statsab/labor.pdf. Accessed April 9, 2007.

[23] Selzer V. Smoking as a risk factor in the health of women. Int J Gynaecol Obstet 2003;82:393–7.

[24] DiFranza JR, Aligne CA, Weitzman M. Prenatal and postnatal environmental tobacco smoke exposure and children's health. Pediatrics 2004;113(4): 1007–15.

[25] Cameron P. The presence of pets and smoking as correlates of perceived disease. J Allergy 1967;40: 12–5.

[26] Cook DG, Strachan DP. Health effects of passive smoking-10: summary of effects of parental smoking on the respiratory health of children and implications for research. Thorax 1999;54: 357–66.

[27] Strachan DP, Cook DG. Health effects of passive smoking 1: parental smoking and lower respiratory illness in infancy and early childhood. Thorax 1997; 52:905–14.

[28] Anderson HR, Cook DG. Health effects of passive smoking 2: passive smoking and sudden infant death syndrome: Review of the epidemiologic evidence. Thorax 1997;52:1003–9.

[29] Strachan DP, Cook DG. Health effects of passive smoking 7: parental smoking and childhood asthma: longitudinal and case-controlled studies. Thorax 1998;53:204–12.

[30] Misra DP, Nguyen RH. Environmental tobacco smoke and low birthweight: a hazard of the workplace? Environ Health Perspect 1999;6765: 897–904.

[31] Windham GC, Eaton A, Hopkins B. Evidence for an association between environmental tobacco smoke exposure and birthweight: a meta-analysis and new data. Paediatr Perinat Epidemiol 1999; 13:35–57.

[32] Neal MS, Hughes EG, Holloway AC, et al. Sidestream smoking is equally as damaging as mainstream smoking on IVF outcomes. Hum Reprod 2005;20(9):2531–5.

[33] Stillman RJ, Rosenberg MJ, Sachs BP. Smoking and reproduction. Fertil Steril 1986;46:545–66.

[34] Sofikitis N, Takenaka M, Kanakas N, et al. Effects of cotinine on sperm mobility, membrane function and fertilizing capacity in vitro. Urol Res 2000; 28(6):370–5.

[35] Shiverick KT, Salatia C. Cigarette smoking and pregnancy. I: ovarian, uterine and placental effects. Placenta 1999;20:265–72.

[36] Hughes EG, Lamont DA, Beccroft MI, et al. Randomized trial of a "state-of-change" oriented smoking cessation intervention in infertile and pregnant women. Fertil Steril 2000;74:498–503.

[37] Gilliland FD, Berhane K, McConnell R, et al. Maternal smoking during pregnancy, environmental tobacco smoke exposure and childhood lung function. Thorax 2000;55:271–6.

[38] Gilliland FD, Li YF, Peters JM. Effects of maternal smoking during pregnancy and environmental tobacco smoke on asthma and wheezing in children. Am J Respir Crit Care Med 2001;163:429–36.

[39] Li YF, Langholz B, Salam MT, et al. Maternal and grandmaternal smoking patterns are associated with early childhood asthma. Chest 2005;127: 1232–41.

[40] Li YF, Gilliland FD, Berhane K, et al. Effects of in utero and environmental tobacco smoke exposure on lung function in boys and girls with and without asthma. Am J Respir Crit Care Med 2000;162: 2097–104.

[41] Skorge TD, Eagan TML, Eide GE, et al. The adult incidence of asthma and respiratory symptoms by passive smoking in utero or in childhood. Am J Respir Crit Care Med 2005;172:61–6.

[42] Svanes C, Omenaas E, Jarvis D, et al. Parental smoking in childhood and adult obstructive lung disease: results from the European Community Respiratory Health Survey. Thorax 2004;59:295–302.

[43] Upton MN, Smith GD, McConnachie A, et al. Maternal and personal cigarette smoking synergize to increase airflow limitation in adults. Am J Respir Crit Care Med 2004;169:479–87.

[44] Larsson ML, Frisk M, Hallstrom J, et al. Environmental tobacco smoke exposure during childhood is associated with increased prevalence of asthma in adults. Chest 2001;120:711–7.

[45] Jaakkola MS, Piipari R, Jaakkola N, et al. Environmental tobacco smoke and adult-onset asthma: a population-based incident case-control study. Am J Public Health 2003;93:2055–60.

[46] Leuenberger P, Schwartz J, Ackermann-Liebrich U, et al. Passive smoking in adults and chronic respiratory symptoms (SAPALDIA Study). Am J Respir Crit Care Med 1994;150:1222–8.

[47] World Health Organization Division of Noncommunicable Disease Tobacco Free Initiative. International conference on environmental tobacco smoke and child health: consultation report. Geneva: WHO; 1999. Available at: http://www.who.int/tob. Accessed April 9, 2007.

[48] Morkjaroenpong V, Rand CS, Butz AM, et al. Environmental tobacco smoke exposure and nocturnal symptoms among inner-city children with asthma. J Allergy Clin Immunol 2002;110:147–53.

[49] Corbo GM, Fuciarelli F, Foresti A, et al. Snoring in children: association with respiratory symptoms and passive smoking. BMJ 1989;299:1491–4.

[50] Huang SW, Giannoni C. The risks of adenoid hypertrophy in children with allergic rhinitis. Ann Allergy Asthma Immunol 2001;87:350–5.

[51] Willatt DJ. Children's sore throats related to parental smoking. Clin Otolaryngol 1996;11:317–21.

[52] Menezes AMB, Victora CG, Perez-Padilla R, the PLATINO Team. The Platino project: methodology of a multicenter prevalence survey of chronic obstructive pulmonary disease in major Latin American cities. BMC Med Res Methodol 2004;4:15.

[53] de Marco R, Accordini S, Cerveri A, et al. An international survey of chronic obstructive pulmonary disease in young adults according to GOLD stages. Thorax 2004;59:120–5.

[54] Center for Disease Control. Asthma mortality and hospitalization among children and young adults-United States, 1980–1993. MMWR Morb Mortal Wkly Rep 1996;45:350–3.

[55] Halfon N, Newacheck PW, Wood DL, et al. Routine emergency department use for sick care by children in the United States. Pediatrics 1996; 98:28–34.

[56] Malveaux FJ, Fletcher-Vincent SA. Environmental risk factors of childhood asthma in urban centers. Environ Health Perspect 1995;103(Suppl 6): 59–162.

[57] Wilson SR, Yamada EG, Sudhakar R, et al. A controlled trial of an environmental tobacco smoke reduction intervention in low-income children with asthma. Chest 2001;120:1709–22.

[58] Gilliland FD, Berhane K, Islam T, et al. Environmental tobacco smoke and absenteeism related to respiratory illness in school-children. Am J Epidemiol 2003;157:861–9.

[59] von Mutius E. Environmental factors influencing the development and progression of pediatric asthma. J Allergy Clin Immunol 2002;109:S525–32.

[60] Colilla S, Nicolae D, Pluzhnikov A, et al. Evidence for gene-environmental interactions in a linkage study of asthma and smoking exposure. J Allergy Clin Immunol 2003;111:840–6.

[61] National Human Genome Research Institiute. National Institutes of Health. LOD Score. Available at: http://www.genome.gov/glossary.cfm. Accessed July 4, 2007.

[62] Olds D. Tobacco exposure and impaired development: a review of the evidence. Ment Retard Dev Disabil Res Rev 1997;3:257–69.

[63] Butler NR, Goldstein H. Smoking in pregnancy and subsequent child development. Br Med J 1973; 4:573–5.

[64] Raintakallio P, Koiranen M. Neurologic handicaps among children whose mothers smoked during pregnancy. Prev Med 1987;16:597–606.

[65] Fogelman KR, Manor O. Smoking in pregnancy and development into early adulthood. BMJ 1988; 297:1233–6.

[66] Fergusson DM, Lloyd M. Smoking during pregnancy and its effects on child cognitive ability from the ages 8 to 12 years. Paediatr Perinat Epidemiol 1991;5:189–200.

[67] McCoe R, Stanton WR. Smoking in pregnancy and child development to age 9. J Paediatr Child Health 1994;30:263–8.

[68] Weitzman M, Byrd RS, Aliqne CA, et al. The effects of tobacco exposure on children's behavioral and cognitive functioning: implications for clinical

and public health policy and future research. Neu-rotoxicol Teratol 2002;24(3):397–406.

[69] Eskenazi B, Castorina R. Association of prenatal maternal or postnatal child environmental tobacco smoke exposure and neurodevelopmental and behavioral problems in children. Environ Health Perspect 1999;107(12):991–1000.

[70] Yolton K, Dietrich K, Auinger P, et al. Exposure to environmental tobacco smoke and cognitive abilities among U.S. children and adolescents. Environ Health Perspect 2005;113(1):98–103.

[71] Warner JO. Worldwide variations in the prevalence of atopic symptoms: what does it all mean? Thorax 1999;54(Suppl 2):S46–51.

[72] Behrendt H, Becker WM, Fritzesche C, et al. Air pollution and allergy: experimental studies on modulation of allergen release from pollen by air pollutants. Int Arch Allergy Immunol 1997;113:69–74.

[73] Bodner C, Godden D, Seaton A. Family size, childhood infections and atopic diseases. The Aberdeen WHEASE Group. Thorax 1998;53:28–32.

[74] Diaz-Sanchez D, Rumold R, Gong H. Challenge with environmental tobacco smoke exacerbates allergic airway disease in human beings. J Allergy Clin Immunol 2006;118:441–6.

[75] Molfino NA. Genetics of COPD. Chest 2004;125:1929–40.

[76] Van der Vaart H, Postma DS, Timens W, et al. Acute effects of cigarette smoke on inflammation and oxidative stress: a review. Thorax 2004;59:713–21.

[77] Saetta M, Finkelstrin R, Cosio MG. Morphological and cellular basis for airflow limitation in smokers. Eur Respir J 1994;7:1505–15.

[78] Eisner MD, Balmes J, Yelin EH, et al. Directly measured secondhand smoke exposure and COPD health outcomes. BMC Pulm Med 2006;6:12. Available at:http://www.biomedcentral.com/1471-2466/6/12. Accessed April 9, 2007.

[79] Whittemore AS, Perlin SA, DiCiccio Y. Chronic obstructive pulmonary disease in lifelong non-smokers: results from NHANES. Am J Public Health 1995;85:702–6.

[80] Behrendt CE. Mild and moderate-to-severe COPD in nonsmokers. Chest 2005;128:1239–44.

[81] Lokke A, Lange P, Scharling H, et al. Developing COPD: a 25 year follow up study of the general population. Thorax 2006;61:935–9.

[82] Lindberg A, Jonsson AC, Ronmark E, et al. Ten-year cumulative incidence of COPD and risk factors for incident disease in a symptomatic cohort. Chest 2005;127:1544–52.

[83] Eisner MD, Balmes J, Katz PP, et al. Lifetime environmental tobacco smoke exposure and the risk of chronic obstructive pulmonary disease. Environ Health 2005;4:7. Available at: http://www.ehjournal.net/content/4/1/7.

[84] Skogstad M, Kjaerheim K, Fladseth G, et al. Cross shift changes in lung function among bar and restaurant workers before and after implementation of a smoking ban. Occup Environ Med 2006;63:482–7.

[85] U.S. Department of Agriculture. Tobacco Outlook. Economic Research Service; April 2005.

[86] He J, Vupputuri S, Allen K, et al. Passive smoking and the risk of coronary artery disease—a meta-analysis of epidemiologic studies. N Engl J Med 1999;340:920–6.

[87] Lam TH, He Y. Passive smoking and coronary heart disease: a brief review. Clin Exp Pharmacol Physiol 1997;24:993–6.

[88] Law MR, Morris JK, Wald NJ. Environmental tobacco smoke exposure and ischemic heart disease: an evaluation of the evidence. Br Med J 1997;315:973–80.

[89] Wells AJ. Passive smoking as a cause of heart disease. J Am Coll Cardiol 1994;24:546–54.

[90] Thun M, Henley J, Apicella L. Epidemiologic studies of fatal and nonfatal cardiovascular disease and ETS exposure from spousal smoking. Environ Health Perspect 1999;107:841–6.

[91] Kaur S, Cohen A, Dolor R, et al. The impact of environmental tobacco smoke on women's risk of dying from heart disease: a meta-analysis. J Women's Health 2004;13:888–97.

[92] Otsuka R, Watanabe H, Hirata K, et al. Acute effects of passive smoking on the coronary circulation in healthy young adults. JAMA 2001;286:436–41.

[93] Enstrom JE, Kabat GC. Environmental tobacco smoke and tobacco related mortality in a prospective study of Californians, 1960–1998. Br Med J 2003;326:1057–63.

[94] Helsing KJ, Sandler DP, Comstock GW, et al. Heart disease mortality in nonsmokers living with smokers. Am J Epidemiol 1988;127:915–8.

[95] Hackshaw AK, Law MR, Wald NJ. The accumulated evidence on lung cancer and environmental tobacco smoke. BMJ 1997;315:980–8.

[96] Vineis P, Alavanja M, Buffler P, et al. Tobacco and cancer: recent epidemiologic evidence. J Natl Cancer Inst 2004;96:99–106. H.

[97] Centers for Disease Control and Prevention. Women and smoking. A report of the Surgeon General (Executive Summary). MMWR 2002;51(No. RR-12):1–30.

[98] Giovino GA. Epidemiology of tobacco use in the United States. Oncogene 2002;21:7326–40.

[99] National Center for Chronic Disease Prevention and Health Promotion. Tobacco Information and Prevention source tips. Updated 01-12-07. Available at: http://www.cdc.gov/tobacco/research_data/environmental/factsheet_ets.htm. Accessed February 3, 2007.

[100] Stockwell HG, Goldman AL, Lyman GH, et al. Environmental tobacco smoke and lung cancer risk in non-smoking women. J Natl Cancer Inst 1992;84(18):1417–22.

[101] Brownson RC, Alavanja MC, Hock ET, et al. Passive smoking and lung cancer in non-smoking women. Am J Public Health 1992;82(11):1525–30.

[102] Frontham ET, Correa P, Reynolds P, et al. Environmantal tobacco smoke and lung cancer in non-smoking women: a multicenter study. JAMA 1994;271:1752–9.

[103] Taylor R, Cumming R, Woodward A, et al. Passive smoking and lung cancer: a cumulative meta-analysis. Aust NZ J Public Health 2001;25(3):203–11.

[104] Zhong L, Goldberg MS, Parent ME, et al. Exposure to environmental tobacco smoke and the risk of lung cancer: a meta-analysis. Lung Cancer 2000;27(1):3–18.

[105] de Andrade M, Ebbert JO, Wampfler JA, et al. Environmental tobacco smoke exposure in women with lung cancer. Lung Cancer 2004;43:127–34.

[106] Boffetta P, Agudo A, Ahrens W, et al. Multicenter case-control study of exposure to environmental tobacco smoke and lung cancer in Europe. J Natl Cancer Inst 1998;90(19):1440–50.

[107] Wang TJ, Zhou BS. Meta-analysis of the potential relationship between exposure to environmental tobacco smoke and lung cancer in non-smoking Chinese women. Lung Cancer 1997;16:145–50.

[108] Vineis P, Airoldi L, Olgiati L, et al. Environmental tobacco smoke and risk of respiratory cancer and chronic obstructive pulmonary disease in former smokers and never smokers in the EPI prospective study. BMJ 2005;doi:10.1136/bmj.38327.648472.82.

[109] Prokopczyk B, Cox JE, Hoffmann D, et al. Identification of tobacco-specific carcinogen in the cervical mucus of smokers and non-smokers. J Natl Cancer Inst 1997;89:868–73.

[110] Trimble CL, Genkinger JM, Burke AE, et al. Active and passive cigarette smoking and the risk of cervical neoplasia. Obstet Gynecol 2005;105:174–81.

[111] Tay SK, Tay KJ. Passive cigarette smoking is a risk factor in cervical neoplasia. Gynecol Oncol 2004;93:116–20.

[112] Lee PN. Environmental tobacco smoke and cancer of sites other than the lung in adult non-smokers. Food Chem Toxicol 2002;40:747–66.

[113] Morabia A. Smoking (active and passive) and breast cancer: epidemiologic evidence up to June 2001. Environ Mol Mutagen 2002;39:89–95.

[114] Gammon MD, Eng SM, Teitelbaum SL, et al. Environmental tobacco smoke and breast cancer incidence. Environ Res 2004;96:176–85.

[115] Hecht SS. Tobacco smoke carcinogens and breast cancer. Environ Mol Mutagen 2002;39:119–26.

[116] Gerhrman CA, Hovell MF. Protecting children from environmental tobacco smoke (ETS) exposure: a critical review. Nicotine Tob Res 2003;5:289–301.

[117] Celli BR, Halbert RJ, Nordyke RJ, et al. Airway obstruction in never smokers: results from the Third National Health and Nutrition Examination Survey. Am J Med 2005;118(12):1364–72.

CLINICS
IN CHEST
MEDICINE

Clin Chest Med 28 (2007) 575–587

Chronic Obstructive Pulmonary Disease in Patients Who Have HIV Infection

Kristina Crothers, MD

*Section of Pulmonary and Critical Care Medicine, Department of Internal Medicine,
Yale University School of Medicine, 333 Cedar Street, TAC 441, PO Box 208057,
New Haven, CT 06520, USA*

Chronic obstructive pulmonary disease (COPD) is currently the fourth leading cause of death worldwide and is projected to increase further as a cause of morbidity and mortality in the coming decades [1,2]. Yet COPD continues to be under-diagnosed [1,3] and risk factors that contribute to the development of COPD are incompletely understood. Cigarette smoking is the major risk factor for the development of COPD. Because not all smokers develop COPD, however, other factors appear to be involved [4]. For example, α_1-antitrypsin deficiency accounts for a small number of cases of COPD. Other genetic factors are under investigation [5]. In addition, studies suggest that COPD susceptibility may vary by gender and race [6–8]. HIV-positive patients may represent another population that has an increased susceptibility to COPD.

This article considers the evidence suggesting an increased risk for COPD, namely emphysema and chronic bronchitis, and the potential increased risk for small airways abnormalities and nonspecific airway hyper-responsiveness among patients who have HIV. Additionally, risk factors for COPD and possible reasons for increased COPD among patients who have HIV infection are discussed. Finally, the management of COPD in HIV-positive patients is reviewed.

Evidence for increased prevalence of chronic obstructive pulmonary disease among HIV-positive patients

COPD is defined in the Global Initiative for Chronic Obstructive Lung Disease (GOLD) guidelines as "a disease state characterized by airflow limitation that is not fully reversible. The airflow limitation is usually both progressive and associated with an abnormal inflammatory response of the lungs to noxious particles or gases" [1]. COPD may result from emphysema, small airways inflammation, bronchoconstriction, excess mucus in the airways, or a combination of these factors. HIV infection is associated with several different manifestations of COPD and airways abnormalities, including features of emphysema [9–11], chronic bronchitis [12], nonspecific airway abnormalities, and bronchial hyper-responsiveness [13,14]. Although separate from COPD and not considered further in this review, bronchiectasis likewise causes an obstructive ventilatory defect and is described in patients who have HIV [15,16].

Somewhat challenging to discern from prior studies is whether HIV infection is an independent risk factor for the development or progression of COPD or whether the increased rates of COPD among patients who have HIV infection may be attributable to the greater rates of smoking, drug abuse, pulmonary infections, and other risk factors for COPD that frequently are encountered in HIV-positive patients. Interpretation of studies reporting increased rates of COPD and airway abnormalities in HIV-positive populations requires careful consideration of the patient populations included and the methods used to control for potential confounders. A summary of the

Funded by National Institutes of Health/National Center for Research Resources (1KL2RR024138).
E-mail address: kristina.crothers@yale.edu

chestmed.theclinics.com

major studies conducted to date of COPD and airway abnormalities in HIV-positive persons is provided in Tables 1 and 2.

One of the major manifestations of COPD, emphysema is described HIV-positive patients in several studies conducted before the advent of highly active antiretroviral therapy (HAART). In studies that included a majority of patients who had a history of prior AIDS-related pulmonary infections, radiographic findings of emphysematous, bullous, or cystic lung disease were encountered in approximately 40% [10,11]. It is unclear if findings such as these share the same pathogenesis as smoking-related emphysema or if they are primarily the result of pneumatoceles and other sequelae of previous infections.

Emphysema is also described, however, in HIV-positive patients who have not had prior AIDS-related pulmonary complications. In one study by Diaz and colleagues, emphysema was found to be the predominant cause of a low diffusing capacity of the lung (DLCO) in HIV-positive patients [17]. In HIV-positive patients who had DLCO values in the bottom 25th percentile (corresponding to values <72% predicted), 50% had detectable emphysema on CT scan. Abnormalities in DLCO in turn were primarily due to decreases in the blood volume component and were accentuated by cigarette smoking, as HIV-positive patients who had the greatest decreases in diffusing capacity had higher mean pack years of cigarette smoking. Decreases in DLCO were not associated with significant obstructive or restrictive ventilatory defects.

An additional study by Diaz and colleagues suggests that HIV infection alone is an independent risk factor for emphysema. In a study of 114 consecutive HIV-positive patients compared with 44 age-, sex-, and smoking-matched HIV-negative controls, 15% of the HIV-positive patients had emphysema on CT scan compared with only 2% of HIV-negative patients ($P = .025$) [9]. DLCO was significantly lower in the HIV-positive patients, although there was no difference in the forced expiratory volume in 1 second (FEV_1), forced vital capacity (FVC), or total lung capacity (TLC) between groups. In patients who had emphysema, the degree of airflow obstruction was mild, with a mean FEV_1/FVC of 69.2%. HIV-positive smokers who had emphysema and underwent bronchoscopy were found to have a significantly higher percentage of cytotoxic lymphocytes compared to HIV-positive smokers who did not have emphysema and to HIV-negative smokers.

In addition to emphysema, HIV infection is associated with an increased frequency of symptoms suggestive of chronic bronchitis, another of the major manifestations of COPD. In one study conducted before HAART, significantly more HIV-positive patients had symptoms of cough and phlegm production "on most days for ≥ 3 months during the year" than HIV-negative persons (approximately 25% HIV-positive versus 12% HIV-negative, $P<.05$) [12]. Although the overall duration is not clear, these symptoms appear consistent with the clinical criteria for chronic bronchitis. The most important predictor of these symptoms was current or former cigarette smoking. In this study, CD4 count was not associated with the presence of airway symptoms, such as cough, phlegm, or wheeze. A low CD4 count, however, was an independent predictor of dyspnea and use of the antiretroviral agent lamivudine was associated with a reduction in dyspnea. Reasons for these findings are unclear, and it is unknown whether a patient's degree of immunosuppression and use of antiretroviral therapy may have any impact on the development or progression of COPD.

Thus far, only one study has examined the association between HIV infection and COPD among patients in the HAART era. This study also suggests that HIV infection may be an independent risk factor for COPD [18]. In an analysis of 1014 HIV-positive and 713 HIV-negative men enrolled in the Veterans Aging Cohort 5 Site Study, conducted at five United States Veterans Affairs medical centers, diagnoses of COPD were determined by *International Classification of Diseases, Ninth Revision* (ICD-9) diagnostic codes and patient self-report on questionnaire. The unadjusted prevalence of COPD by ICD-9 codes was 10% in HIV-positive patients and 9% in HIV-negative patients ($P = .4$) and by patient self-report was 15% and 12%, respectively ($P = .04$). In both HIV-positive and HIV-negative patients, the prevalence of COPD increased according to pack years of smoking and age. The HIV-positive patients were younger and had fewer pack years of smoking than the HIV-negative controls. After adjusting for differences in age, smoking, race/ethnicity, and other potential confounders such as injection drug use and alcohol abuse, HIV-positive patients were approximately 50% to 60% more likely to have COPD than HIV-negative patients by ICD-9 codes or patient self-report. Thus, combined data from the above studies suggest that the risk for COPD is increased as a result of HIV infection, as the prevalence of COPD remains significantly greater among HIV-positive patients after controlling for smoking, age, and other common risk factors for COPD.

Evidence for increased prevalence of airway abnormalities in HIV-positive patients

HIV infection may also be associated with an increased prevalence of small airways abnormalities, expiratory flow abnormalities, and bronchial hyper-responsiveness, particularly in smokers (see Table 2). Nonspecific focal air trapping with decreased expiratory flow rates were significantly more common among HIV-positive patients compared with HIV-negative patients who did not have prior AIDS-related pulmonary complications [19]. In this study, the presence of focal air trapping was more likely in patients who had a longer duration of HIV infection. Bronchial dilatation in the absence of significant airflow obstruction has also been described in HIV-positive patients [20]. Bronchial dilatation was found to correlate with increased neutrophilia in bronchoalveolar lavage specimens, suggesting the presence of increased airways inflammation. In another study, a decreased expiratory flow rate or a significant response to inhaled bronchodilator was encountered in 44% of 99 HIV-positive patients, many of whom had a history of *Pneumocystis* pneumonia (PCP) or systemic Kaposi's sarcoma [14].

Data regarding the association of HIV infection with bronchial hyper-responsiveness is conflicting. Although more HIV-positive subjects tended to have bronchial hyper-responsiveness to methacholine challenge than HIV-negative subjects in a study from the Pulmonary Complications of HIV Infection Study Cohort (19.3% HIV positive versus 12.9% HIV negative), this difference was not statistically significant [21]. Of the HIV-positive patients who had airway hyper-responsiveness, however, 70% had no prior history of asthma. In contrast, another investigation of 236 HIV-positive and 236 HIV-negative men found significantly increased bronchial hyper-responsiveness to methacholine challenge in HIV-positive compared to HIV-negative subjects [13]. Smoking status influenced bronchial hyper-responsiveness, as bronchial hyper-responsiveness was significantly greater only among HIV-positive current smokers compared with HIV-negative current smokers (30% versus 13%, $P < .05$) but

was not significantly different for the comparison of HIV-positive nonsmokers to HIV-negative nonsmokers (20% versus 15%). As bronchial hyper-responsiveness is a risk factor for progressive COPD [22], these data suggest that an interaction between smoking and HIV infection could enhance susceptibility to the progression of COPD.

Taken together, these data support that COPD is increased in prevalence among HIV-positive patients and suggest that HIV infection may increase the risk for COPD independently, apart from smoking. Data is limited, however, in understanding whether or not the pathogenesis of COPD and the progression of COPD are similar in HIV-positive and in HIV-negative patients. How HIV infection might alter the course of established COPD is also unknown. Further, whether COPD described in HIV-positive patients is primarily in the form of emphysema, chronic bronchitis, small airways disease, or even asthma or a combination of these abnormalities is unclear. Nonetheless, these retrospective and cross-sectional data do not definitively rule out the possibility that the greater prevalence of COPD among HIV-positive patients may be the result of residual confounding, related to the generally greater prevalence of other known risk factors for COPD in HIV-positive populations, such as smoking or infection, which are discussed later in further detail.

Risk factors for chronic obstructive pulmonary disease among HIV-positive patients

Exposures to a variety of substances are associated with risk for COPD. Cigarette smoking, the most potent risk factor for COPD, is highly prevalent in HIV-positive populations [23]. Previous studies reported that nearly 75% of HIV-positive patients have ever smoked [23,24] and approximately 40% to 50% are current smokers [24–26]. In contrast, the prevalence of current smoking in the general HIV-uninfected population in the United States is approximately 21% [27].

Additional potential risk factors for COPD that tend to be more common in HIV-positive compared with HIV-negative populations include inhaled and intravenous substance abuse [12,28]. The use of inhaled drugs, such as marijuana, cocaine, and heroin, are variably reported to be associated with airflow obstruction [29]. Although use of these drugs is clearly associated with increased frequency of respiratory symptoms, it

Table 1
Evidence for increased emphysema and chronic bronchitis in HIV-positive patients

Author, year	Design and population	Findings	Relationship to smoking and other factors
Kuhlman et al [11], 1989	Retrospective chart review of 55 HIV+ patients who had AIDS and 50 neutropenic patients who had acute leukemia.	42% of HIV+ patients compared with 16% of leukemia patients had bullous changes on CT scan ($P < .01$).	70% of patients who have premature bullous damage had prior or recurrent pulmonary infections, with 61% having prior PCP; no difference in smoking or injection drug use in AIDS patients ± bullous damage; overall prevalence of smoking not stated.
Guillemi et al [10], 1996	Cross-sectional evaluation of 32 consecutive HIV+ men who had AIDS referred for initiation of PCP prophylaxis; 78% had ever smoked.	60% with unexpected lung lesions on CT scan; nearly half consisted of emphysematous or cystic changes.	No patients had history of intravenous drug use; patients who had prior lung infections were not excluded; no difference in smoking between patients ± lung abnormalities.
Diaz et al [17], 1999	Baseline, cross-sectional analysis of prospective cohort of 243 HIV+ patients and 30 HIV− controls; 67% HIV+ and 63% HIV− group were smokers.	Of the 95 HIV+ patients who underwent HRCT, emphysema was found to correlate with decreased DLco, which primarily was due to decreases in the capillary blood volume component; HIV+ patients who had decreased DLco had significantly decreased VC and FEV$_1$, although still within normal ranges, with preserved TLC and no significant difference in FEV$_1$/FVC ratio. Of patients who had DLco < 25th percentile, 50% had CT evidence of emphysema.	Patients who had prior AIDS-related pulmonary complications were excluded; HIV+ subjects who had DLco below the 25th percentile (<72% predicted) had greater pack years of smoking than HIV+ subjects who had DLco > 25th percentile. No significant difference between groups in occupational exposures, family history of COPD, or diagnoses of pneumonia.
Diaz et al [9], 2000	Cross-sectional sample of larger prospective cohort study included 114 consecutive HIV+ patients and 44 age-, sex-, and smoking-matched HIV− controls. 60% of HIV+ and 56% of HIV− patients were smokers.	Radiographic emphysema observed in 15% of HIV+ compared with 2% of HIV− patients; no difference in FEV$_1$, FVC overall between HIV+ and HIV−, although DLco was significantly lower among HIV+ patients ($P = .03$). Only mild airflow obstruction in HIV+ patients who had emphysema (FEV$_1$/FVC 69.2%). HIV+ emphysema had higher % cytotoxic lymphocytes on BAL compared with HIV+ without emphysema and HIV− smokers without emphysema.	Patients who had prior AIDS-related pulmonary complications were excluded; approximately 10% of HIV+ and HIV− patients had a history of injection drug use; <10% of patients were on protease inhibitors. Age and smoking controlled for by matching.

Diaz et al [12], 2003	Baseline, cross-sectional analysis of respiratory symptoms in a prospective cohort study of 327 HIV+ patients and 52 HIV− patients. 54% of HIV+ and 50% of HIV− were current smokers.	Significantly increased cough, phlegm, wheeze, and dyspnea in HIV+ compared with HIV− patients; specifically, both increased cough and phlegm production "on most days for ≥3 months during the year" (approximately 25% HIV + versus 12% HIV−, $P<.05$). Use of lamivudine associated with less dyspnea.	Patients who had prior AIDS-related pulmonary complications were excluded; greater prevalence of intravenous drug use among HIV+; smoking was significantly associated with all respiratory symptoms; unclear if symptom duration of cough/phlegm was ≥2 years, required for chronic bronchitis diagnosis.
Crothers et al [18], 2006	Baseline cross-sectional analysis of a prospective cohort study included 1014 HIV+ and 713 HIV− men; 75% of both HIV+ and HIV− patients had ever smoked.	HIV+ patients 50%–60% more likely to have COPD, adjusting for age, race/ethnicity, pack years of smoking, injection drug use, and alcohol abuse (OR 1.5 for diagnosis of COPD by ICD-9 codes and 1.6 for patient self-report, $P<.05$).	Patients who had prior lung disease were not excluded; COPD was based on ICD-9 codes and patient self-report; approximately 80% of HIV+ patients were on HAART. Smoking and injection drug use controlled for in multivariate analyses. Women were excluded in these analyses due to low percentage in overall study.

Abbreviations: BAL, bronchoalveolar lavage; HIV−, HIV negative; HIV+, HIV positive; HRCT, high-resolution chest CT; OR, odds ratio; VC, vital capacity; ±, with and without.

Table 2
Evidence for increased airway abnormalities in HIV-positive patients

Author, year	Design and population	Findings	Relationship to smoking and other factors
O'Donnell et al [14], 1988	Retrospective chart review of 99 HIV+ patients who had AIDS referred for pulmonary physiologic assessment in PFT laboratory; 35% were smokers.	44% with abnormal airway function: decreased airflow in 33% (defined as an FEV_1, FVC, or FEF 25-75 of 1.65 standard deviations below predicted values) and significant response to bronchodilator in 31% (defined as increase in the FEV_1 of $\geq 12\%$ or if the FEF 25-75 increased $\geq 25\%$ with a change in VC of $<10\%$).	54% of patients had PCP and 29% had systemic KS within 3 months before testing; abnormal airway function was found in 8 of 18 (44%) patients who had KS, 9 of 42 (21%) of those who had PCP, 7 of 11 (64%) of those who had PCP and KS, and 20 of 28 (71%) of those who did not have PCP or KS. No difference in airflow abnormalities according to smoking status.
King et al [20], 1997	Cross-sectional subset of prospective cohort study, included 50 HIV+ and 11 HIV− patients; 69% had ever smoked.	36% of HIV+ and none of HIV− patients had bronchial dilatation on CT; significantly decreased D_{LCO} but no difference in airflow obstruction in subjects $\pm$ bronchial dilatation. BAL neutrophilia ($>4\%$) in 22% of HIV+ compared with 9% of HIV− patients; BAL neutrophil counts significantly higher in those who had bronchial dilatation ($P = .014$).	Patients who had prior AIDS-related pulmonary complications were excluded; no significant difference in smoking history between HIV+ and HIV− patients, in those $\pm$ bronchial dilatation, and in those $\pm$ BAL neutrophilia. No pulmonary infections diagnosed on BAL. Significantly longer duration of HIV infection in those who had bronchial dilatation.
Wallace et al [21], 1997	Cross-sectional substudy of prospective cohort study, consisting of 62 HIV+ and 62 HIV− patients matched by age, gender, race, smoking, prior asthma, and baseline FEV_1; 52% of each group had ever smoked.	Hyper-responsiveness to methacholine challenge detected in 19.3% of HIV+ and 12.9% of HIV− ($P > .1$).	HIV− controls were selected from another cohort study; study underpowered to detect a difference of this magnitude. Smoking controlled for by matching.
Gelman et al [19], 1999	Cross-sectional subset of prospective cohort study included 48 consecutive HIV+ and 11 consecutive HIV− patients; 54% of HIV+ and 55% of HIV− patients were current smokers.	63% of HIV+ and 27% of HIV− patients had focal air trapping on expiratory HRCT scan ($P = .03$); subjects who had air trapping had lower mean FEV_1, FEF 25-75, and D_{LCO} than those who had normal HRCT ($P < .05$). Air trapping was associated significantly with bronchial dilatation.	Patients who had prior AIDS-related pulmonary complications and coexistent lung disease, including bronchiectasis and emphysema, were excluded; no difference in current smoking and pack years of smoking according to presence of focal air trapping or HIV. Significantly longer duration of HIV infection in those who had focal air trapping.

| Poirier et al [13], 2001 | Cross-sectional study of 248 HIV+ and 236 healthy HIV− men, ages 20–44 years. 62% of HIV+ compared with 35% of HIV− men were current smokers ($P<.05$). | Hyper-responsiveness to methacholine challenge found in 26.2% of HIV+ and 14.4% of HIV− patients ($P<.05$); when stratified by current smoking, bronchial hyper-responsiveness significantly different in HIV+ current smokers compared with HIV− current smokers only (30.3% versus 13.3%, $P<.05$). | Subjects required to have a normal chest x-ray, no respiratory infections in the 6 weeks, and no PCP in the 3 months before study participation. Although not statistically significant, 17.3% of HIV+ patients reported a history of asthma compared with 12.3% of HIV− patients. Subjects stratified by smoking status in analyses; no data on other drug use or occupational exposures. |

Abbreviations: BAL, bronchoalveolar lavage; FEF 25-75, forced mid-expiratory flow; HIV−, HIV negative; HIV+, HIV positive; HRCT, high-resolution chest CT; KS, Kaposi's sarcoma; PFT, pulmonary function test; VC, vital capacity; ±, with and without.

is not entirely clear whether or not they are associated independently with the development of airflow obstruction or emphysema after controlling for concomitant cigarette smoking [30–32]. For example, a recent systematic review on the pulmonary complications of marijuana found that although marijuana smoking was associated with increased respiratory symptoms, no clear association with long-term abnormalities in pulmonary function testing was demonstrated [33]. The effects of intravenous drug use on the lung are also varied. Although associated more commonly with talc granulomatosis, restrictive ventilatory defects, and pulmonary hypertension, the intravenous use of illicit drugs—particularly of methylphenidate—also can be associated with the development of precocious emphysema [29]. Although data on the association of alcohol abuse with obstructive lung disease is conflicting [34,35], alcohol abuse is also prevalent in HIV-positive patients [28]. Whether or not alcohol plays a greater role in the susceptibility to COPD in patients who have HIV infection has not been investigated.

Other possible risk factors to consider in HIV-infected populations that may have an impact on the development or progression of COPD but that have been addressed incompletely in prior studies include occupational or environmental exposures [36] and low socioeconomic status [37,38]. In addition, recurrent pulmonary infections or colonization with microorganisms in the respiratory tract may influence the course of COPD. Although the pathogenic role of microorganisms in the course of COPD is controversial [39–41], increased airflow obstruction subsequent to episodes of bacterial pneumonia and PCP has been documented in HIV-positive patients [42]. It is as yet unknown whether or not CD4 count, HIV viral load, or HAART influences the development or clinical course of COPD.

Potential mechanisms of increased risk for chronic obstructive pulmonary disease in HIV

Pathophysiologic studies offer several potential observations as to why HIV may increase susceptibility to COPD. CD8+ T cells are believed to play a critical role in the development of COPD [43,44], and HIV infection can result in intense infiltration of CD8+ T cells in the lung, particularly in early to mid stages of disease [45,46]. These T cells are shown to secrete interferon-γ (IFN-γ) [45]. Although it is unclear whether or not the lymphocytic alveolitis and expression of IFN-γ play any role in the development of COPD in HIV-positive persons, overexpression of IFN-γ is shown to cause emphysema in animal models [43].

Chronic viral infections are also believed to be involved in the pathogenesis of COPD [47]. Latent adenoviral infections in the lung are postulated to play a role in amplifying the development of cigarette smoke-induced emphysema. The local consequences of HIV infection in the pathogenesis of COPD are unknown, however, and the impact of immune reconstitution and HAART on the development and progression of COPD has not been investigated.

Additionally, episodes of clinical pneumonia or colonization with respiratory organisms may contribute to airway obstruction [42–49], which may be of particular relevance to the pathogenesis of COPD in immunosuppressed persons who have HIV disease. For example, a history of bacterial pneumonia or PCP is associated with significant expiratory airflow limitation in subjects who have HIV infection [42]. In addition, colonization with *Pneumocystis jirovecii*, the organism responsible for human PCP, is associated with the presence and severity of COPD in HIV-negative patients [41]. *P jirovecii* has also been identified in the sputum of asymptomatic HIV-negative patients who have chronic bronchitis [50] and has been detected with higher frequency in HIV-positive smokers compared with nonsmokers in the absence of active PCP [51].

Oxidative stress may play a key role in the development and progression of COPD, particularly in patients who have HIV. Increased oxidative stress is demonstrated systemically and in the lungs of patients who have COPD and asthma above that seen in healthy smokers [52]. A decreased ability to maintain an antioxidant defense may enhance susceptibility to COPD [53]. HIV-positive patients have evidence of abnormal systemic and lung oxidant/antioxidant balance, as demonstrated by decreased antioxidant defenses, most notably superoxide dismutase and glutathione [54,55], and elevated serum levels of lipid peroxidation products, such as malondialdehyde and hydroperoxide [56]. Smoking may enhance this oxidative stress, further depleting antioxidant defenses systemically and in the lung that already are abnormal in HIV-positive patients [57]. Further work is needed to elucidate which, if any, of these processes plays a causal role either alone or in conjunction with cigarette smoking or other risk factors in the pathogenesis of COPD in HIV-positive persons.

Clinical impact of chronic obstructive pulmonary disease in HIV

Given the high frequency of smoking [23], increasing age, and greater prevalence of COPD in patients who have HIV infection [9,18], COPD is emerging as an important clinical problem in HIV-positive patients in the era of HAART. This is likely to be true particularly in areas of the world with access to HAART, such as in the United States, where an estimated 1 million people are living with HIV. Overall, noninfectious complications and comorbid illnesses in HIV-positive patients have generally increased in frequency as survival has improved among those on HAART [58–60]. Consistent with this, COPD is the second most frequently encountered new pulmonary condition after bacterial pneumonia in a cohort of HIV-positive veterans studied in the HAART era [61]. This is in contrast to the pre-HAART era, when infectious complications, such as bacterial pneumonia and PCP, were the two most common lung complications among HIV-positive patients [62].

Furthermore, the chronic complications from smoking now contribute significantly to morbidity and mortality of HIV-positive patients, whereas studies before HAART had conflicting conclusions regarding the association of smoking with mortality [63]. Compared to those who have never smoked, current smokers who have HIV have a significantly increased prevalence of COPD and a greater mortality [63]. These findings, in turn, raise the possibility that the increased mortality may be attributable in part to COPD and underscore the increasing importance of COPD and other noninfectious comorbid conditions among HIV-positive patients on effective HAART.

Management of chronic obstructive pulmonary disease in HIV-positive patients

To date, no studies have addressed the management of COPD specifically in HIV-positive patients. Given the absence of such data, current therapy should follow the COPD management guidelines proposed for HIV-uninfected patients [64]. Special consideration should be given, however, to a few key aspects of COPD management for HIV-positive patients. First, the use of inhaled steroids for COPD in HIV-positive patients requires careful follow-up. Given the risks for oral candidiasis and the recently identified concern for an increased risk for bacterial pneumonia

associated with high-dose inhaled steroids [65], providers should monitor for infectious complications, particularly in patients who have low CD4 T-cell counts. Likewise, the regular use of systemic steroids preferably should be avoided in HIV-positive patients. In addition, providers should review vaccination records with their HIV-positive patients to ensure that all patients have received the recommended pneumococcal and yearly influenza vaccine.

Second, smoking cessation is of paramount importance, as current smoking is associated with increased respiratory symptoms, COPD, bacterial pneumonia, mortality, and decreased quality of life in HIV-positive patients [63]. Rates of current smoking are nearly twofold higher in most HIV-positive compared with HIV-negative populations [27]. Health care providers, however, of HIV-positive patients may be less aware of current smoking and less confident in their ability to counsel their patients regarding smoking cessation [66]. These findings highlight the need to increase efforts at smoking cessation among patients who have HIV. Although the number of studies is limited, data suggest that smoking cessation interventions can be effectively applied in HIV-positive populations [67–69]. One study combining the nicotine patch and counseling found a smoking cessation rate of 50% after 8 months among HIV-positive smokers [69]. Another study using cellular telephones for counseling in HIV-positive smokers increased cessation rates to 37% compared with 10% in the usual care group [68]. These results are similar to those from a study of HIV-negative patients using telephone intervention [70].

Third, as with HIV-negative patients, HIV-positive patients who have COPD should be considered for participation in pulmonary rehabilitation programs. In HIV-positive veterans, COPD or asthma was among the top comorbid conditions independently associated with self-reported increased physical disability [71]. In studies of HIV-negative patients who have COPD, physical functioning can be improved significantly with participation in pulmonary rehabilitation programs [72].

Referral for pulmonary rehabilitation thus should be considered early in HIV-positive patients who have COPD, as the systemic and skeletal manifestations encountered in HIV-negative patients who have COPD may potentially be exaggerated and associated with even greater decrements in physical capacity in patients who have HIV.

Possible reasons for this include the concomitant skeletal muscle dysfunction and mitochondrial abnormalities related to HIV infection and its treatment superimposed on those associated with COPD alone [73]. Furthermore, peak aerobic capacity is decreased in HIV-positive patients: a 41% decrease in the maximal oxygen consumption was noted in HIV-positive patients compared with expected values from age- and gender-matched healthy sedentary HIV-negative controls [74]. Respiratory muscle function also may be affected in HIV, as another study found decreased respiratory muscle strength in otherwise healthy HIV-positive patients compared with HIV-negative patients [75]. No studies to date have investigated the systemic manifestations of COPD in HIV-positive patients or have compared the anatomic or functional features of skeletal muscle dysfunction in HIV to those found in HIV-negative patients who have COPD. Although studies support the safety and potential benefit of exercise training in HIV-positive patients [76,77], further studies are needed to determine the role and optimal type of exercise training in HIV-positive patients, in particular those who have concomitant comorbid diseases such as COPD.

Summary

HIV-positive patients appear to have an increased risk for COPD, although whether this represents increased emphysema, chronic bronchitis, other obstructive lung diseases including asthma, or a combination of these disorders has not been evaluated fully. Although some of the increased COPD may be attributable to the greater rates of smoking and drug abuse in HIV-positive populations, the apparent risk for COPD remains elevated in HIV-positive patients even after controlling for these and other potential confounders [9,18]. It also remains unclear whether HIV infection accelerates the course of COPD. Further work is needed to elucidate the pathogenesis of COPD in HIV-positive persons, and can provide insights relevant to understanding COPD in HIV-negative patients as well.

Given the increasing age of HIV-positive patients as survival has improved for those on HAART combined with the high prevalence of smoking, health care providers are likely to encounter a substantial number of HIV-positive patients who have COPD. Increased awareness of COPD among health care providers of HIV-positive patients is warranted. Identification of COPD is important, as undiagnosed airway obstruction is associated with impaired health and functional status [78]. Appropriate management of COPD is associated with health benefits, such as decreased symptoms and COPD exacerbations, and improved smoking cessation, exercise capacity, and quality of life [79,80]. Additional studies are needed to determine whether or not the pharmacologic and nonpharmacologic management strategies for COPD should differ in HIV-positive patients versus HIV-negative to best maintain patient health over time.

References

[1] 2006 Update: global strategy for the diagnosis, management, and prevention of COPD. Available at: www.goldcopd.com. Accessed May 31, 2007.

[2] Murray CJ, Lopez AD. Alternative projections of mortality and disability by cause 1990–2020: global burden of disease study. Lancet 24 1997;349(9064): 1498–1504.

[3] Mannino DM, Homa DM, Akinbami LJ, et al. Chronic obstructive pulmonary disease surveillance–United States, 1971–2000. MMWR Surveill Summ 2002;51(6):1–16.

[4] Mannino DM. COPD: epidemiology, prevalence, morbidity and mortality, and disease heterogeneity. Chest 2002;121(Suppl 5):121S–6S.

[5] Sandford AJ, Silverman EK. Chronic obstructive pulmonary disease. 1: susceptibility factors for COPD the genotype-environment interaction. Thorax 2002;57(8):736–41.

[6] Chapman KR. Chronic obstructive pulmonary disease: are women more susceptible than men? Clin Chest Med 2004;25(2):331–41.

[7] Silverman EK, Weiss ST, Drazen JM, et al. Gender-related differences in severe, early-onset chronic obstructive pulmonary disease. Am J Respir Crit Care Med 2000;162(6):2152–8.

[8] Petty TL, Weinmann GG. Building a national strategy for the prevention and management of and research in chronic obstructive pulmonary disease. National heart, lung, and blood institute workshop summary. Bethesda, Maryland, August 29–31, 1995. JAMA 1997;277(3):246–53.

[9] Diaz PT, King MA, Pacht ER, et al. Increased susceptibility to pulmonary emphysema among HIV-seropositive smokers. Ann Intern Med 2000;132(5):369–72.

[10] Guillemi SA, Staples CA, Hogg JC, et al. Unexpected lung lesions in high resolution computed tomography (HRTC) among patients with advanced HIV disease. Eur Respir J 1996;9(1):33–6.

[11] Kuhlman JE, Knowles MC, Fishman EK, et al. Premature bullous pulmonary damage in AIDS: CT diagnosis. Radiology 1989;173(1):23–6.

[12] Diaz PT, Wewers MD, Pacht E, et al. Respiratory symptoms among HIV-seropositive individuals. Chest 2003;123(6):1977–82.

[13] Poirier CD, Inhaber N, Lalonde RG, et al. Prevalence of bronchial hyperresponsiveness among HIV-infected men. Am J Respir Crit Care Med 2001;164(4):542–5.

[14] O'Donnell CR, Bader MB, Zibrak JD, et al. Abnormal airway function in individuals with the acquired immunodeficiency syndrome. Chest 1988;94(5): 945–8.

[15] McGuinness G, Naidich DP, Garay S, et al. AIDS associated bronchiectasis: CT features. J Comput Assist Tomogr 1993;17(2):260–6.

[16] Bard M, Couderc LJ, Saimot AG, et al. Accelerated obstructive pulmonary disease in HIV infected patients with bronchiectasis. Eur Respir J 1998;11(3): 771–5.

[17] Diaz PT, King MA, Pacht ER, et al. The pathophysiology of pulmonary diffusion impairment in human immunodeficiency virus infection. Am J Respir Crit Care Med 1999;160(1):272–7.

[18] Crothers K, Butt AA, Gibert CL, et al. Increased COPD among HIV-positive compared to HIV-negative veterans. Chest 2006;130(5):1326–33.

[19] Gelman M, King MA, Neal DE, et al. Focal air trapping in patients with HIV infection: CT evaluation and correlation with pulmonary function test results. AJR Am J Roentgenol 1999;172(4):1033–8.

[20] King MA, Neal DE, St John R, et al. Bronchial dilatation in patients with HIV infection: CT assessment and correlation with pulmonary function tests and findings at bronchoalveolar lavage. AJR Am J Roentgenol 1997;168(6):1535–40.

[21] Wallace JM, Stone GS, Browdy BL, et al. Nonspecific airway hyperresponsiveness in HIV disease. Pulmonary complications of HIV infection study group. Chest 1997;111(1):121–7.

[22] Tashkin DP, Altose MD, Connett JE, et al. Methacholine reactivity predicts changes in lung function over time in smokers with early chronic obstructive pulmonary disease. The lung health study research group. Am J Respir Crit Care Med 1996;153(6 Pt 1): 1802–11.

[23] Niaura R, Shadel WG, Morrow K, et al. Human immunodeficiency virus infection, AIDS, and smoking cessation: the time is now. Clin Infect Dis 2000;31(3): 808–12.

[24] Gritz ER, Vidrine DJ, Lazev AB, et al. Smoking behavior in a low-income multiethnic HIV/AIDS population. Nicotine Tob Res 2004;6(1):71–7.

[25] Page-Shafer K, Delorenze GN, Satariano WA, et al. Comorbidity and survival in HIV-infected men in the San Francisco men's health survey. Ann Epidemiol 1996;6(5):420–30.

[26] Galai N, Park LP, Wesch J, et al. Effect of smoking on the clinical progression of HIV-1 infection. J Acquir Immune Defic Syndr Hum Retrovirol 1997;14(5):451–8.

[27] Centers for Disease Control and Prevention (CDC). Cigarette smoking among adults—United States, 2004. MMWR Morb Mortal Wkly Rep 2005; 54(44):1121–4.

[28] Justice AC, Dombrowski E, Conigliaro J, et al. Veterans Aging Cohort Study (VACS): overview and description. Med Care 2006;44(8 Suppl 2):S13–24.

[29] Wolff AJ, O'Donnell AE. Pulmonary effects of illicit drug use. Clin Chest Med 2004;25(1):203–16.

[30] Haim DY, Lippmann ML, Goldberg SK, et al. The pulmonary complications of crack cocaine. A comprehensive review. Chest 1995;107(1):233–40.

[31] Moore BA, Augustson EM, Moser RP, et al. Respiratory effects of marijuana and tobacco use in a U.S. sample. J Gen Intern Med 2005;20(1):33–7.

[32] Tashkin DP. Airway effects of marijuana, cocaine, and other inhaled illicit agents. Curr Opin Pulm Med 2001;7(2):43–61.

[33] Tetrault JM, Crothers K, Moore BA, et al. Effects of marijuana smoking on pulmonary function and respiratory complications: a systematic review. Arch Intern Med 2007;167(3):221–8.

[34] Cohen BH, Celentano DD, Chase GA, et al. Alcohol consumption and airway obstruction. Am Rev Respir Dis 1980;121(2):205–15.

[35] Lange P, Groth S, Mortensen J, et al. Pulmonary function is influenced by heavy alcohol consumption. Am Rev Respir Dis 1988;137(5):1119–23.

[36] Balmes J, Becklake M, Blanc P, et al. American Thoracic Society Statement: occupational contribution to the burden of airway disease. Am J Respir Crit Care Med 2003;167(5):787–97.

[37] Prescott E, Vestbo J. Socioeconomic status and chronic obstructive pulmonary disease. Thorax 1999;54(8):737–41.

[38] Chen Y, Breithaupt K, Muhajarine N. Occurrence of chronic obstructive pulmonary disease among Canadians and sex-related risk factors. J Clin Epidemiol 2000;53(7):755–61.

[39] Sethi S. Bacterial infection and the pathogenesis of COPD. Chest 2000;117(5 Suppl 1):286S–91S.

[40] Hogg JC. Role of latent viral infections in chronic obstructive pulmonary disease and asthma. Am J Respir Crit Care Med 2001;164(10 Pt 2):S71–5.

[41] Morris A, Sciurba FC, Lebedeva IP, et al. Association of chronic obstructive pulmonary disease severity and Pneumocystis colonization. Am J Respir Crit Care Med 2004;170(4):408–13.

[42] Morris AM, Huang L, Bacchetti P, et al. Permanent declines in pulmonary function following pneumonia in human immunodeficiency virus-infected persons. The pulmonary complications of HIV infection study group. Am J Respir Crit Care Med 2000;162(2 Pt 1):612–6.

[43] Wang Z, Zheng T, Zhu Z, et al. Interferon gamma induction of pulmonary emphysema in the adult murine lung. J Exp Med 2000;192(11):1587–600.

[44] Saetta M, Baraldo S, Corbino L, et al. CD8+ve cells in the lungs of smokers with chronic obstructive

pulmonary disease. Am J Respir Crit Care Med 1999;160(2):711–7.

[45] Twigg HL 3rd, Spain BA, Soliman DM, et al. Production of interferon-gamma by lung lymphocytes in HIV-infected individuals. Am J Physiol 1999; 276(2 Pt 1):L256–62.

[46] Twigg HL, Soliman DM, Day RB, et al. Lymphocytic alveolitis, bronchoalveolar lavage viral load, and outcome in human immunodeficiency virus infection. Am J Respir Crit Care Med 1999;159(5 Pt 1): 1439–44.

[47] Hogg JC, Hegele RG. Adenovirus and Epstein-Barr virus in lung disease. Semin Respir Infect 1995;10(4): 244–53.

[48] Seemungal T, Harper-Owen R, Bhowmik A, et al. Respiratory viruses, symptoms, and inflammatory markers in acute exacerbations and stable chronic obstructive pulmonary disease. Am J Respir Crit Care Med 2001;164(9):1618–23.

[49] Wilkinson TM, Patel IS, Wilks M, et al. Airway bacterial load and FEV1 decline in patients with chronic obstructive pulmonary disease. Am J Respir Crit Care Med 2003;167(8):1090–5.

[50] Calderon E, de la Horra C, Medrano FJ, et al. Pneumocystis jiroveci isolates with dihydropteroate synthase mutations in patients with chronic bronchitis. Eur J Clin Microbiol Infect Dis 2004;23(7):545–9.

[51] Morris A, Kingsley LA, Groner G, et al. Prevalence and clinical predictors of Pneumocystis colonization among HIV-infected men. AIDS 2004;18(5):793–8.

[52] MacNee W. Oxidants/antioxidants and COPD. Chest 2000;117(5 Suppl 1):303S–17S.

[53] MacNee W. Pulmonary and systemic oxidant/antioxidant imbalance in chronic obstructive pulmonary disease. Proc Am Thorac Soc 2005;2(1):50–60.

[54] Treitinger A, Spada C, Verdi JC, et al. Decreased antioxidant defence in individuals infected by the human immunodeficiency virus. Eur J Clin Invest 2000;30(5):454–9.

[55] Buhl R. Imbalance between oxidants and antioxidants in the lungs of HIV-seropositive individuals. Chem Biol Interact 1994;91(2–3):147–58.

[56] Revillard JP, Vincent CM, Favier AE, et al. Lipid peroxidation in human immunodeficiency virus infection. J Acquir Immune Defic Syndr 1992;5(6):637–8.

[57] Pacht ER, Diaz P, Clanton T, et al. Alveolar fluid glutathione decreases in asymptomatic HIV-seropositive subjects over time. Chest 1997;112(3):785–8.

[58] Braithwaite RS, Justice AC, Chang CC, et al. Estimating the proportion of patients infected with HIV who will die of comorbid diseases. Am J Med 2005;118(8):890–8.

[59] Krentz HB, Kliewer G, Gill MJ. Changing mortality rates and causes of death for HIV-infected individuals living in Southern Alberta, Canada from 1984 to 2003. HIV Med 2005;6(2):99–106.

[60] Crum NF, Riffenburgh RH, Wegner S, et al. Comparisons of causes of death and mortality rates among HIV-infected persons: analysis of the pre-,

early, and late HAART (highly active antiretroviral therapy) eras. J Acquir Immune Defic Syndr 2006; 41(2):194–200.

[61] Crothers K, Justice AC, Rimland D, et al. Increased infectious and non-infectious pulmonary diseases among HIV positive compared to HIV negative veterans. Proc Am Thorac Soc 2006;3:A477.

[62] Wallace JM, Hansen NI, Lavange L, et al. Respiratory disease trends in the pulmonary complications of HIV infection study cohort. Pulmonary complications of HIV infection study group. Am J Respir Crit Care Med 1997;155(1):72–80.

[63] Crothers K, Griffith TA, McGinnis KA, et al. The impact of cigarette smoking on mortality, quality of life, and comorbid illness among HIV-positive veterans. J Gen Intern Med 2005; 20(12):1142–5.

[64] Celli BR, MacNee W. Standards for the diagnosis and treatment of patients with COPD: a summary of the ATS/ERS position paper. Eur Respir J 2004;23(6):932–46.

[65] Calverley PM, Anderson JA, Celli B, et al. Salmeterol and fluticasone propionate and survival in chronic obstructive pulmonary disease. N Engl J Med 2007; 356(8):775–89.

[66] Crothers K, Goulet JL, Rodriguez-Barradas MC, et al. Decreased awareness of current smoking among health care providers of HIV-positive compared to HIV-negative veterans. J Gen Intern Med 2007;22(6):749–54.

[67] Cummins D, Trotter G, Moussa M, et al. Smoking cessation for clients who are HIV-positive. Nurs Stand 2005;20(12):41–7.

[68] Vidrine DJ, Arduino RC, Lazev AB, et al. A randomized trial of a proactive cellular telephone intervention for smokers living with HIV/AIDS. AIDS 2006;20(2):253–60.

[69] Wewers ME, Neidig JL, Kihm KE. The feasibility of a nurse-managed, peer-led tobacco cessation intervention among HIV-positive smokers. J Assoc Nurses AIDS Care 2000;11(6):37–44.

[70] An LC, Zhu SH, Nelson DB, et al. Benefits of telephone care over primary care for smoking cessation: a randomized trial. Arch Intern Med 2006;166(5):536–42.

[71] Oursler KK, Goulet JL, Leaf DA, et al. Association of comorbidity with physical disability in older HIV-infected adults. AIDS Patient Care STDS 2006; 20(11):782–91.

[72] Nici L, Donner C, Wouters E, et al. American Thoracic Society/European Respiratory Society statement on pulmonary rehabilitation. Am J Respir Crit Care Med 2006;173(12):1390–413.

[73] Authier FJ, Chariot P, Gherardi RK. Skeletal muscle involvement in human immunodeficiency virus (HIV)-infected patients in the era of highly active antiretroviral therapy (HAART). Muscle Nerve 2005;32(3):247–60.

[74] Oursler KK, Sorkin JD, Smith BA, et al. Reduced aerobic capacity and physical functioning in older

HIV-infected men. AIDS Res Hum Retroviruses 2006;22(11):1113–21.

[75] Schulz L, Nagaraja HN, Rague N, et al. Respiratory muscle dysfunction associated with human immunodeficiency virus infection. Am J Respir Crit Care Med 1997;155(3):1080–4.

[76] Nixon S, O'Brien K, Glazier RH, Tynan AM. Aerobic exercise interventions for adults living with HIV/AIDS. Cochrane Database Syst Rev 2005;2: CD001796.

[77] O'Brien K, Nixon S, Glazier RH, Tynan AM. Progressive resistive exercise interventions for adults living with HIV/AIDS. Cochrane Database Syst Rev 2004;4:CD004248.

[78] Coultas DB, Mapel D, Gagnon R, et al. The health impact of undiagnosed airflow obstruction in a national sample of United States adults. Am J Respir Crit Care Med 2001;164(3):372–7.

[79] Sin DD, McAlister FA, Man SF, et al. Contemporary management of chronic obstructive pulmonary disease: scientific review. JAMA 2003;290(17):2301–12.

[80] Tomas LH, Varkey B. Improving health-related quality of life in chronic obstructive pulmonary disease. Curr Opin Pulm Med 2004;10(2):120–7.

CLINICS
IN CHEST
MEDICINE

Clin Chest Med 28 (2007) 589–607

Update on the Pharmacologic Therapy for Chronic Obstructive Pulmonary Disease

Nicola A. Hanania, MD, MS[a],*, Amir Sharafkhaneh, MD[b]

[a]Asthma Clinical Research Center, Section of Pulmonary and Critical Care Medicine, Baylor College of Medicine, 1504 Taub Loop, Houston, TX 77030, USA
[b]Section of Pulmonary and Critical Care Medicine, Baylor College of Medicine, 1504 Taub Loop, Houston, TX 77030, USA

Chronic obstructive pulmonary disease (COPD) is a growing worldwide problem [1,2]. The most distressing symptoms for patients who have COPD are dyspnea, exercise intolerance, and the progressive inability to engage in activities of daily living. These clinical manifestations of COPD ultimately lead to poor health-related quality of life. As with many other chronic diseases, a multimodality approach to the management of COPD is advocated in several published, evidence-based guidelines [3,4]. The main goals of management of COPD are focused on relieving symptoms, improving health status, preventing lung function decline, improving exercise performance, preventing exacerbations, and decreasing mortality. Furthermore, these goals should be reached with minimal side effects from treatment. Traditional COPD therapies have focused on symptom control with the aim of alleviating the problems of reduced airflow and declining lung function. With improved knowledge about the multicomponent nature of the disease, however, recent therapeutic approaches aim to target the symptoms and the inflammation that underlie and drive COPD [5].

Current treatment recommendations

Evidence-based guidelines for COPD emphasize a comprehensive and stepwise approach to the management of COPD and stipulate that all patients who are symptomatic merit a trial of pharmacologic intervention (Table 1) [3,4]. Short-acting bronchodilators given when needed are recommended for patients who have intermittent symptoms, such as cough, wheeze, or exertional dyspnea. Maintenance therapy should be initiated, however, in patients who have persistent daily symptoms, such as dyspnea or nighttime awakenings, despite use of as-needed short-acting agents. In this setting, maintenance treatment should be initiated with a long-acting bronchodilator or, alternatively, a short-acting agent given 4 times per day. Rescue therapy with albuterol should be continued as needed. If the benefit of treatment is limited, then a bronchodilator from another drug class or a combination of two drug classes (eg, long-acting bronchodilator plus inhaled corticosteroid [ICS]) should be attempted. The addition of regular ICS therapy should be considered in patients who have forced expiratory volume in 1 second (FEV_1) less than 50% of predicted who have had disease exacerbations requiring a course of oral steroids or antibiotic at least once in the preceding year.

Current medications used for COPD can reduce or abolish symptoms and the number and severity of exacerbations and can improve exercise capacity and health status [6]. However, several recent surveys also show that patients who have COPD tend to be undertreated with maintenance medications. For example, the Confronting COPD survey, a telephone interview of 447 patients who had mild to moderate COPD in the United States, showed that only 67% of patients reported taking prescription medications for treatment of COPD, which most commonly included short-acting β_2-agonists (44% of patients), followed by ICS (31%), anticholinergics (26%), and theophylline (12%) [7].

* Corresponding author.
E-mail address: hanania@bcm.edu (N.A. Hanania).

0272-5231/07/$ - see front matter © 2007 Elsevier Inc. All rights reserved.
doi:10.1016/j.ccm.2007.06.007

Table 1
Stepwise approach to the pharmacologic management of chronic obstructive pulmonary disease

Severity	Spirometric findings	Intervention
Stage I: mild	$FEV_1/FVC < 70\%$ $FEV_1 \geq 80\%$	Add a short-acting bronchodilator to be used when needed; anticholinergic or β_2-adrenoceptor agonist
Stage II: moderate	$FEV_1/FVC < 70\%$ $50\% \leq FEV1 < 80\%$	Add one or more long-acting bronchodilators on a scheduled basis. Consider pulmonary rehabilitation.
Stage III: severe	$FEV_1/FVC < 70\%$ $30\% \leq FEV_1 < 50\%$	Add inhaled steroids if repeated exacerbations.
Stage IV: very severe	$FEV_1/FVC < 70\%$ $FEV_1 < 30\%$	Evaluate for adding oxygen. Consider surgical options.

Assessing response to therapy in chronic obstructive pulmonary disease

Assessment of lung function in COPD is important in the diagnosis, staging, and determination of the prognosis of the disease but it should not be used as the sole measure to assess clinical response to treatment of COPD medications. In addition to spirometry measures (FEV_1, forced vital capacity [FVC], and FEV_1/FVC), several other physiologic measures should be considered to determine a response to therapy [8–10]. These include improvement in lung volumes (inspiratory capacity) and improvement in exercise tolerance. Other outcome measures that are important in determining if a treatment is effective include improvement in health status, decrease in exacerbation rate or severity, improvement in dyspnea, and improvement of exercise tolerance. Ultimately, the long-term effectiveness of a treatment usually is assessed by determining its effect on the decline in lung function or on mortality.

Pharmacologic interventions for smoking cessation

Smoking cessation is the single most effective and cost-effective intervention to reduce the progression of COPD and should be attempted in all patients [11]. Unfortunately, even with the best intervention strategies, less than a third of smokers become sustained quitters [12]. Furthermore, once individuals develop demonstrable airflow obstruction, their symptoms and airway inflammation may persist even after smoking cessation [13,14]. Several effective therapies for tobacco dependence are available and should be considered in those patients interested in quitting smoking (Table 2)

[15–17]. Nicotine replacement therapy can be delivered by many routes: oral, inhaled, sublingual, or transdermal, and its use with or without the antidepressant, bupropion, is shown to increase 1-year smoking cessation rates in clinical trials. Other antidepressants, such as nortriptyline and clonidine, also have been studied with limited efficacy data. More recently, varenicline, an $\alpha4\beta2$ nicotinic receptor partial agonist, was approved for smoking cessation in the United States [18,19]. Although clinical studies on its use in COPD are ongoing, its efficacy in diminishing withdrawal symptoms and achieving a smoking cessation status is described in the general population in several recent studies [20–23]. A total of 3659 patients was included in these studies, which showed that this medication was superior to bupropion and to nicotine patches. The current approved course of therapy with varenicline is for 12 weeks; however, the use of additional 12 weeks of maintenance therapy in those who were successful in quitting showed a reduction in the relapse rate.

Bronchodilator therapy

General considerations

Bronchodilators are believed to work primarily through their direct relaxation effect on airway smooth muscle cells, although many have non-bronchodilator activities, which may contribute to their beneficial effects in COPD. Three classes of bronchodilators—β_2-agonists, anticholinergics, and theophylline—currently are available and can be used individually or in combination (Table 3). Several issues need to be considered when assessing the response to bronchodilator therapy. First, the lack of acute response to one class of

Table 2
Pharmacologic therapies for smoking cessation

	Dose	Frequency
Oral		
Nicotine polacrilex	2 mg, 4 mg	10–20 mg/d
		Every 1–2 hours
Nicotine lozenges/tablets	1 mg, 2 mg	10–20 mg/d
		1 piece every hour
Buproprion sustained release	150 mg	150 mg for 3 days, then 300 mg each day
Varenicline	1 mg	Initial 1-week dose titration, then 1 mg twice daily for 12 weeks
Patch		
Transdermal nicotine, three types	21, 14, 7 mg	Over 24 hours
	15, 10, 5 mg	Over 16 hours
	22, 11 mg	Over 24 hours
Inhaled		
Nasal nicotine spray	0.5 mg/inhalation	10–40 mg/d in hourly or as-needed dosing
Nicotine inhaler	10 mg/ampule	6–10 ampule/d

bronchodilator does not imply nonresponsiveness to another. Donohue [24] reported that 73% of 813 patients who had COPD increased their FEV_1 by greater than or equal to 12% or 200 mL after long-term salmeterol treatment. However, 11% of patients showed a similar increase in FEV_1 after acute administration of ipratropium, 27% after albuterol, and 35% with

Table 3
Pharmacologic agents used commonly for chronic obstructive pulmonary disease

Short-acting agents	Long-acting agents
β-Adrenoceptor agonists	β-Adrenoceptor agonists
Albuterol (MDI, NS)	Salmeterol (DPI)
Levalbuterol (MDI, NS)	Formoterol (DPI, NS)
Pirbuterol (MDI)	Arformoterol (NS)
Anticholinergic	Anticholinergic
Ipratropium bromide	Tiotropium bromide
(MDI, NS)	(DPI)
Fixed combination	Fixed combination
Albuterol/ipratropium	Salmeterol/vluticasone[a]
(MDI, NS)	(DPI, MDI)
	Formoterol/budesonide[b]
	(DPI, MDI)
	Methylxanthines
	Theophylline (PO)

Abbreviations: NS, nebulized solution; PO, oral preparation.
[a] Only one dose formulation (250/50) approved for COPD in the United States.
[b] Currently not approved for COPD in United States.

both drugs combined. One further consideration is that a patient's FEV_1 response to acute bronchodilator therapy does not predict long-term response to bronchodilator therapy and may vary from day to day. Calverley and colleagues [25] performed acute bronchodilator testing using albuterol, ipratropium bromide, or a combination of the two on 660 patients who had COPD who had been classified according to European Respiratory Society and American Thoracic Society (ATS) spirometric criteria. Over the 2-month study period, 55% of patients classified as having "irreversible" airflow obstruction by ATS criteria changed to "reversible" status on at least one of the visits. In summary, the acute response to short-acting bronchodilators is of limited value in deciding future response to long-acting agents. In addition, studies that stratify patients as "responders" versus "nonresponders" consistently demonstrate a similar trend in the response to the therapeutic agent being investigated in both groups. The clinical efficacy of bronchodilators traditionally has been assessed by the degree of improvement FEV_1. Other physiologic measures, however, such as the change in inspiratory capacity, correlate better with change in symptoms, such as dyspnea and exercise tolerance [26]. This suggests that assessment of bronchodilator treatment using indices of hyperinflation or air trapping may provide a better indicator of efficacy [27]. Although changes in lung volumes are independent of changes in FEV_1, several studies have demonstrated that the more sustained airway patency offered by long-acting bronchodilators reduces air trapping [28,29]. Several other outcome measures also are used to assess response to bronchodilator therapy. COPD exacerbation is an important but occasionally overlooked parameter [30,31]. The use of long-acting β2-adrenoceptor agonists and long-acting anticholinergic agents reduces the frequency of exacerbation and severity of individual exacerbations [32–34].

The effects of long-acting bronchodilators on health status also are well documented in several clinical trials [32,34–37]. Dyspnea is a common and troublesome manifestation of COPD and its relief is another important goal of bronchodilator therapy. Instruments available to assess dyspnea can either discriminate the level of dyspnea (discriminative) or evaluate dyspnea over time (evaluative). An instrument that is used widely is the Baseline and Transition Dyspnea Index, which assesses breathlessness in domains related to functional impairment, magnitude of task, and magnitude of effort. This instrument is shown responsive to a variety of therapeutic modalities, such as long-acting bronchodilator use. More recently, self-administered versions of this instrument have been described, which may eliminate interviewer bias and decrease the time needed for questionnaire administration. Exercise limitation is another significant problem for patients who have COPD, and it can be assessed using several different techniques. The simplest method to assess exercise tolerance is the 6-minute walk distance, commonly used to assess the functional status of patients who have COPD [38]. It is a reliable, objective, inexpensive, and easy-to-apply tool, regardless of a patient's age or educational level. Other methods to assess exercise tolerance include incremental and steady state cardiopulmonary exercise testing (CPET). CPET is helpful in evaluating mechanisms of improvement in dyspnea secondary to pharmacologic agents, such as long-acting bronchodilators [39–41].

The long-term effects of bronchodilators used currently are not well known and long-term studies will contribute to understanding their effects on the natural history of the disease. The long-term effects of the long-acting β-agonist, salmeterol, and salmeterol/fluticasone propionate combination (SFC) on all-cause mortality and other outcomes over 3 years have been investigated in a recently published trial (Towards a Revolution in COPD Health [TORCH]) [42,43]. Another trial, now underway, will examine the effect of tiotropium on the decline in postbronchodilator FEV_1 over 4 years (the Understanding of Potential Long-term Impact on Function with Tiotropium [UPLIFT] trial) [44].

To achieve maximal benefit, a bronchodilator must be delivered correctly to the airway using proper technique. Inhaled bronchodilators traditionally have been delivered to the lung using a metered-dose inhaler (MDI). A significant number of patients who have COPD cannot coordinate their breathing effectively using a MDI. This problem may be remedied by the use of a dry powder inhaler (DPI), a MDI with a spacer device or a nebulizer. The results of a systematic review of 59 randomized controlled trials in which the same drug (bronchodilator or ICS) was delivered using different delivery devices (MDI with or without a spacer, DPI, or a nebulizer) in patients who had asthma or COPD recently were published [45]. This review concludes, "for the treatment of COPD in the outpatient setting, the MDI, with or without spacer/holding chamber, the nebulizer, and the DPI were all appropriate for the delivery of inhaled β2-agonists and anticholinergic agents."

β2-Adrenoceptor agonists

Pharmacology

β2-adrenoceptor agonists act by binding to the β2-adrenoceptor (β2-AR), which is a member of the seven transmembrane domains, G protein–coupled family of receptors [46]. Although β2-ARs are present in high density in airway smooth muscle cells, they also are present in submucosal glands, vascular endothelium, ciliated epithelium, mast cells, circulating inflammatory cells (such as eosinophils and lymphocytes), Clara cells, type II pneumocytes, and cholinergic ganglia. Upon agonist binding to receptor, adenylyl cyclase is activated via the signal transducing G_s protein, which results in a rise in cellular cyclic adenosine monophosphate (cAMP) levels and activation of protein kinase A (PKA). The precise PKA phosphorylation targets mediating bronchial smooth muscle relaxation are not understood fully but likely include myosin light chain kinase and Ca^{++}-dependent K^+ channels [46]. β2-adrenoceptor agonists are delivered through the inhaled or oral route, although the later is limited because of the increased risk for adverse systemic effects. There are several important pharmacologic differences among the existing agents [46,47]. First, the onset of action is similar for albuterol and formoterol (1–3 minutes) but it is more prolonged with salmeterol. This difference in onset of action is related to the lipophilicity of each of these agents and their ability to activate the β_2-AR in the aqueous phase (albuterol and formoterol). Albuterol has a short duration of action lasting less than 6 hours, whereas the duration of action of salmeterol and formoterol is approximately 12 hours. Second, these agents differ significantly in their ability to activate the β_2-AR (intrinsic efficacy). The efficacy of β_2-AR activation by these agents is dependent on their affinity and potency [46]. Although formoterol has a high intrinsic efficacy (ie, is a strong agonist), albuterol and salmeterol have a very low intrinsic efficacy (ie, are weak agonists). The clinical relevance of this difference needs to be explored further in future trials. The majority of β_2-adrenoceptor agonists currently used are racemic compounds, which contain a 50-50 mixture of the (R)- and (S)-enantiomers of the agonist. Recently, the (R)-enantiomer of albuterol (levalbuterol) [48,49] and the (R,R)-enantiomer of formoterol (arformoterol) were approved for clinical use in the management of COPD [50,51]. Much of the pharmacologic activity of the agonist usually resides in the effects of the (R)-enantiomer; the (S)-enantiomer is believed to have no bronchodilator effects but may induce deleterious effects. Data from an in vitro study indicate that (S,S)-formoterol is not biologically inert, such that in racemic mixtures, it inhibits the beneficial effects of (R,R)-formoterol on proliferation, anti-inflammatory cellular surface marker expression, and cytokine secretion [52]. The effectiveness and cost-effectiveness of isomeric versus racemic β_2-adrenoceptor agonists in the management of airway diseases, such as COPD, however, need to be explored further and remain controversial [53,54].

Clinical benefits

Short-acting β_2-adrenoceptor agonists have a rapid onset of action and are effective for rescue of symptoms in COPD. Albuterol is the agent used most commonly. In addition to their bronchodilatory properties, these agents are effective in increasing mucociliary clearance. A systematic review showed that regular use of short-acting β_2-adrenoceptor agonists in COPD was associated with improvement in lung function and dyspnea [55]. The two currently available long-acting β_2-adrenoceptor agonists (LABAs)—salmeterol and formoterol—are shown to improve lung function, health status, and symptom reduction significantly compared with placebo [28,56–58] and ipratropium [34,59]. In addition, because of formoterol's

fast onset of action, it has a potential role in the management of acute COPD exacerbation either as a sole medication or in combination with another bronchodilator [60,61] and for use as a rescue and maintenance medication [62]. A recent study demonstrated a superior effect of formoterol compared with tiotropium bromide in improving FEV_1 in the first 2 hours after administration; however, the area under the curve FEV_1 over 12 hours was similar in these two agents [63]. Several systematic reviews of LABAs reveal that these agents can reduce the rate of COPD exacerbations by approximately 15% to 20% [32,64]. In a study of 634 patients who have COPD, the administration of salmeterol for 12 months improved health outcomes, including exacerbations, especially in patients who complied with therapy [65].

Nonbronchodilator effects of β_2-adrenoceptor agonists

Although the major action of β_2-adrenoceptor agonists on airways is relaxation of airway smooth muscles, they also exert several effects mediated through the activation of β_2-ARs expressed on resident airway cells, such as epithelial cells, mast cells, and circulating inflammatory cells, such as eosinophils and neutrophils [66,67]. These effects include inhibition of airway smooth muscle cell proliferation and inflammatory mediator release and nonsmooth muscle effects, such as stimulation of mucociliary transport [68], cytoprotection of the respiratory mucosa, and attenuation of neutrophil recruitment and activation [67]. Many of these effects are described within in vitro studies, however, and in vivo studies are needed to explore these effects fully. More recently, the physiologic and clinical benefits of LABAs have been shown to be enhanced when administered in conjunction with ICSs [69–72], which may translate to clinical benefits (discussed later).

Anticholinergic bronchodilators

Parasympathetic activity in the large- and medium-sized airways is mediated through the muscarinic receptors (M_1 and M_3) and results in airways smooth-muscle contraction, mucus secretion, and possibly increased ciliary activity. M_2 receptors are located on the postganglionic parasympathetic nerves and inhibit acetylcholine release from the nerve terminals. Increased cholinergic tone is important in the pathogenesis of COPD, contributing to increased bronchial smooth muscle tone and to mucus hypersecretion [73,74]. Thus, anticholinergic agents reduce airway tone and improve expiratory flow limitation, hyperinflation, and exercise capacity in patients who have COPD. Two anticholinergic bronchodilators currently are available for clinical use in the United States. The short-acting anticholinergic agent, ipratropium bromide, acts on all three muscarinic receptors. Its short duration of action requires dosing every 6 hours.

The longer-acting anticholinergic agent, tiotropium bromide (dosed once daily), binds to all three receptor subtypes; however, it dissociates rapidly from M_2 receptors. In contrast, its prolonged dissociation half-life from M_3 receptors of nearly 35 hours results in a prolonged bronchodilatory effect. Peak bronchodilation occurs within 1 to 3 hours and continues for up to 32 hours, with a dip between 16 and 24 hours related to circadian change. The bronchoprotective effect of tiotropium against a bronchospastic agent continues, however, up to 48 hours [75].

Clinical benefits

The short-acting ipratropium has been used for many years either as monotherapy or in combination with albuterol in the maintenance therapy for COPD [27,76,77]. Several studies show, however, that the use of long-acting bronchodilators is superior in improving health outcomes. The use of tiotropium in patients who have COPD results in improved health status, dyspnea, and exercise capacity and reduced hyperinflation and COPD exacerbation rate in patients who have moderate to severe COPD relative to placebo [36,40,78] and ipratropium [37]. Data from large long-term trials showed that trough FEV_1 increased by 100 to 150 mL and the peak FEV_1 increased by 150 to 200 mL above the trough level after inhalation of 18 micrograms of tiotropium. No loss of efficacy was seen over the course of 1 year of regular treatment with tiotropium. Furthermore, in a multicenter Veterans Administration trial involving 1829 patients who had severe COPD, the addition of tiotropium to other COPD therapies reduced acute COPD exacerbations significantly and reduced COPD hospitalizations when compared with placebo [33]. Data from three more recent studies, specifically designed to explore the potential differences between tiotropium and salmeterol, seem to indicate a greater efficacy of tiotropium [79–81]. An ongoing large clinical trial will evaluate the effect of tiotropium on the decline of lung function over a 4-year period [44].

Nonbronchodilator effects of anticholinergics

Some nonbronchodilator effects of the existing anticholinergic agents are reported [82]. Furthermore, results from a recent study performed on sputum cells obtained from patients who had COPD demonstrate that muscarinic receptors may be involved in airway inflammation in subjects who have COPD through acetylcholine-induced, ERK1/2-dependent leukotriene B4 (LTB_4) release [83]. These results suggest that anticholinergic therapy may contribute to reduced neutrophilic inflammation in COPD; however, these findings need to be evaluated further in humans.

Methylxanthines

Theophylline is a nonselective phosphodiesterase inhibitor that acts as a weak bronchodilator and a respiratory stimulant. It is shown to improve diaphragmatic contractility and has some anti-inflammatory properties [84]. Because of its potential ability to activate the histone deacetylase system, theophylline may have the ability of enhancing the effects of ICSs in patients who have COPD [85,86]. Several studies demonstrate beneficial effects of theophylline when added to other treatment in patients who have COPD [87,88]. Because of potential adverse effects and a narrow therapeutic index, however, theophylline should be used only when symptoms persist despite optimal alternate bronchodilator therapy.

Safety of bronchodilator therapy

Although the safety of LABAs as monotherapy in asthma recently has been questioned [89], the use of these medications in COPD generally is described as safe. In general, short-acting β_2-agonists are well tolerated, apart from occasional episodes of tachycardia and tremor. It is reported that the continued use of β_2-agonists may be associated with an increase in cardiovascular risk compared with placebo [90]. A recent meta-analysis (N = 2853) of data from seven clinical trials examining the effects of salmeterol in patients who had COPD, however, showed no clinically significant difference in the incidence of cardiovascular events between salmeterol and placebo [91]. It also is suggested that tolerance to the bronchodilator effects of LABAs may occur with their prolonged use in COPD [79,92]. A study examining the bronchodilator effect of long-term use of salmeterol, however, demonstrated a sustained bronchodilator effect for salmeterol administered for 6 months [58]. Data from the recently completed TORCH study suggest that 3-year chronic use of salmeterol as monotherapy in patients who had COPD produced no increase in mortality [43], as was suggested by the Salmeterol Multicenter Asthma Research Trial (SMART) in patients who had asthma [89]. Nevertheless, β-agonists should be used with caution in patients who have underlying cardiac disorders, including ischemic heart disease or unstable cardiac arrhythmia [90,93].

The use of anticholinergics may be associated with class-related side effects, such as dry mouth, an increased risk for glaucoma, and urinary retention. When used in recommended doses, however, agents used currently generally are safe, as the quaternary nitrogen atom prevents them from being absorbed systemically. These agents, however, should be used with caution in patients who have bladder neck obstruction resulting from prostatism and in patients who have glaucoma. The long-term safety of tiotropium over 4 years is being investigated in the UPLIFT study, currently underway [44]. A recent meta-analysis [94], which included randomized controlled trials of at least 3 months' duration that evaluated anticholinergic or β_2-agonist use compared with placebo or each other in patients who had COPD, documented that although inhaled anticholinergics significantly reduced severe exacerbations and respiratory deaths in patients who had COPD, β_2-adrenoceptor agonists were associated with an increased risk for respiratory deaths. As highlighted by the investigators themselves, however, this meta-analysis had several methodologic limitations that limited the validity of its results.

Theophylline is associated with tremors and nausea and, less frequently, with cardiac arrhythmias and seizures [95]. The risk for such adverse events can be reduced by monitoring the drug's plasma levels and reducing the dose accordingly.

Anti-inflammatory therapy

Increasingly, COPD is recognized as an inflammatory disorder and the severity of airway inflammation is related directly to the severity of the underlying COPD [96]. Airway inflammation is present even in smokers who are physiologically "normal" and in those who quit smoking. Corticosteroids are the only anti-inflammatory medications available for use in selected patients who have COPD.

Given the prominence of airway inflammation in COPD, highly potent but nonspecific anti-inflammatory agents, such as corticosteroids, could be expected to have some effects on lung function and health outcomes of patients who have COPD. Although these agents seem to have minimal significant effects on key inflammatory chemoattractants, such as interleukin (IL)-8, tumor necrosis factor α (TNF-α), and matrix metalloproteinases (MMPs) [97], there are data to suggest an association with reduced neutrophil chemotaxis [98]. The clinical relevance of this observation remains uncertain. During exacerbations, where there is a large increase in the concentrations of proinflammatory cells, including neutrophils, systemic corticosteroids improve lung function significantly, shorten hospital stays, and reduce the risk for relapses as compared with placebo [99,100].

Current guidelines recommend the use of regular treatment with ICS for symptomatic patients who suffer frequent exacerbations and whose FEV_1 is less than 50% of predicted [3,4]. Several, large, 3-year, randomized trials have failed to show a significant effect of ICS on the rate of decline of FEV_1 compared with placebo [101–104]. These trials excluded patients who had any significant bronchodilator reversibility, however, a subpopulation of patients who have COPD who theoretically may benefit most from ICS. Moreover, a meta-analysis by Sutherland and colleagues [105] showed that high-dose ICS did reduce the rate of decline in FEV_1 by 9.9 mL per year compared with placebo ($P = .01$). In a recent pooled analysis of seven studies, ICS therapy was shown more effective in ex-smokers than in current smokers and in women compared with men who had COPD in improving lung function in the first 6 months of therapy. After 6 months, however, ICS therapy did not modify the decline in FEV_1 among those who completed these randomized clinical trials [106]. Whether or not this short-term effect on lung function is important clinically remains unresolved. It is generally agreed, however, that ICSs have a positive influence on clinical endpoints in patients who have COPD. In the Inhaled Steroids in Obstructive Lung Disease (ISOLDE) trial, the median exacerbation rate was reduced by 25% with fluticasone propionate compared with placebo, with a concomitant significant reduction in health status deterioration [107,108]. These effects on reduction of exacerbations and improvement in health status also were observed in several other studies, including the recently published 3-year study (TORCH) [32,43,109]. Furthermore, withdrawal from treatment with ICS was associated with a more rapid onset and increased recurrence of exacerbations and with a significant deterioration in health status [110,111]. Observational studies suggested reductions in morbidity and possibly even mortality from long-term ICS therapy [109,112–114]; many of these studies, however, did not correct for the immortal time bias in their analyses [115]. Furthermore, there was no effect of ICS on survival in the prospective 3-year study (TORCH) [43].

Combination therapy

Bronchodilator combination therapy

Current guidelines highlight the fact that for patients whose conditions are not controlled with bronchodilator monotherapy, the use of a combination of more than one class of bronchodilators may be more effective than the use of single agents with respect to improvements in lung function and symptoms and reducing the risk for adverse events [116–118].

In particular, the use of an inhaled anticholinergic with a β_2-adrenoceptor agonist seems to be a convenient way of delivering treatment and obtaining better results. Large studies have demonstrated that the combination of the short-acting β_2-adrenoceptor agonist, albuterol, with the short-acting anticholinergic, ipratropium, is superior to either single agent alone [119]. Some trials have highlighted that the addition of LABAs to ipratropium is more effective than either agent used alone [120,121]. In a 12-week trial, ZuWallack and colleagues [122] showed that salmeterol plus theophylline caused significantly greater improvements in pulmonary function and symptoms than either single agent. Considering that formoterol provides a greater degree of early bronchodilation (in the first 2 hours) than tiotropium and comparable bronchodilation over 12 hours [63], the bronchodilatory effects of single doses of formoterol (12 μg) and tiotropium (18 μg) versus formoterol (12 μg) plus tiotropium (18 μg) given together were examined in stable COPD [123]. Formoterol and tiotropium appeared complementary. More recently, van Noord and colleagues [124] explored these effects elicited by 6 weeks of treatment with tiotropium (18 μg once daily in the morning), or formoterol (12 μg twice a day) versus tiotropium (18 μg) versus formoterol (12 μg once daily in the morning) in patients suffering from moderate to severe COPD. Patients receiving combination treatment had a greater improvement in FEV_1 and FVC compared with those receiving the individual agents over 24 hours. Tiotropium was superior to formoterol for FEV_1 response over 0 to 12 hours (owing to significant differences from 8 to 12 hours), but the two treatments were not significantly different for FEV_1 over 12 to 24 hours or 0 to 24 hours. A similar observation was documented in a more recently published 2-week study of tiotropium alone or tiotropium plus formoterol once or twice daily after a 2-week pretreatment period with tiotropium. In this study, the use of an additional evening dose of formoterol had a clear added benefit compared with once-a-day formoterol [125].

Inhaled corticosteroid/long-acting β_2-agonist combination therapy

Although corticosteroids and LABAs are effective by themselves in improving lung function and reducing exacerbations, their beneficial effects are amplified when they are given together. There is a large and growing body of experimental and clinical evidence supporting the use of combination therapy with ICSs and LABAs for the long-term treatment of patients who have COPD who have moderate to severe disease. The use of ICS and LABA combination products are shown to improve lung function, symptoms, and health status and to reduce exacerbations in patients who have moderate to severe COPD [126–129].

The rationale for using a combination of ICS and a long-acting β_2-agonist may be secondary to their complementary effects at the receptor level. Corticosteroids can modulate β_2-receptors and their function by several mechanisms, including protection against desensitization and development of tolerance, increased efficiency of receptor coupling, and protection against inflammation-induced receptor down-regulation and uncoupling. At the same time, studies have shown that translocation of the glucocorticoid receptor from the cell cytosol to the nucleus, a fundamental step in the anti-inflammatory activity of corticosteroids, is increased by the addition of a β_2-agonist [70,130,131].

A study of fluticasone propionate (250 μg) plus salmeterol (50 μg) showed improvement in lung function in patients who have COPD compared with either therapy alone [126]. In another pivotal study (N = 1465), Calverley and colleagues [128] reported that treatment for 12 months with a SFC improved pretreatment FEV_1 significantly compared with placebo or either single agent alone. A clinically significant improvement in health status and a reduction in daily symptoms also were observed with combination treatment together with a significant reduction in exacerbations [128,129]. A similar effect on improvement in several health outcomes was demonstrated in two 1-year studies using the budesonide/formoterol combination [129,132]. A more recent study, specifically designed and powered to detect changes in annualized exacerbations in nearly 1000 patients who had COPD, showed that 44 weeks of treatment with the SFC (50/500 µg twice daily) was significantly more effective than salmeterol (50 µg twice daily) in reducing the total number and annualized rates of severe exacerbations [133]. Moreover, the number needed to treat (NNT) with SFC versus salmeterol to prevent one moderate/severe exacerbation per year was 2.08. More recently, the TORCH study (n = 6112) demonstrated a significant effect of therapy with SFC over 3 years on several COPD outcomes [43]. SFC had a 2.6% absolute risk reduction in all-cause mortality compared with placebo ($P =$ .052) and was significantly superior to placebo and both component drugs in reducing moderate to severe exacerbations and improving health status ($P < .001$). Over the 3-year treatment period, patients taking SFC experienced a 25% reduction in the annual rate of moderate to severe exacerbations compared with placebo ($P < .001$; NNT = 4 to prevent one exacerbation in 1 year), a 12% reduction compared with salmeterol ($P = .002$), and a 9% reduction compared with fluticasone propionate ($P = .024$). SFC also reduced the annual rate of exacerbations leading to hospitalization by 17% versus placebo ($P = .03$; NNT = 32 to prevent one hospitalization in 1 year). Although the exact mechanism for the clinical benefits observed with the ICS/LABA combination is not well understood, a recent study demonstrated a significant effect of therapy with this combination in patients who had COPD on markers of airway inflammation, including sputum neuutrophils and airway CD8 lymphocytes [69].

Safety of long-acting β2-adrenoceptor agonists plus inhaled corticosteroid combination therapy

Oropharyngeal candidiasis was reported as the most common adverse event for the use of the LABA/ICS combination relative to placebo over a period of 24 to 52 weeks, with headache, upper respiratory tract infection, and musculoskeletal pain reported less frequently. Moreover, data from TORCH show that neither SFC, salmeterol alone, or fluticasone propionate alone leads to increased cardiac disorders, ophthalmic adverse events, or increased probability of bone fractures over a 3-year treatment period [43]. An unexpected safety finding was an increased incidence of pneumonia reported in patients taking fluticasone propionate and SFC; however, this did not lead to increased mortality and did not compromise the overall benefits of SFC treatment. This finding does, however, merit further investigation.

Inhaled corticosteroid/long-acting β2-adrenoceptor agonist/anticholinergic combination therapy

Emerging evidence from in vitro studies suggests an interaction between corticosteroid and muscarinic receptors, which may provide a rationale for the use of anticholinergic/corticosteroid combination therapies [71]. The clinical effects of such interaction need to be investigated in future clinical trials. A recent trial investigating the effect of triple combination of tiotropium and SFC over 1 year demonstrated a borderline effect of such a combination compared with tiotropium alone on time to first COPD exacerbation but a significant effect in improving lung function and health status and in reducing hospitalization [134].

Long-term oxygen therapy

Supplemental oxygen therapy is associated with a variety of beneficial effects in patients who have severe COPD and who are hypoxemic while breathing room air. These include prolonged survival [112], reduced secondary polycythemia, improved cardiac function during rest and exercise [135], reduction in the oxygen cost of ventilation [136], and improved exercise tolerance [137]. Patients who have PaO_2 less than 55 mm Hg (SaO_2 < 88%), whose disease is stable despite receiving otherwise comprehensive medical treatment, are candidates to receive long-term oxygen therapy (LTOT). Patients whose PaO_2 is 55 to 59 mm Hg are eligible to receive LTOT if they show signs of pulmonary hypertension, cor pulmonale, erythrocytosis, edema from right heart failure, or impaired mental state. If oxygen desaturation occurs only during exercise or sleep, oxygen therapy should be considered for use specifically under those conditions. Although LTOT may lead to hypercapnia with resulting respiratory acidosis [138], this usually can be minimized by titrating the oxygen flow to maintain the Pao_2 at 60 to 65 mm Hg. A multicenter study is underway to investigate the role of LTOT in patients who have COPD and who demonstrate mild to moderate hypoxemia while breathing room air.

Other therapies

Augmentation therapy for α_1-antitrypsin deficiency

Replacement therapy with α_1-proteinase inhibitor is approved for patients who have emphysema resulting from α_1-antiprotease deficiency. Given in weekly infusions to patients who have ZZ or null AAT phenotypes, therapy can increase serum levels above the target threshold of 11 mmol and can provide protective levels within the epithelial lining of the lung. There are three approved AAT augmentation therapies currently marketed in the United States. Although AAT augmentation therapy has a sound theoretic basis, proof of its efficacy has been difficult to document. Available evidence, however, supports the use of this therapy in patients who have AAT serum levels less than 11 mmol and FEV_1 between 30% and 65% predicted but may not be useful in other subsets of patients who have COPD [139,140].

Antibiotics

Although empiric treatment with antibiotics has been shown to be of benefit in COPD exacerbations, the role of antibiotics in chronic management is not well defined and currently not recommended. The role of chronic macrolide therapy in COPD is under investigation, as this group of antibiotics may have an additional anti-inflammatory effect on airway inflammation.

Mucolytic agents

Mucus impaction contributes to worsening of symptoms of patients who have COPD. Several studies investigating the role of mucolytics, however, such as potassium iodide and guaifenesin, failed to demonstrate significant clinical efficacy of these agents in the management of patients who have COPD, although some have shown some decrease in COPD exacerbations [141]. A variety of new agents addressing mucociliary clearance/mucus production are under investigation [142].

Pharmacologic therapy for acute exacerbations of chronic obstructive pulmonary disease

COPD is characterized by periods of acute worsening of respiratory symptoms, such as increased dyspnea, cough, and sputum production. The deterioration in symptoms is beyond day-to-day variation of a patient's symptoms and usually requires a change in therapy [31]. Although infection of the tracheobronchial tree and air pollution are the major causes of exacerbations, some exacerbations are idiopathic [143]. The differential diagnosis of exacerbations includes pneumonia, pulmonary embolism, pleural effusion, and acute cardiovascular pathology, including congestive heart failure and cardiac arrhythmias. Treatment failures account for many of the 120,000 COPD deaths in this country each year. Some exacerbations are mild and may not be reported by patients, but others produce striking clinical deterioration and require hospitalization. The severity and impact of an exacerbation depends on patients' baseline health status and baseline lung function, ventilation and oxygenation, and presence of comorbid conditions. In addition to baseline severity of COPD, management decisions depend on severity of dyspnea, presence of signs of acute respiratory insufficiency, lung parenchymal infection, pulmonary embolism, and simultaneous acute decompensation of other organs, in particular the cardiovascular system.

Management of exacerbations is aimed at minimizing air flow obstruction via bronchodilation, reducing inflammation, treating infection, providing supportive care (including ventilation and oxygen), and minimizing nonrespiratory-related symptoms, including anxiety and sleep disturbances that may accompany exacerbations [99].

Bronchodilators

Short-acting bronchodilators with fast onset of action improve airflow limitation and dyspnea in patients who have COPD and may prove helpful during exacerbations. β-Agonists and anticholinergics are recommended for use [31]. Medication delivered by MDI (and spacer) is as effective as nebulized forms, although patients who have severe COPD and difficulty performing inspiratory maneuvers may prefer the latter. Long-acting bronchodilators are not recommended for use in the management of acute exacerbation of COPD, although the efficacy of formoterol, used alone [61,144] or in combination with other bronchodilators [61] or ICS [145], is documented in several studies.

Systemic corticosteroids

The use of systemic corticosteroids is discouraged and may lead to systemic side effects in stable patients who have COPD. Systemic corticosteroids, however, do play a role in the management of acute exacerbations of COPD. Systemic corticosteroid therapy improves various outcomes, including lung function, symptoms, and oxygenation, and reduces treatment failure and length of hospital stay in patients who have acute exacerbations of COPD and who have severely or very severely impaired FEV_1 [146–148]. The maximum benefit from these agents is obtained during the first 2 weeks of therapy, and longer duration of therapy or the use of doses larger than 40 to 60 mg of prednisone per day do not confer any added benefits.

Antibiotics

Antibiotics may improve outcomes in exacerbations of COPD [149]. Patients who present with dyspnea and increased sputum volume or purulence or patients who require mechanical ventilation benefit from a 3- to 7-day course of oral or parenteral antibiotics [150]. The causative organism for the exacerbation may be difficult to identify. Sputum Gram's stain and culture often are nondiagnostic, because many of these patients' airways are colonized with different bacteria. Furthermore, blood cultures usually are negative. The type of the organisms present and the antibiotics used may differ with severity of COPD, however. Patients who have milder stages of COPD tend to be colonized and get lower respiratory tract infections with *Haemophilus influenza*, *Streptococcus pneumonia*, or *Moraxella catarrhalis*, whereas patients who have severe COPD, prior hospital admission, and frequent antibiotics use also may have pseudomonas [151,152]. Thus, the selection of empiric antibiotics to treat acute exacerbations should depend on the severity of the underlying disease and severity of COPD exacerbations. Oral β-lactam antibiotics, tetracycline, trimethopim-sulfamethoxazole, and macrolides are recommended for milder exacerbations. Therapy for more severe exacerbations should include coverage of antibiotic-resistant bacteria, such as *Pseudomonas* or methicillin-resistant *Stapholococcus aureus*. In such patients, fluoroquinolones, β-lactam/β-lactamase

inhibitors, second- or third-generation cephalosporins, or vancomycin can be considered [3,31].

Novel therapeutic targets for chronic obstructive pulmonary diasease

A variety of novel pharmacologic agents that target different aspects of the pathogenesis of COPD are under clinical development (Table 4) [153,154].

Novel bronchodilators

Novel β2-adrenoceptor agonists

A variety of β-agonists with longer half-lives are under development, with the hope of achieving once-daily dosing [155]. These include carmoterol; indacaterol; GSK-159,797; GSK-597,901; GSK-159,802; GSK-642,444; and GSK-678,007. These compounds mainly are (R, R)-enantiomers and have high intrinsic efficacy and quick onset of action. Although a quick onset of action and a prolonged 24-hour effect are desirable in the management of COPD, the use of agonists with high intrinsic efficacy theoretically may be associated with a rapid onset of tolerance, a fact that may limit their clinical use [46]. This needs to be taken into consideration in the evaluation of new agents under development. It is likely, however, that once-daily dosing of a LABA will lead to enhancement of compliance with therapy and may have advantages leading to improved overall clinical outcomes in patients who have COPD.

Novel anticholinergics

Several new long-acting anticholinergic agents are under development, including LAS-34,273 (aclidinium); LAS-35,201; GSK-656,398; GSK-233,705; and NVA-237 (glycopyrrolate). Although clinical details still are not available, potential advantages of such agents over tiotropium may include a quicker onset of action and a better safety profile.

Novel anti-inflammatory agents

Phosphodiesterase-4 inhibitors

Phosphodiesterase 4 (PDE4) metabolizes cAMP in airway smooth muscle cells and in many inflammatory cells that play a major role in the inflammatory cascade of COPD. Several PDE4 inhibitors are in various stages of development [156]. Selective inhibition of PDE4 has been shown to cause smooth muscle relaxation and anti-inflammatory effects. Although the bronchodilator effects of these agents are modest, their

Table 4
Novel therapies for chronic obstructive pulmonary disease in clinical development

Products in late-phase development	Products in early-phase development
• Bronchodilators • Ultra-LABAs • Indacaterol • Carmoterol • LAMAs • LAS 34,273 (aclidinium) • PDE4 inhibitors • Roflumilast • Cilomilast • Combination therapy • ICS/LABA • Budesonide + formoterol[a] • Mometasone + indacaterol • Mometasone + formoterol • Bronchodilator combination • LABA/LAMA/ICS combination	• Smoking cessation • Nicotine vaccines/ inhibitors • Broncodilators • Ultra-LABAs • GSK 159,797; 597,901; 159,802; 642,444; 678,007 • LAMAs • NVA 237 (glycopyrrolate) • GSK 656,398 • GSK 233,705 • LAS 35,201 • Combination • Carmoterol + tiotropium • Salmeterol + tiotropium • Indacaterol + NVA 237 • Others • Anti-inflammatory • P38 MAPK, other PDE4 inhibitors, PPAR-γ agonists • Mediator antagonists • LTB4, IL-8, and related chemokines inhibitors • TNF-α inhibitors • Antioxidants • Fibrosis inhibitors • TGF-β inhibitors • Protease inhibitors • Cathepsin • MMP inhibitors • Alveolar repair • Retinoids • Stem cells • Mucoregulators • EGFR inhibitors • CACC inhibitors

Abbreviations: LAMA, long-acting antimuscurinic (anticholinergic); ultra-LABA, once-a-day LABA.

[a] Approved for asthma in the United States.

combined anti-inflammatory and bronchodilator effects make them appealing. Although these agents generally have a better safety profile than theophylline, their use may be limited by gastrointestinal adverse effects in some patients. Preliminary studies have been published on the clinical efficacy and safety of roflumilast [157–159] and cilomilast [160,161] in COPD, although none of these compounds currently is approved for clinical use in the United States.

Leukotriene inhibitors/receptor antagonists

Leukotrienes C4, D4, and E4 play a major role in asthma; however, blocking their receptor (CysLT1 receptor) by antagonists, such as zafirlukast and montelukast, is not effective in COPD. LTB$_4$, however, is a key chemoattractant of neutrophils, thereby making it an attractive target for therapeutic intervention in COPD. Antagonists of the two subtypes of LTB$_4$ receptor (eg, LY29311 [162] and SB201146 [163]) are at the early stages of clinical development and are shown to inhibit sputum-induced neutrophil chemotaxis. Alternatively, inhibitors of LTB$_4$ synthesis (eg, BAYx1005) produce a modest reduction in sputum LTB$_4$ concentrations [164], although the clinical relevance of this result remains to be established. Leukotriene inhibitors, such as zileuton, may be effective in some patients who have COPD; however, their role in this disease needs further study.

Cytokine and chemokine inhibitors

There are several chemokines and cytokines that play important roles in mediating inflammation in COPD and, therefore, are potential therapeutic targets. For example, IL-8 recruits and activates neutrophils via the chemokine receptors, CXCR1 and CXCR2, and it can be inhibited by the small-molecule CXCR1/CXCR2 antagonist, repertaxin [165]. In addition, CXCR2-specific antagonists, such as SB 225,002, block the CXCR2 receptor, which is required for the recruitment of neutrophils [162]. An alternative means of intercepting the IL-8 pathway is to use a human anti–IL-8 monoclonal antibody [166].

Concentrations of TNF-α are raised in the sputum of patients who have COPD. TNF-α augments inflammation and induces IL-8 and other chemokines in airway cells via activation of the transcription factor, nuclear factor κB. The severe wasting in some patients who have advanced COPD could be the result of increased release of TNF-α. Humanized monoclonal antibody to TNF (infliximab) and to soluble TNF receptor (etanercept) are effective in other inflammatory disorders and may play a role in COPD. A recently published prospective randomized study failed to demonstrate, however, any beneficial effects of infliximab infusion in patients who have moderate to severe COPD [167].

Antioxidants

Oxidative stress is increased in patients who have COPD, particularly during exacerbations. The use of N-acetylcysteine (NAC), to provide intracellular cysteine for the production of the endogenous antioxidant glutathione is one of several treatment options under investigation. The role of NAC has been described in a metanal-ysis, which demonstrated a statistically significant (23%) reduction in exacerbation rates with its use in patients who have chronic bronchitis [168]. The results of this meta-analysis, however, were lim-ited because of the differing definitions of chronic bronchitis, patient selection criteria, differing dosing regimens, and lack of information regard-ing concurrently administered bronchodilators. A more recent randomized controlled trial failed to show that the addition of NAC to treatment with corticosteroids, and bronchodilators can modify the outcome in acute exacerbations of COPD [169]. In a recently published 3-year study, the yearly rate of decline in FEV_1 and the annual number of exacerbations did not differ between patients assigned to NAC and those assigned to placebo [170]. Subgroup analysis suggested that the exacerbation rate might be reduced with in pa-tients not treated with ICSs and secondary analy-sis was suggestive of an effect on hyperinflation.

Antiproteinases

Proteinase/antiproteinase imbalance is a major mechanism that explains the tissue destruction that occurs in COPD, particularly in emphysema. Synthetic antiproteinases other than α_1-antitrypsin are under development and may be useful in treat-ment of emphysema.

In terms of restoring the balance between proteases and protease inhibitors in COPD, the development of small-molecular inhibitors of proteinases, especially those that show elastolytic activity, is another promising area.

Retinoids

Proteolytic destruction of lung parenchyma leads to loss of elastic recoil in patients who have emphysema. Retinoic acid has been shown in the rat model to increase proliferation of alveoli after elastase-induced lung injury [171]. No defin-itive clinical benefits related to the administration of retinoids were observed in a recently published

feasibility study [172]. Time- and dose-dependent changes in diffusion capacity of lung for carbon monoxide, CT density mask score, and health status, however, were observed in subjects treated with all-trans retinoic acid, suggesting the possi-bility of exposure-related biologic activity that warrants further investigation [172]. A longer study is underway to investigate the role of retinoic acid analogs in patients who have emphsyema.

Summary

COPD is a treatable disease. Current pharma-cotherapy aims at improvement of symptoms, exercise tolerance, and health status and decrease in exacerbations. Prevention of disease progres-sion and reduction in mortality are the ultimate goals of such therapy. All symptomatic patients who have COPD should receive pharmacologic intervention. Inhaled short-acting bronchodila-tors are recommended for rescue of symptoms in patients who have mild disease, whereas inhaled long-acting bronchodilators are recommended as first-line agents for maintenance therapy in pa-tients who have moderate and severe disease and those who have daily symptoms. When symptoms are not controlled sufficiently by the use of one bronchodilator, combining bronchodilators of different classes may be a more effective approach. In addition, combining a long-acting β_2-agonist with an ICS is shown more effective than the use of either agent alone. Several novel therapies are now in different stages of development for use either alone or in combination with other agents.

References

[1] Halbert RJ, Natoli JL, Gano A, et al. Global bur-den of COPD: systematic review and meta-analysis. Eur Respir J 2006;28(3):523–32.

[2] Chapman KR, Mannino DM, Soriano JB, et al. Epidemiology and costs of chronic obstructive pul-monary disease. Eur Respir J 2006;27(1):188–207.

[3] Celli BR, Macnee W. Standards for the diagnosis and treatment of patients with COPD: a summary of the ATS/ERS position paper. Eur Respir J 2004; 23(6):932–46.

[4] Rabe KF, Hurd S, Anzueto A, et al. Global strat-egy for the diagnosis, management, and prevention of COPD - 2006 update. Am J Respir Crit Care Med 2007, in press.

[5] Agusti AG. COPD, a multicomponent disease: im-plications for management. Respir Med 2005;99(6): 670–82.

[6] Hanania NA, Ambrosino N, Calverley P, et al. Treatments for COPD. Respir Med 2005;99 (Suppl B):S28–40.

[7] Halpern MT, Stanford RH, Borker R. The burden of COPD in the U.S.A.: results from the confronting COPD survey. Respir Med 2003;97 (Suppl C):S81–9.

[8] Make B, Casaburi R, Leidy NK. Interpreting results from clinical trials: understanding minimal clinically important differences in COPD outcomes. COPD 2005;2(1):1–5.

[9] Tashkin DP. The role of patient-centered outcomes in the course of chronic obstructive pulmonary disease: how long-term studies contribute to our understanding. Am J Med 2006;119(10 Suppl 1): 63–72.

[10] Gross NJ. Outcome measures for COPD treatments: a critical evaluation. COPD 2004;1(1):41–57.

[11] Fiore MC. US public health service clinical practice guideline: treating tobacco use and dependence. Respir Care 2000;45(10):1200–62.

[12] Anthonisen NR, Connett JE, Kiley JP, et al. Effects of smoking intervention and the use of an inhaled anticholinergic bronchodilator on the rate of decline of FEV1. The Lung Health Study. JAMA 1994;272(19):1497–505.

[13] Gamble E, Grootendorst DC, Hattotuwa K, et al. Airway mucosal inflammation in COPD is similar in smokers and ex-smokers: a pooled analysis. Eur Respir J 2007, in press.

[14] Rutgers SR, Postma DS, Ten Hacken NH, et al. Ongoing airway inflammation in patients with COPD who do not currently smoke. Thorax 2000; 55(1):12–8.

[15] Foulds J, Burke M, Steinberg M, et al. Advances in pharmacotherapy for tobacco dependence. Expert Opin Emerg Drugs 2004;9(1):39–53.

[16] Frishman WH. Smoking cessation pharmacotherapy—nicotine and non-nicotine preparations. Prev Cardiol 2007;10(2 Suppl 1):10–22.

[17] Henningfield JE, Fant RV, Buchhalter AR, et al. Pharmacotherapy for nicotine dependence. CA Cancer J Clin 2005;55(5):281–99.

[18] Coe JW, Brooks PR, Vetelino MG, et al. Varenicline: an alpha4beta2 nicotinic receptor partial agonist for smoking cessation. J Med Chem 2005;48 (10):3474–7.

[19] Tonstad S. Varenicline for smoking cessation. Expert Rev Neurother 2007;7(2):121–7.

[20] Gonzales D, Rennard SI, Nides M, et al. Varenicline, an alpha4beta2 nicotinic acetylcholine receptor partial agonist, vs sustained-release bupropion and placebo for smoking cessation: a randomized controlled trial. JAMA 2006;296(1):47–55.

[21] Jorenby DE, Hays JT, Rigotti NA, et al. Efficacy of varenicline, an alpha4beta2 nicotinic acetylcholine receptor partial agonist, vs placebo or sustained-release bupropion for smoking cessation: a randomized controlled trial. JAMA 2006;296(1):56–63.

[22] Tonstad S, Tonnesen P, Hajek P, et al. Effect of maintenance therapy with varenicline on smoking cessation: a randomized controlled trial. JAMA 2006;296(1):64–71.

[23] Williams KE, Reeves KR, Billing CB Jr, et al. A double-blind study evaluating the long-term safety of varenicline for smoking cessation. Curr Med Res Opin 2007;23(4):793–801.

[24] Donohue JF. Therapeutic responses in asthma and COPD. Bronchodilators. Chest 2004;126(2 Suppl): 125S–37S.

[25] Calverley PM, Burge PS, Spencer S, et al. Bronchodilator reversibility testing in chronic obstructive pulmonary disease. Thorax 2003;58(8):659–64.

[26] O'Donnell DE, Webb KA. Exertional breathlessness in patients with chronic airflow limitation. The role of lung hyperinflation. Am Rev Respir Dis 1993;148(5):1351–7.

[27] O'Donnell DE, Lam M, Webb KA. Spirometric correlates of improvement in exercise performance after anticholinergic therapy in chronic obstructive pulmonary disease. Am J Respir Crit Care Med 1999;160(2):542–9.

[28] Ramirez-Venegas A, Ward J, Lentine T, et al. Salmeterol reduces dyspnea and improves lung function in patients with COPD. Chest 1997;112(2): 336–40.

[29] Celli B, ZuWallack R, Wang S, et al. Improvement in resting inspiratory capacity and hyperinflation with tiotropium in COPD patients with increased static lung volumes. Chest 2003;124(5): 1743–8.

[30] Niewoehner DE. The impact of severe exacerbations on quality of life and the clinical course of chronic obstructive pulmonary disease. Am J Med 2006;119(10 Suppl 1):38–45.

[31] Celli BR, Barnes PJ. Exacerbations of chronic obstructive pulmonary disease. Eur Respir J 2007; 29(6):1224–38.

[32] Sin DD, McAlister FA, Man SF, et al. Contemporary management of chronic obstructive pulmonary disease: scientific review. JAMA 2003;290(17): 2301–12.

[33] Niewoehner DE, Rice K, Cote C, et al. Prevention of exacerbations of chronic obstructive pulmonary disease with tiotropium, a once-daily inhaled anticholinergic bronchodilator: a randomized trial. Ann Intern Med 2005;143(5):317–26.

[34] Mahler DA, Donohue JF, Barbee RA, et al. Efficacy of salmeterol xinafoate in the treatment of COPD. Chest 1999;115(4):957–65.

[35] Barr RG, Bourbeau J, Camargo CA, et al. Tiotropium for stable chronic obstructive pulmonary disease: a meta-analysis. Thorax 2006;61(10): 854–62.

[36] Casaburi R, Mahler DA, Jones PW, et al. A long-term evaluation of once-daily inhaled tiotropium in chronic obstructive pulmonary disease. Eur Respir J 2002;19(2):217–24.

[37] Vincken W, van Noord JA, Greefhorst AP, et al. Improved health outcomes in patients with COPD during 1 yr's treatment with tiotropium. Eur Respir J 2002;19(2):209–16.

[38] Okudan N, Gok M, Gokbel H, et al. Single dose of tiotropium improves the 6-minute walk distance in chronic obstructive pulmonary disease. Lung 2006; 184(4):201–4.

[39] O'Donnell DE, Sciurba F, Celli B, et al. Effect of fluticasone propionate/salmeterol on lung hyperinflation and exercise endurance in COPD. Chest 2006;130(3):647–56.

[40] O'Donnell DE, Fluge T, Gerken F, et al. Effects of tiotropium on lung hyperinflation, dyspnoea and exercise tolerance in COPD. Eur Respir J 2004; 23(6):832–40.

[41] O'Donnell DE, Voduc N, Fitzpatrick M, et al. Effect of salmeterol on the ventilatory response to exercise in chronic obstructive pulmonary disease. Eur Respir J 2004;24(1):86–94.

[42] Vestbo J. The TORCH (towards a revolution in COPD health) survival study protocol. Eur Respir J 2004;24(2):206–10.

[43] Calverley PM, Anderson JA, Celli B, et al. Salmeterol and fluticasone propionate and survival in chronic obstructive pulmonary disease. N Engl J Med 2007;356(8):775–89.

[44] Decramer M, Celli B, Tashkin DP, et al. Clinical trial design considerations in assessing long-term functional impacts of tiotropium in COPD: the UPLIFT trial. COPD 2004;1(2):303–12.

[45] Dolovich MB, Ahrens RC, Hess DR, et al. Device selection and outcomes of aerosol therapy: evidence-based guidelines: American College of Chest Physicians/American College of Asthma, Allergy, And Immunology. Chest 2005;127(1):335–71.

[46] Hanania NA, Sharafkhaneh A, Barber R, et al. Beta-agonist intrinsic efficacy: measurement and clinical significance. Am J Respir Crit Care Med 2002;165(10):1353–8.

[47] Lotvall J. Pharmacology of bronchodilators used in the treatment of COPD. Respir Med 2000; 94(Suppl E):S6–10.

[48] Costello J. Prospects for improved therapy in chronic obstructive pulmonary disease by the use of levalbuterol. J Allergy Clin Immunol 1999;104 (2 Pt 2):S61–8.

[49] Truitt T, Witko J, Halpern M. Levalbuterol compared to racemic albuterol: efficacy and outcomes in patients hospitalized with COPD or asthma. Chest 2003;123(1):128–35.

[50] Arformoterol: (R,R)-eformoterol, (R,R)-formoterol, arformoterol tartrate, eformoterol-sepracor, formoterol-sepracor, R,R-eformoterol, R,R-formoterol. Drugs R D 2004;5(1):25–7.

[51] Baumgartner RA, Hanania NA, Calhoun WJ, et al. Nebulized arformoterol in patients with COPD: A 12-week, multicenter, randomized, double-blind, double-dummy, placebo- and active-controlled trial. Clin Ther 2007;29(2):261–78.

[52] Steinke JW, Baramki D, Borish L. Opposing actions of (R,R)-isomers and (S,S)-isomers of formoterol on T-cell function. J Allergy Clin Immunol 2006;118(4):963–5.

[53] Barnes PJ. Treatment with (R)-albuterol has no advantage over racemic albuterol. Am J Respir Crit Care Med 2006;174(9):969–72.

[54] Ameredes BT, Calhoun WJ. (R)-albuterol for asthma: pro [a.k.a. (S)-albuterol for asthma: con]. Am J Respir Crit Care Med 2006;174(9):965–9.

[55] Sestini P, Renzoni E, Robinson S, et al. Short-acting beta 2 agonists for stable chronic obstructive pulmonary disease. Cochrane Database Syst Rev 2002;4:CD001495.

[56] Boyd G, Morice AH, Pounsford JC, et al. An evaluation of salmeterol in the treatment of chronic obstructive pulmonary disease (COPD). Eur Respir J 1997;10(4):815–21.

[57] Cazzola M, Matera MG, Santangelo G, et al. Salmeterol and formoterol in partially reversible severe chronic obstructive pulmonary disease: a dose-response study. Respir Med 1995;89(5):357–62.

[58] Hanania NA, Kalberg C, Yates J, et al. The bronchodilator response to salmeterol is maintained with regular, long-term use in patients with COPD. Pulm Pharmacol Ther 2005;18(1):19–22.

[59] Dahl R, Greefhorst LA, Nowak D, et al. Inhaled formoterol dry powder versus ipratropium bromide in chronic obstructive pulmonary disease. Am J Respir Crit Care Med 2001;164(5):778–84.

[60] Cazzola M, Santus P, Matera MG, et al. A single high dose of formoterol is as effective as the same dose administered in a cumulative manner in patients with acute exacerbation of COPD. Respir Med 2003;97(5):458–62.

[61] Di MF, Verga M, Santus P, et al. Effect of formoterol, tiotropium, and their combination in patients with acute exacerbation of chronic obstructive pulmonary disease: a pilot study. Respir Med 2006; 100(11):1925–32.

[62] Campbell M, Eliraz A, Johansson G, et al. Formoterol for maintenance and as-needed treatment of chronic obstructive pulmonary disease. Respir Med 2005;99(12):1511–20.

[63] Richter K, Stenglein S, Mucke M, et al. Onset and duration of action of formoterol and tiotropium in patients with moderate to severe COPD. Respiration 2006;73(4):414–9.

[64] Stockley RA, Whitehead PJ, Williams MK. Improved outcomes in patients with chronic obstructive pulmonary disease treated with salmeterol compared with placebo/usual therapy: results of a meta-analysis. Respir Res 2006;7(1):147.

[65] Stockley RA, Chopra N, Rice L. Addition of salmeterol to existing treatment in patients with COPD: a 12 month study. Thorax 2006;61(2):122–8.

[66] Johnson M, Rennard S. Alternative mechanisms for long-acting beta(2)-adrenergic agonists in COPD. Chest 2001;120(1):258–70.

[67] Hanania NA, Moore RH. Anti-inflammatory activities of beta2-agonists. Curr Drug Targets Inflamm Allergy 2004;3(3):271–7.

[68] Bennett WD, Almond MA, Zeman KL, et al. Effect of salmeterol on mucociliary and cough clearance in chronic bronchitis. Pulm Pharmacol Ther 2006; 19(2):96–100.

[69] Barnes NC, Qiu YS, Pavord ID, et al. Antiinflammatory effects of salmeterol/fluticasone propionate in chronic obstructive lung disease. Am J Respir Crit Care Med 2006;173(7):736–43.

[70] Johnson M. Interactions between corticosteroids and beta2-agonists in asthma and chronic obstructive pulmonary disease. Proc Am Thorac Soc 2004; 1(3):200–6.

[71] Johnson M. Corticosteroids: potential beta2-agonist and anticholinergic interactions in chronic obstructive pulmonary disease. Proc Am Thorac Soc 2005;2(4):320–5.

[72] Sin DD, Johnson M, Gan WQ, et al. Combination therapy of inhaled corticosteroids and long-acting beta2-adrenergics in management of patients with chronic obstructive pulmonary disease. Curr Pharm Des 2004;10(28):3547–60.

[73] Gross NJ, Co E, Skorodin MS. Cholinergic bronchomotor tone in COPD. Estimates of its amount in comparison with that in normal subjects. Chest 1989;96:984–7.

[74] Gross NJ, Skorodin MS. Role of the parasympathetic system in airway obstruction due to emphysema. N Engl J Med 1984;311:421–5.

[75] O'Connor BJ, Towse LJ, Barnes PJ. Prolonged effect of tiotropium bromide on methacholine-induced bronchoconstriction in asthma. Am J Respir Crit Care Med 1996;154:876–80.

[76] Appleton S, Jones T, Poole P, et al. Ipratropium bromide versus long-acting beta-2 agonists for stable chronic obstructive pulmonary disease. Cochrane Database Syst Rev 2006;3:CD006101.

[77] Ayers ML, Mejia R, Ward J, et al. Effectiveness of salmeterol versus ipratropium bromide on exertional dyspnoea in COPD. Eur Respir J 2001;17(6): 1132–7.

[78] Anzueto A, Tashkin D, Menjoge S, et al. One-year analysis of longitudinal changes in spirometry in patients with COPD receiving tiotropium. Pulm Pharmacol Ther 2005;18(2):75–81.

[79] Donohue JF, van Noord JA, Bateman ED, et al. A 6-month, placebo-controlled study comparing lung function and health status changes in COPD patients treated with tiotropium or salmeterol. Chest 2002;122(1):47–55.

[80] Brusasco V, Hodder R, Miravitlles M, et al. Health outcomes following treatment for six months with once daily tiotropium compared with twice daily salmeterol in patients with COPD. Thorax 2003; 58(5):399–404.

[81] Briggs DD Jr, Covelli H, Lapidus R, et al. Improved daytime spirometric efficacy of tiotropium compared with salmeterol in patients with COPD. Pulm Pharmacol Ther 2005;18(6):397–404.

[82] Belmonte KE. Cholinergic pathways in the lungs and anticholinergic therapy for chronic obstructive pulmonary disease. Proc Am Thorac Soc 2005;2(4): 297–304.

[83] Profita M, Giorgi RD, Sala A, et al. Muscarinic receptors, leukotriene B4 production and neutrophilic inflammation in COPD patients. Allergy 2005;60(11):1361–9.

[84] Barnes PJ. Theophylline for COPD. Thorax 2006; 61(9):742–4.

[85] Barnes PJ. Targeting histone deacetylase 2 in chronic obstructive pulmonary disease treatment. Expert Opin Ther Targets 2005;9(6):1111–21.

[86] Cosio BG, Tsaprouni L, Ito K, et al. Theophylline restores histone deacetylase activity and steroid responses in COPD macrophages. J Exp Med 2004; 200(5):689–95.

[87] Cazzola M, Gabriella MM. The additive effect of theophylline on a combination of formoterol and tiotropium in stable COPD: a pilot study. Respir Med 2006;101(5):952–62.

[88] Man GC, Champman KR, Ali SH, et al. Sleep quality and nocturnal respiratory function with once-daily theophylline (Uniphyl) and inhaled salbutamol in patients with COPD. Chest 1996; 110(3):648–53.

[89] Nelson HS, Weiss ST, Bleecker ER, et al. The salmeterol multicenter asthma research trial: a comparison of usual pharmacotherapy for asthma or usual pharmacotherapy plus salmeterol. Chest 2006;129(1):15–26.

[90] Salpeter SR. Cardiovascular safety of beta(2)-adrenoceptor agonist use in patients with obstructive airway disease: a systematic review. Drugs Aging 2004;21(6):405–14.

[91] Ferguson GT, Funck-Brentano C, Fischer T, et al. Cardiovascular safety of salmeterol in COPD. Chest 2003;123(6):1817–24.

[92] Donohue JF, Menjoge S, Kesten S. Tolerance to bronchodilating effects of salmeterol in COPD. Respir Med 2003;97(9):1014–20.

[93] Cazzola M, Matera MG, Donner CF. Inhaled beta2-adrenoceptor agonists: cardiovascular safety in patients with obstructive lung disease. Drugs 2005;65(12):1595–610.

[94] Salpeter SR, Buckley NS, Salpeter EE. Meta-analysis: anticholinergics, but not beta-agonists, reduce severe exacerbations and respiratory mortality in COPD. J Gen Intern Med 2006;21(10): 1011–9.

[95] Barnes PJ. Current therapies for asthma. Promise and limitations. Chest 1997;111(2 Suppl):17S–26S.

[96] Hogg JC, Chu F, Utokaparch S, et al. The nature of small-airway obstruction in chronic obstructive pulmonary disease. N Engl J Med 2004;350(26): 2645–53.

[97] Barnes PJ. Inhaled corticosteroids are not beneficial in chronic obstructive pulmonary disease. Am J Respir Crit Care Med 2000;161(2 Pt 1):342–4.

[98] Confalonieri M, Mainardi E, Della PR, et al. Inhaled corticosteroids reduce neutrophilic bronchial inflammation in patients with chronic obstructive pulmonary disease. Thorax 1998;53(7):583–5.

[99] Rodriguez-Roisin R. COPD exacerbations.5: management. Thorax 2006;61(6):535–44.

[100] Niewoehner DE. Systemic corticosteroids for chronic obstructive pulmonary disease: benefits and risks. Monaldi Arch Chest Dis 1999;54(5):422–6.

[101] Burge S. Should inhaled corticosteroids be used in the long term treatment of chronic obstructive pulmonary disease? Drugs 2001;61(11):1535–44.

[102] Vestbo J, Sorensen T, Lange P, et al. Long-term effect of inhaled budesonide in mild and moderate chronic obstructive pulmonary disease: a randomised controlled trial. Lancet 1999;353(9167): 1819–23.

[103] Pauwels RA, Lofdahl CG, Laitinen LA, et al. Long-term treatment with inhaled budesonide in persons with mild chronic obstructive pulmonary disease who continue smoking. European Respiratory Society Study on chronic obstructive pulmonary disease. N Engl J Med 1999;340(25):1948–53.

[104] Effect of inhaled triamcinolone on the decline in pulmonary function in chronic obstructive pulmonary disease. N Engl J Med 2000;343(26):1902–9.

[105] Sutherland ER, Allmers H, Ayas NT, et al. Inhaled corticosteroids reduce the progression of airflow limitation in chronic obstructive pulmonary disease: a meta-analysis. Thorax 2003;58(11):937–41.

[106] Soriano JB, Sin DD, Zhang X, et al. A pooled analysis of FEV1 decline in COPD patients randomized to inhaled corticosteroids or placebo. Chest 2007; 131(3):682–9.

[107] Burge PS, Calverley PM, Jones PW, et al. Randomised, double blind, placebo controlled study of fluticasone propionate in patients with moderate to severe chronic obstructive pulmonary disease: the ISOLDE trial. Br Med J 2000;320(7245): 1297–303.

[108] Spencer S, Calverley PM, Sherwood BP, et al. Health status deterioration in patients with chronic obstructive pulmonary disease. Am J Respir Crit Care Med 2001;163(1):122–8.

[109] Alsaeedi A, Sin DD, McAlister FA. The effects of inhaled corticosteroids in chronic obstructive pulmonary disease: a systematic review of randomized placebo-controlled trials. Am J Med 2002;113(1): 59–65.

[110] van der Valk P, Monninkhof E, van der Palen J, et al. Effect of discontinuation of inhaled corticosteroids in patients with chronic obstructive pulmonary

disease: the COPE study. Am J Respir Crit Care Med 2002;166(10):1358–63.

[111] Wouters EF, Postma DS, Fokkens B, et al. Withdrawal of fluticasone propionate from combined salmeterol/fluticasone treatment in patients with COPD causes immediate and sustained disease deterioration: a randomised controlled trial. Thorax 2005;60(6):480–7.

[112] Nocturnal Oxygen Therapy Trial Group. Continuous or nocturnal oxygen therapy in hypoxemic chronic obstructive lung disease: a clinical trial. Nocturnal oxygen therapy trial group. Ann Intern Med 1980;93(3):391–8.

[113] Sin DD, Tu JV. Inhaled corticosteroids and the risk of mortality and readmission in elderly patients with chronic obstructive pulmonary disease. Am J Respir Crit Care Med 2001;164(4):580–4.

[114] Sin DD, Wu L, Anderson JA, et al. Inhaled corticosteroids and mortality in chronic obstructive pulmonary disease. Thorax 2005;60(12):992–7.

[115] Suissa S. Effectiveness of inhaled corticosteroids in chronic obstructive pulmonary disease: immortal time bias in observational studies. Am J Respir Crit Care Med 2003;168(1):49–53.

[116] Fabbri L, Pauwels RA, Hurd SS. Global strategy for the diagnosis, management, and prevention of chronic obstructive pulmonary disease: gold executive summary updated 2003. COPD 2004;1(1): 105–41.

[117] Global Initiative for Chronic Obstructive Lung Disease. Global strategy for the diagnosis, management, and prevention of chronic obstructive pulmonary disease—2004 update. 2005. Available at: http://www.goldcopd.com. Accessed April 24, 2005.

[118] Donohue JF. Combination therapy for chronic obstructive pulmonary disease: clinical aspects. Proc Am Thorac Soc 2005;2(4):272–81.

[119] COMBIVENT Inhalation Aerosol Study Group. In chronic obstructive pulmonary disease, a combination of ipratropium and albuterol is more effective than either agent alone. An 85-day multicenter trial. Chest 1994;105(5):1411–9.

[120] D'Urzo AD, De Salvo MC, Ramirez-Rivera A, et al. In patients with COPD, treatment with a combination of formoterol and ipratropium is more effective than a combination of salbutamol and ipratropium: a 3-week, randomized, double-blind, within-patient, multicenter study. Chest 2001; 119(5):1347–56.

[121] van Noord JA, de Munck DR, Bantje TA, et al. Long-term treatment of chronic obstructive pulmonary disease with salmeterol and the additive effect of ipratropium. Eur Respir J 2000;15(5):878–85.

[122] ZuWallack RL, Mahler DA, Reilly D, et al. Salmeterol plus theophylline combination therapy in the treatment of COPD. Chest 2001;119(6):1661–70.

[123] Cazzola M, Di MF, Santus P, et al. The pharmacodynamic effects of single inhaled doses of formoterol, tiotropium and their combination in patients

with COPD. Pulm Pharmacol Ther 2004;17(1): 35–9.

[124] van Noord JA, Aumann JL, Janssens E, et al. Comparison of tiotropium once daily, formoterol twice daily and both combined once daily in patients with COPD. Eur Respir J 2005;26(2):214–22.

[125] van Noord JA, Aumann JL, Janssens E, et al. Effects of tiotropium with and without formoterol on airflow obstruction and resting hyperinflation in patients with COPD. Chest 2006;129(3):509–17.

[126] Hanania NA, Darken P, Horstman D, et al. The efficacy and safety of fluticasone propionate (250 microg)/salmeterol (50 microg) combined in the diskus inhaler for the treatment of COPD. Chest 2003;124(3):834–43.

[127] Mahler DA, Wire P, Horstman D, et al. Effectiveness of fluticasone propionate and salmeterol combination delivered via the diskus device in the treatment of chronic obstructive pulmonary disease. Am J Respir Crit Care Med 2002;166(8):1084–91.

[128] Calverley P, Pauwels R, Vestbo J, et al. Combined salmeterol and fluticasone in the treatment of chronic obstructive pulmonary disease: a randomised controlled trial. Lancet 2003;361(9356): 449–56.

[129] Calverley PM, Boonsawat W, Cseke Z, et al. Maintenance therapy with budesonide and formoterol in chronic obstructive pulmonary disease. Eur Respir J 2003;22(6):912–9.

[130] Eickelberg O, Roth M, Lorx R, et al. Ligand-independent activation of the glucocorticoid receptor by beta2-adrenergic receptor agonists in primary human lung fibroblasts and vascular smooth muscle cells. J Biol Chem 1999;274(2):1005–10.

[131] Usmani OS, Ito K, Maneechotesuwan K, et al. Glucocorticoid receptor nuclear translocation in airway cells after inhaled combination therapy. Am J Respir Crit Care Med 2005;172(6):704–12.

[132] Szafranski W, Cukier A, Ramirez A, et al. Efficacy and safety of budesonide/formoterol in the management of chronic obstructive pulmonary disease. Eur Respir J 2003;21(1):74–81.

[133] Kardos P, Wencker M, Glaab T, et al. Impact of salmeterol/fluticasone propionate versus salmeterol on exacerbations in severe chronic obstructive pulmonary disease. Am J Respir Crit Care Med 2007; 175(2):144–9.

[134] Aaron SD, Vandemheen KL, Fergusson D, et al. Tiotropium in combination with placebo, salmeterol, or fluticasone-salmeterol for treatment of chronic obstructive pulmonary disease: a randomized trial. Ann Intern Med 2007;146(8):545–55.

[135] Zielinski J. Effects of long-term oxygen therapy in patients with chronic obstructive pulmonary disease. Curr Opin Pulm Med 1999;5(2):81–7.

[136] Mannix ET, Manfredi F, Palange P, et al. Oxygen may lower the O2 cost of ventilation in chronic obstructive lung disease. Chest 1992;101(4):910–5.

[137] Somfay A, Porszasz J, Lee SM, et al. Dose-response effect of oxygen on hyperinflation and exercise endurance in nonhypoxaemic COPD patients. Eur Respir J 2001;18(1):77–84.

[138] Dunn WF, Nelson SB, Hubmayr RD. Oxygen-induced hypercarbia in obstructive pulmonary disease. Am Rev Respir Dis 1991;144(3 Pt 1): 526–30.

[139] Stoller JK, Fallat R, Schluchter MD, et al. Augmentation therapy with alpha1-antitrypsin: patterns of use and adverse events. Chest 2003;123 (5):1425–34.

[140] American Thoracic Society/European Respiratory Society statement: standards for the diagnosis and management of individuals with alpha-1 antitrypsin deficiency. Am J Respir Crit Care Med 2003; 168(7):818–900.

[141] Poole PJ, Black PN. Oral mucolytic drugs for exacerbations of chronic obstructive pulmonary disease: systematic review. BMJ 2001;322(7297): 1271–4.

[142] Barnes PJ. Current and future therapies for airway mucus hypersecretion. Novartis Found Symp 2002; 248:237–49.

[143] White AJ, Gompertz S, Stockley RA. Chronic obstructive pulmonary disease. 6: the aetiology of exacerbations of chronic obstructive pulmonary disease. Thorax 2003;58(1):73–80.

[144] Cazzola M, Matera MG. Long-acting beta(2) agonists as potential option in the treatment of acute exacerbations of COPD. Pulm Pharmacol Ther 2003;16(4):197–201.

[145] Cazzola M, Noschese P, De MF, et al. Effect of formoterol/budesonide combination on arterial blood gases in patients with acute exacerbation of COPD. Respir Med 2006;100(2):212–7.

[146] Thompson WH, Nielson CP, Carvalho P, et al. Controlled trial of oral prednisone in outpatients with acute COPD exacerbation. Am J Respir Crit Care Med 1996;154(2 Pt 1):407–12.

[147] Niewoehner DE, Erbland ML, Deupree RH, et al. Effect of systemic glucocorticoids on exacerbations of chronic obstructive pulmonary disease. Department of Veterans Affairs Cooperative Study Group. N Engl J Med 1999;340(25): 1941–7.

[148] Aaron SD, Vandemheen KL, Hebert P, et al. Outpatient oral prednisone after emergency treatment of chronic obstructive pulmonary disease. N Engl J Med 2003;348(26):2618–25.

[149] Saint S, Bent S, Vittinghoff E, et al. Antibiotics in chronic obstructive pulmonary disease exacerbations. A meta-analysis. JAMA 1995;273(12): 957–60.

[150] Anthonisen NR, Manfreda J, Warren CP, et al. Antibiotic therapy in exacerbations of chronic obstructive pulmonary disease. Ann Intern Med 1987;106(2):196–204.

[151] Sethi S. Coinfection in exacerbations of COPD: a new frontier. Chest 2006;129(2):223–4.

[152] Sethi S, Evans N, Grant BJ, et al. New strains of bacteria and exacerbations of chronic obstructive pulmonary disease. N Engl J Med 2002;347(7): 465–71.

[153] Barnes PJ. Chronic obstructive pulmonary disease * 12: new treatments for COPD. Thorax 2003; 58(9):803–8.

[154] Barnes PJ. Emerging targets for COPD therapy. Curr Drug Targets Inflamm Allergy 2005;4(6):675–83.

[155] Cazzola M, Matera MG, Lotvall J. Ultra long-acting beta 2-agonists in development for asthma and chronic obstructive pulmonary disease. Expert Opin Investig Drugs 2005;14(7):775–83.

[156] Soto FJ, Hanania NA. Selective phosphodiesterase-4 inhibitors in chronic obstructive lung disease. Curr Opin Pulm Med 2005;11(2):129–34.

[157] Calverley PM, Sanchez-Toril F, McIvor A, et al. Effect of one year treatment with roflumilast in severe chronic obstructive pulmonary disease. Am J Respir Crit Care Med 2007;176(2):154–61.

[158] Antoniu SA. Roflumilast for the treatment of chronic obstructive pulmonary disease. Curr Opin Investig Drugs 2006;7(5):412–7.

[159] Rabe KF, Bateman ED, O'Donnell D, et al. Roflumilast—an oral anti-inflammatory treatment for chronic obstructive pulmonary disease: a randomised controlled trial. Lancet 2005;366(9485): 563–71.

[160] Gamble E, Grootendorst DC, Brightling CE, et al. Antiinflammatory effects of the phosphodiesterase-4 inhibitor cilomilast (Ariflo) in chronic obstructive pulmonary disease. Am J Respir Crit Care Med 2003;168(8):976–82.

[161] Rennard SI, Schachter N, Strek M, et al. Cilomilast for COPD: results of a 6-month, placebo-controlled study of a potent, selective inhibitor of phosphodiesterase 4. Chest 2006;129(1):56–66.

[162] Donnelly LE, Rogers DF. Therapy for chronic obstructive pulmonary disease in the 21st century. Drugs 2003;63(19):1973–98.

[163] Beeh KM, Kornmann O, Buhl R, et al. Neutrophil chemotactic activity of sputum from patients with COPD: role of interleukin 8 and leukotriene B4. Chest 2003;123(4):1240–7.

[164] Gompertz S, Stockley RA. A randomized, placebo-controlled trial of a leukotriene synthesis inhibitor in patients with COPD. Chest 2002; 122(1):289–94.

[165] Bertini R, Allegretti M, Bizzarri C, et al. Noncompetitive allosteric inhibitors of the inflammatory chemokine receptors CXCR1 and CXCR2: prevention of reperfusion injury. Proc Natl Acad Sci USA 2004;101(32):11791–6.

[166] Mahler DA, Huang S, Tabrizi M, et al. Efficacy and safety of a monoclonal antibody recognizing interleukin-8 in COPD: a pilot study. Chest 2004;126(3): 926–34.

[167] Rennard SI, Fogarty C, Kelsen S, et al. The safety and efficacy of infliximab in moderate to severe chronic obstructive pulmonary disease. Am J Respir Crit Care Med 2007;175(9):926–34.

[168] Sutherland ER, Crapo JD, Bowler RP. N-acetylcysteine and exacerbations of chronic obstructive pulmonary disease. COPD 2006;3(4): 195–202.

[169] Black PN, Morgan-Day A, McMillan TE, et al. Randomised, controlled trial of N-acetylcysteine for treatment of acute exacerbations of chronic obstructive pulmonary disease. BMC Pulm Med 2004; 4(1):13.

[170] Decramer M, Rutten-van MM, Dekhuijzen PN, et al. Effects of N-acetylcysteine on outcomes in chronic obstructive pulmonary disease (Bronchitis Randomized on NAC Cost-Utility Study, BRONCUS): a randomised placebo-controlled trial. Lancet 2005;365(9470):1552–60.

[171] Massaro GD, Massaro D. Retinoic acid treatment abrogates elastase-induced pulmonary emphysema in rats. Nat Med 1997;3(6):675–7.

[172] Roth MD, Connett JE, D'Armiento JM, et al. Feasibility of retinoids for the treatment of emphysema study. Chest 2006;130(5):1334–45.

ELSEVIER
SAUNDERS

Clin Chest Med 28 (2007) 609–616

CLINICS
IN CHEST
MEDICINE

Disease Modification in Chronic Obstructive Pulmonary Disease

Antonio Anzueto, MD[a,b,*]

[a]Department of Medicine, University of Texas Health Science Center, 7400 Merton Minter Boulevard,
111 East, San Antonio, TX 78229, USA
[b]Pulmonary Diseases Section, South Texas Veterans Health Care System,
Audie L. Murphy Memorial Veterans Hospital, 7400 Merton Minter Boulevard,
111 East, San Antonio, TX 78229, USA

In their consensus statements, the American Thoracic Society and European Respiratory Society and the Global Initiative for Chronic Obstructive Lung Disease (GOLD) statement emphasize that chronic obstructive pulmonary disease (COPD) is a preventable and treatable disease state characterized by airflow limitation that is not fully reversible and usually progressive [1,2]. Although the airflow limitation is associated with an abnormal inflammatory response of the lungs to noxious particles, the impact of COPD is not restricted to the lungs, as significant systemic consequences also are produced. The lung function impairment, characterized by expiratory flow limitation leading to air trapping, or hyperinflation, is worsened by periodic disease exacerbations. Together, lung function impairment and disease exacerbations promote a cycle of decline that includes dyspnea, reduced exercise endurance, physical inactivity, and deconditioning, leading to disease progression. and, consequently, to disability, poor health-related quality of life (HRQOL) and premature mortality (Fig. 1).

Changing the clinical course of chronic obstructive pulmonary disease

Disease modification in COPD can be viewed in terms of patient-centered outcomes such as

symptoms and HRQOL, or in terms of reduced decline in lung function over time and reduced morbidity and mortality. The impact of smoking cessation and pharmacotherapies for COPD on these outcomes is discussed.

Smoking cessation

Cigarette smoking is the main cause of COPD. As shown in the landmark study of London transit workers by Fletcher and Peto [3], lung function evaluated by forced expiratory volume in 1 second (FEV_1) declines naturally with aging, but in susceptible smokers, the rate of decline is accelerated greatly (Fig. 2). It is recognized that baseline FEV_1 is predictive of mortality in patients who have COPD [4–6]. Age and baseline FEV_1 were the most accurate predictors of death in a 3-year survival study of 985 patients who had COPD [4]. The prognostic significance of FEV_1 was particularly evident at baseline values less than 30% of predicted. Smoking cessation changes the clinical course of COPD by preserving lung function. The earlier the age of smoking cessation, the greater the lung function that is preserved. In the Lung Health Study, smoking cessation resulted in a significant impact on FEV_1 even in patients with stage I COPD, with normal lung function [5]. Over an 11-year period, the rate of FEV_1 decline among continuing smokers was more than twice the rate of decline among those who were sustained quitters (Fig. 3). This benefit of smoking cessation was evident in both men (66.1 mL/y decline in smokers versus 30.2 mL/y decline in nonsmokers) and women (54.2 mL/y

* Audie L. Murphy Memorial Veterans Hospital, 7400 Merton Minter Boulevard, 111 East, San Antonio, TX 78229.
   E-mail address: anzueto@uthscsa.edu

0272-5231/07/$ - see front matter © 2007 Elsevier Inc. All rights reserved.
doi:10.1016/j.ccm.2007.05.001

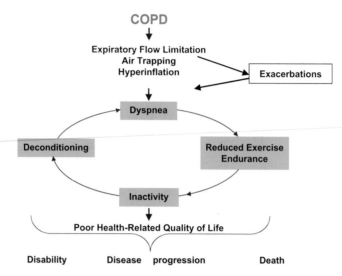

Fig. 1. The chronic obstructive pulmonary disease (COPD) cycle of decline. Lung function impairment and disease exacerbations promote a cycle of dyspnea, reduced exercise endurance, physical inactivity, and deconditioning, leading to disease progression, and, consequently, to disability, poor health-related quality of life, and premature mortality. (*Data from* Cooper C. The connection between chronic obstructive pulmonary disease symptoms and hyperinflation and its impact on the exercise and function. Am J Med 2006;119:S21–31.)

decline in smokers versus 21.5 mL/y decline in nonsmokers). In addition, FEV_1 fell below 60% of predicted after 11 years in more continuing smokers than sustained quitters (38% versus 10%, respectively).

In a recent analysis from this study conducted at 14.5 years, patients randomly assigned to the smoking cessation intervention had a significant 18% reduction in all-cause mortality compared with usual care (no smoking cessation intervention) ($P = .03$) [6]. When the cause of death was considered in the Lung Health Study, patients allocated to the smoking cessation intervention

had lower rates of death because of coronary heart disease (CHD), cerebrovascular disease, lung cancer, and respiratory disease other than lung cancer as compared with those assigned to usual care (continue to smoke) (Fig. 4A) [6]. The death rates were higher in all groups receiving usual care compared with those receiving the smoking cessation intervention. The difference associated with the smoking cessation intervention reached statistical significance only for deaths from respiratory disease not related to lung cancer

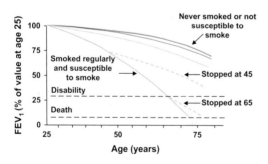

Fig. 2. Decline of forced expiratory volume in 1 second (FEV_1) with age and smoking history according to model of Fletcher and Peto. (*Reprinted from* Fletcher C, Peto R. The natural history of chronic airflow obstruction. Br Med J 1977;1:1645–8; with permission.)

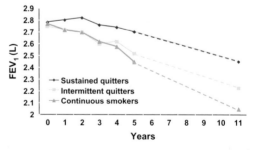

Fig. 3. Smoking cessation reduces the rate of decline in lung function in patients with mild chronic obstructive pulmonary disease. Data from the Lung Health Study at 11 years. (*Data from* Anthonisen NR, Connett JE, Murray RP. Smoking and lung function of Lung Health Study participants after 11 years. Am J Respir Crit Care Med 2002;166:675–9.)

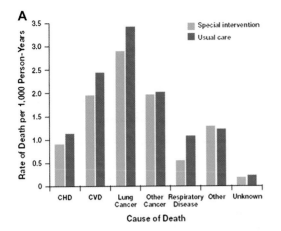

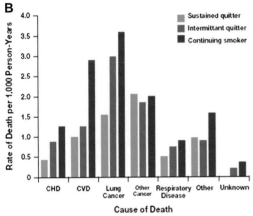

Fig. 4. Effect of smoking cessation on mortality cause at 14.5 years in the Lung Health Study. (*A*) Comparison of smoking cessation intervention with usual care. (*B*) Comparison according to smoking status. Data from the Lung Health Study at 14.5 years. *Abbreviations:* CHD, coronary heart disease; CVD, cardiovascular disease. (*Reprinted from* Anthonisen NR, Skeans MA, Wise RA, et al. The effects of a smoking cessation intervention on 14.5-year mortality: a randomized clinical trial. Ann Intern Med 2005;142:233–9; with permission.)

that smoking cessation has a beneficial impact on lung function and mortality. Therefore, smoking cessation must be an essential part of any COPD treatment plan. In addition, the Lung Health Study provides information on disease progression, disease prevention, and the systemic aspects of disease. It demonstrates that COPD is associated with other major medical comorbidities, such as CHD and other cerebrovascular diseases. In addition, although patients who quit smoking intermittently may have some reduction in mortality risk, the greatest benefits—primarily in terms of reduced mortality from cardiovascular disease, lung cancer and smoking-related diseases, including COPD—are achieved only by those who stop smoking on a sustained basis.

Pharmacotherapy of chronic obstructive pulmonary disease: long-acting beta-agonists

The current treatment guidelines recommend that the first phase of maintenance therapy in COPD for patients with moderate to severe disease involves treatment with one or more long-acting bronchodilators [1,2]. Long-acting β_2-agonists (LABA) (salmeterol, Serevent, and formoterol, Foradil) have been shown to be effective in patients who have stable COPD. These drugs have a prolonged bronchodilator effect, decrease nocturnal symptoms, reduce the frequency of exacerbations, and improve the patient's quality of life and exercise capacity [1,2]. A study in 674 patients who had COPD showed salmeterol administered for 16 weeks significantly improved both daily and nighttime symptoms compared with placebo. During treatment with salmeterol, FEV_1 improved significantly, and patients experienced significantly less breathlessness as measured by the 6-minute walk distance test [7]. In another study comparing formoterol with salmeterol in 47 patients with moderate to severe COPD, both treatments produced increases in inspiratory capacity , suggesting reduction in lung hyperinflation [8]. In addition, when compared with the short-acting bronchodilators ipratropium or theophylline, both formoterol and salmeterol improve symptoms, spirometric indices, exacerbations, and quality of life of patients with COPD [9]. Thus, overall existing data do show that LABA can modify COPD by improving parameters such as lung function, reducing symptoms and exacerbations. These agents, however, have not been shown to alter the rate of decline in lung function over time.

($P = .01$) (see Fig. 4A). Regardless of whether patients received the smoking cessation intervention or usual care, however, the death rates for CHD, cerebrovascular disease, and lung cancer were related significantly to smoking status (continuing smoker, intermittent quitter, or sustained quitter). Sustained quitters had significantly lower death rates for CHD ($P = .02$), cardiovascular disease ($P \leq .001$), and lung cancer ($P = .001$) (Fig. 4B).

The results of the Lung Health Study prospectively validated the model proposed by Fletcher and Peto [3] and clearly demonstrated

Pharmacotherapy of chronic obstructive pulmonary disease: tiotropium

The most recently approved maintenance therapy for the treatment of stable COPD is the once-daily anticholinergic tiotropium (Spiriva). Tiotropium is an anticholinergic bronchodilator maintenance treatment with a long duration of action, attributed to slow dissociation from airway M_3 muscarinic receptors that allow once-daily dosing. Two large, long-term, 1-year, placebo-controlled studies conducted in the United States have shown that once-daily inhalation with tiotropium (18 μg once daily) significantly improves airflow and forced vital capacity over 24 hours in patients who have COPD. Additionally, these benefits were maintained consistently over the year [10]. Furthermore, these and other studies have shown consistently that patients treated with tiotropium have significant improvements in dyspnea, decreases in exacerbations, and improvements in HRQOL [10,11].

To date, intervention, with the exception of smoking cessation, has been proven to decrease the rate of FEV_1 decline in COPD. Recent data, however, suggest that tiotropium bromide also may effect a positive change on the clinical course of the disease. In an analysis of two identical 1-year, randomized, double-blind, double-dummy studies involving 535 patients who had COPD, tiotropium (18 μg once daily) increased trough FEV_1 by 120 mL at the end of the trial, whereas treatment with ipratropium (40 μg four times daily) was associated with a 30 mL reduction in trough FEV_1 ($P < .001$) [11]. A post hoc analysis was performed using data from 921 ambulatory COPD patients who participated in the two 1-year, randomized, controlled registration trials of tiotropium [12]. Patients reached steady state on tiotropium therapy within 8 days. The change in trough FEV_1 from day 8 to day 344 was approximately 12.4 mL/y in the tiotropium group and approximately 58.0 mL/y in the placebo group ($P=.005$) (Fig. 5). Further analysis of the patient subgroups most likely to respond to long-acting bronchodilators was conducted. In the tiotropium subgroup with moderate COPD (GOLD stratification: $FEV_1/FVC < 70\%$ and $50\% \leq FEV_1 \leq 80\%$ predicted), the trough FEV_1 increased from baseline by 117 mL/y, primarily within the first few days. This increase was sustained between day 8 and day 344. In the placebo group, trough FEV_1 declined by 86.5 mL ($P < .001$). By the end of the year, the mean change from baseline in peak FEV_1 with tiotropium

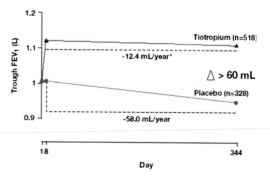

Fig. 5. Rate of decline in trough forced expiratory volume in 1 second from day 8 to day 344 in a post hoc analysis of chronic obstructive pulmonary disease patients in the tiotropium registration trials. *$P=.005$ tiotropium versus placebo (mean regression slopes). (*Data from* Anzueto A, Tashkin D, Menjoge S, et al. One-year analysis of longitudinal changes in spirometry in patients with COPD receiving tiotropium. Pulm Pharmacol Ther 2005;18:75–81.)

relative to placebo was > 200 mL for all severities combined. When patients were divided by disease severity, FEV_1 improvements above placebo were: mild patients 210 plus or minus 40 mL, moderate patients 270 plus or minus 30 mL, and severe patients 180 plus or minus 30 mL ($P < .001$ compared with placebo) [12]. Similar results were observed in former and current smokers. In former smokers, the change in trough FEV_1 from day 8 to day 344 was approximately 17.0 mL with tiotropium and approximately 67.9 mL with placebo ($P = .011$), whereas in smokers, the changes in trough FEV_1 were approximately 3.8 mL and approximately 40.5 mL, respectively ($P = .19$). The lack of statistically significant differences for FEV_1 in smokers may be because of the small number of patients when the analysis was stratified by smoking status. The mean baseline FEV_1 was lower in the former smokers, however; thus, it is possible that those who stopped smoking were patients with more rapidly progressing disease, such that continued smoking was no longer tolerable [12].

The sustained improvement in lung function seen during these 1-year studies with tiotropium [11–13] suggests that tiotropium may slow the decrease in lung function over time and subsequently change the clinical course of the disease. A longer-term study named UPLIFT [14] is underway to examine these potential effects.

In patients who have COPD, both airflow limitation and deconditioning lead to reduced exercise tolerance. Pulmonary rehabilitation (PR) has been shown to improve exercise tolerance and dyspnea [15,16]. A placebo-controlled trial tested the hypothesis that improvements in ventilatory mechanics resulting from tiotropium use would permit enhanced ability to train muscles of ambulation and, therefore, augment exercise tolerance benefits of PR. Tiotropium (18 μg once daily) was given to 93 patients who had moderate to severe COPD participating in 8 weeks of PR. Treatments were administered 5 weeks before, 8 weeks during, and 12 weeks following PR. Tiotropium in combination with PR improved endurance of a constant work rate treadmill task and produced clinically meaningful improvements in dyspnea and health status compared with PR alone. Furthermore, following PR completion, improvements with tiotropium were sustained for 3 months [17].

Pharmacotherapy of chronic obstructive pulmonary disease: inhaled corticosteroids and long-acting β$_2$-agonists–inhaled corticosteroids in combination

Data from studies where patients have received inhaled corticosteroids (ICS) or the fixed combination of long-acting bronchodilators and inhaled corticosteroids also have shown an improvement in spirometry, dyspnea, and reduction in the frequency of exacerbations [18–21].

In one clinical study, 691 patients who had COPD received the combination of fluticasone and salmeterol (500 μg/50 μg), salmeterol (50 μg), fluticasone (500 μg), or placebo twice daily for 24 weeks. At the end of the trial, lung function significantly improved with all treatments compared with placebo ($P < .05$); however, the combination of fluticasone and salmeterol provided significantly greater improvement compared with either treatment alone ($P < .05$). The combination also significantly improved dyspnea compared with fluticasone ($P = .033$), salmeterol ($P < .001$), and placebo ($P < .0001$). In this trial, health status and symptoms also were improved significantly [18]. Similar results were observed in another trial with fluticasone and salmeterol combination (250 μg/50 μg) [19].

Another combination of ICS and LABA, budesonide and formoterol, also has been studied. In a 1-year trial, patients who had COPD received budesonide/formoterol (320 μg of budesonide and 9 μg of formoterol) had fewer exacerbations, a prolonged time to first exacerbation, and maintained higher FEV$_1$, compared with placebo. The combination also improved HRQOL. The combination of budesonide/formoterol was more effective than either of the individual treatments alone [20]. Another trial with the combination budesonide/formoterol showed significant decrease in all symptom scores and use of short-acting β$_2$-agonists compared with placebo and budesonide, and also improved quality of life versus placebo [21].

Furthermore, the impact of combination therapy (fluticasone propionate/salmeterol) on patients' mortality, frequency of exacerbations, and long-term effects on lung function has been reported recently. TORCH (TOward a Revolution in COPD Health) trial is the first and largest study to prospectively investigate the potential for combination therapy (fluticasone propionate/salmeterol) to impact survival in patients who have COPD. TORCH is a 3-year, multicenter, randomized, double-blind, parallel group, placebo-controlled study [22,23]. Approximately 6112 patients were randomized into four study groups: placebo, salmeterol, fluticasone propionate (500 μg), and fluticasone propionate/salmeterol (500/50 μg). The primary end point was the reduction in all-cause mortality, comparing fluticasone propionate/salmeterol with placebo. Secondary end points included COPD morbidity (rate of exacerbations) and quality of life assessment. The study showed a 17% relative reduction in mortality over 3 years for patients receiving fluticasone propionate/salmeterol as compared with placebo ($P = .052$); 25% reduction in exacerbations compared with placebo ($P < .001$); and significant improvement in quality of life measured by the St. George's Respiratory Questionnaire ($P < .001$) [23]. Taken together, existing data suggest that combination LABA/inhaled corticosteroid therapy modifies COPD by improving bronchodilatation, symptoms, HRQOL, and reducing exacerbations. Importantly, this therapy also may alters the course of the disease by reducing mortality.

Implications for chronic obstructive pulmonary disease management

GOLD [2] recommends a stepwise increase in treatment depending on the severity of COPD, which is based on the degree of symptoms and airflow limitation. In assessing the patient for therapy, the frequency and severity of exacerbations also should be considered, as well as comorbidities and health status. The use of drug therapy is designed to control symptoms, reduce exacerbations, and improve exercise tolerance and health status. The GOLD guidelines recommend short-acting β_2-agonists on an as-needed basis for patients who have mild COPD, and regular long-acting bronchodilator therapy for patients who have more severe disease or greater symptoms [2]. Clinical decision-making in COPD management, however, typically is based on patient symptomatology. Thus, the ATS/ERS guidelines recommend that the use of bronchodilators be based on patients' symptoms and response to therapy [1]. The important threshold is whether patients can tolerate and control intermittent symptoms with as-needed β_2-agonist or short-acting anticholinergic use, or whether they have persistent symptoms that necessitate maintenance treatment with longer-acting bronchodilators and/or inhaled corticosteroids.

Regardless of whether the treatment paradigm is driven by symptoms or spirometry, an important issue is whether regular treatment with long-acting bronchodilators and/or the combination of LABA-inhaled corticosteroids should be initiated at an earlier stage of the disease. This issue was examined in a subanalysis of patients who were diagnosed with COPD but were not on chronic therapy (naïve patients; some patients received short-acting β_2-agonists in the preceding year) identified retrospectively from the tiotropium registration trials [24]. The trough FEV_1 increased by approximately 150 mL from baseline in the tiotropium group ($P < .001$ versus placebo) (Fig. 6) [25]. Over the course of 1 year, the increase in trough FEV_1 remained constant in the tiotropium group, while it declined in the placebo group. Peak FEV_1, dyspnea score, and HRQOL measured by the St. George's Respiratory Questionnaire (SGRQ) were all significantly greater with tiotropium compared with placebo ($P < .05$). Notably, the naïve patients responded to tiotropium to a much greater extent compared with previously diagnosed patients who already were receiving treatment. The benefit of tiotropium on HRQOL (SGRQ) was evident in the naïve patients after 6 months of therapy, and was significant at the end of the year compared with placebo ($P < .05$). In the placebo group, changes in HRQOL (SGRQ) were seen initially (day 92) but returned to baseline by the end of the year [24].

A similar analysis of 378 patients diagnosed with COPD ($40\% < FEV_1 < 65\%$ of predicted; $FEV_1/FVC < 70\%$) but naïve to COPD therapy also was performed with ICS or ICS plus

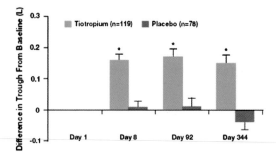

Fig. 6. Change in trough forced expiratory volume in 1 second during 1 year in post hoc analysis of naïve chronic obstructive pulmonary disease patients participating in the tiotropium registration trials. $*P < .001$ versus placebo. (*Reprinted from* Adams SG, Anzueto A, Briggs DD, et al. Tiotropium in COPD patients not previously receiving maintenance respiratory medications. Respir Med 2006;100:1495–1503; with permission.)

long-acting beta-antagonist (LABA) therapy [26]. Over a 24-week period, these patients received either the fixed-dose combination fluticasone/salmeterol (250/50 µg twice daily), fluticasone (250 µg twice daily), salmeterol (50 µg twice daily), or placebo. Trough FEV_1 increased in the fixed-dose combination group ($P \leq .044$ versus placebo and salmeterol). Over the 24 weeks, the increase in trough FEV_1 remained constant in the fluticasone/salmeterol group. Peak FEV_1 was also significantly greater with the combination therapy compared with placebo or fluticasone alone ($P \leq .0068$ for both). Dyspnea score and HRQOL measured by the Chronic Respiratory Disease Questionnaire (CRDQ) also improved [25]. These data showed that the efficacy of initial maintenance therapy with fluticasone/salmeterol (250/50 µg twice daily) in patients naïve to COPD maintenance therapy was consistent, with efficacy results seen in the overall study population [19]. These results also demonstrate that there is still much work to be done to diagnose COPD patients earlier in their disease and to understand more how the disease is affecting their day-to-day activity.

Further work also is needed to determine whether initiation of maintenance therapy with long-acting bronchodilators or combination therapy at early stages of disease can improve long-term clinical outcomes to a greater degree than therapy started when the disease is already moderate or severe. Just as arterial hypertension is treated as early as possible with the expectation of preventing future strokes and other cardiovascular events, perhaps COPD needs to be treated at an early stage with the expectation of preventing or delaying lung function deterioration, exacerbations, future deconditioning and disability, and hence the progression of disease. It remains to be determined whether continuous maintenance therapy will help to avoid airway remodeling and further decline in lung function over time, beyond 1 year. The results of ongoing placebo-controlled trials, UPLIFT with tiotropium [12,14,27] and recent data obtained from the TORCH study with fluticasone, salmeterol, or the fixed-dose combination of fluticasone plus salmeterol, are providing answers to some of these questions (Fig. 7) [23].

It is important to point out that these therapies have shown a significant reduction in COPD exacerbations. This effect may be of particular importance in disease modification, given that exacerbations are associated with increased loss in lung function, increased symptoms, worsening HRQOL, disability, and mortality [27,28].

Better methods are needed for the detection of patients with early COPD who may benefit from early intervention. One approach is to perform screening spirometry in patients over 50 years of age whose risk of COPD is increased because they smoke cigarettes. It may be wise to question newly-diagnosed patients about their activity levels so that signs of avoidance or reduction of activity can be identified and acted upon before the cycle of deconditioning advances too far. Regular maintenance therapy should be instituted at an early stage before symptoms restrict activity

levels. As the approach to the diagnosis and treatment of COPD changes, there is a need of long-term prospective, randomized, controlled trials that evaluate the impact of early therapy in the evolution of this disease.

Summary

Patients who have COPD are clearly a population at risk, as lung function eventually will decline at an increased rate as the disease progresses. COPD management needs to focus on modifying the course of the disease by focus on four major areas:

Earlier diagnosis of the disease
Risk reduction through smoking cessation
Treatment with pharmacotherapy and pulmonary rehabilitation to improve daily and long-term functioning
Decrease in complications by reducing exacerbations and improving pulmonary function with drug therapy

Intervention with regular, pharmacologic maintenance therapy at an earlier mild stage of COPD may be beneficial to patients as suggested by an analysis of naïve patients (ie, treated as mild with β-agonists as needed). Currently, only smoking cessation intervention has been proven to change the clinical course of the disease by preserving lung function. Whether pharmacologic interventions can change the long-term clinical course of disease remains to be demonstrated. The results of ongoing long-term studies soon may provide evidence that in addition to improving lung function and patient-centered outcomes, specific pharmacologic therapies also may alter the clinical course of COPD.

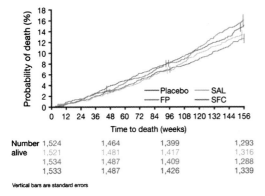

Fig. 7. TORCH study: probability of all-cause mortality in all treatment groups. (*Adapted from* Calverley PM, Anderson JA, Celli B, et al. Salmetrol and fluticasone propionate and survival in chronic obstructive pulmonary disease. N Engl J Med 2007;356(8):781; with permission.)

References

[1] Celli BR, MacNee W. Standards for the diagnosis and treatment of patients with COPD: a summary of the ATS/ERS position paper. Eur Respir J 2004;23:932–46.

[2] GOLD. Global initiative for chronic obstructive lung disease. Global strategy for the diagnosis, management, and prevention of chronic obstructive pulmonary disease—updated November 2006. J Resp Crit Care Med 2007, in press. Available at: www.gold. org. Accessed January 26, 2007.

[3] Fletcher C, Peto R. The natural history of chronic airflow obstruction. Br Med J 1977;1:1645–8.

[4] Anthonisen NR, Wright EC, Hodgkin JE. Prognosis in chronic obstructive pulmonary disease. Am Rev Respir Dis 1986;133:14–20.

[5] Anthonisen NR, Connett JE, Murray RP. Smoking and lung function of Lung Health Study participants after 11 years. Am J Respir Crit Care Med 2002;166: 675–9.

[6] Anthonisen NR, Skeans MA, Wise RA, et al. The effects of a smoking cessation intervention on 14.5-year mortality: a randomized clinical trial. Ann Intern Med 2005;142:233–9.

[7] Boyd G, Morice AH, Pounsford JC, et al. An evaluation of salmeterol in the treatment of chronic obstructive pulmonary disease (COPD). Eur Respir J 1997;10:815–21.

[8] Bouros D, Kottakis J, Le Gros V, et al. Effects of formoterol and salmeterol on resting inspiratory capacity in COPD patients with poor FEV(1) reversibility. Curr Med Res Opin 2004;20:581–6.

[9] Dougherty JA, Didur BL, Aboussouan LS. Long-acting inhaled beta 2-agonists for stable COPD. Ann Pharmacother 2003;37:1247–55.

[10] Casaburi R, Mahler DA, Jones PW, et al. A long-term evaluation of once-daily inhaled tiotropium in chronic obstructive pulmonary disease. Eur Respir J 2002;19:217–24.

[11] Vincken W, van Noord JA, Greefhorst AP, et al. Improved health outcomes in patients with COPD during 1 yr's treatment with tiotropium. Eur Respir J 2002;19:209–16.

[12] Anzueto A, Tashkin D, Menjoge S, et al. One-year analysis of longitudinal changes in spirometry in patients with COPD receiving tiotropium. Pulm Pharmacol Ther 2005;18:75–81.

[13] Kesten S, Flanders J, Menjoge SS, et al. Tiotropium in patients with mild, moderate, and severe COPD in one-year placebo-controlled clinical trials. Chest 2001;120:170S.

[14] Decramer M, Celli B, Tashkin DP, et al. Clinical trial design considerations in assessing long-term functional impacts of tiotropium in COPD: the UPLIFT trial. COPD 2004;1:303–12.

[15] Sewell L, Singh SJ, Williams JE, et al. How long should outpatient pulmonary rehabilitation be? A randomised controlled trial of 4 weeks versus 7 weeks. Thorax 2006;61(9):767–71.

[16] Ries AL, Bauldoff G, Carlin BW, et al. Pulmonary rehabilitation executive summary. Chest 2007;131: 15–35.

[17] Casaburi R, Kukafka D, Cooper CB, et al. Improvement in exercise tolerance with the combination of tiotropium and pulmonary rehabilitation in patients with COPD. Chest 2005;127:809–17.

[18] Mahler DA, Wire P, Horstman D, et al. Effectiveness of fluticasone propionate and salmeterol combination delivered via the Diskus device in the treatment of chronic obstructive pulmonary disease. Am J Respir Crit Care Med 2002;166:1084–91.

[19] Hanania NA, Darken P, Horstman D, et al. The efficacy and safety of fluticasone propionate (250 microg)/salmeterol (50 microg) combined in the Diskus inhaler for the treatment of COPD. Chest 2003;124:834–43.

[20] Calverley PM, Boonsawat W, Cseke Z, et al. Maintenance therapy with budesonide and formoterol in chronic obstructive pulmonary disease. Eur Respir J 2003;22:912–9.

[21] Szafranski W, Cukier A, Ramirez A, et al. Efficacy and safety of budesonide/formoterol in the management of chronic obstructive pulmonary disease. Eur Respir J 2003;21:74–81.

[22] Vestbo J. The TORCH (TOwards a Revolution in COPD Health) survival study protocol. Eur Respir J 2004;24:206–10.

[23] Calverley P, Anderson JA, Celli B, et al. The TORCH (TOwards a Revolution in COPD Health). N Engl J Med 2007;356:775–89.

[24] Anzueto A, Kesten S. Effects of tiotropium in COPD patients only treated with PRN albuterol. Proc Am Thorac Soc 2004;1:A611.

[25] Adams SG, Anzueto A, Briggs DD, et al. Tiotropium in COPD patients not previously receiving maintenance respiratory medications. Respir Med 2006;100:1495–503.

[26] Anzueto A, Sense W, Yates J, et al. Efficacy of Advair Diskus 250/50 (fluticasone propionate/salmeterol) in patients previously naive to COPD maintenance therapy. Chest 2004;126:808S.

[27] Donaldson GC, Seemungal TAR, Bhomik A, et al. Relationship between exacerbation frequency and lung function decline in chronic obstructive pulmonary disease. Thorax 2002;57:847–52.

[28] Soler-Cataluna JJ, Martinez-Garcia MA, Roman Sanchez P, et al. Severe acute exacerbations and mortality in patients with chronic obstructive pulmonary disease. Thorax 2005;60:925–31.

ELSEVIER
SAUNDERS

Clin Chest Med 28 (2007) 617–628

CLINICS
IN CHEST
MEDICINE

Self-Management Strategies in Chronic Obstructive Pulmonary Disease

Jean Bourbeau, MD[a,b],*, Diane Nault, RN, MSc[c]

[a]Division of Pulmonary Medicine, McGill University, Montréal, Québec, Canada
[b]COPD Clinic and Pulmonary Rehabilitation, Montréal Chest Institute, McGill University Health Center,
3650 St., Urbain, Room K1.30, Montréal, Québec H2X 2P4, Canada
[c]Service Régional de Soins Respiratoires à Domicile, Hôpital Maisonneuve-Rosemont,
Centre Affilié à l'Université de Montréal, 5199, Sherbrook East, Bureau 4150,
Montréal, Québec, H1T 3X2, Canada

Chronic obstructive pulmonary disease (COPD) is a chronic illness for which no cure exists; however, health and illness can coexist. The meaning of health is largely the patient's ability to manage and cope with illness. In the trajectory of a chronic illness, patient and family are in a constant process of learning new skilled behaviors that are needed for appropriate disease management.

Many interventions [1,2], such as pulmonary rehabilitation [3], are known to be beneficial to patients who have COPD. These short-term interventions are too often used with the philosophy of an acute care approach, however, in which the physician makes the diagnosis, provides treatment, and reacts to medical complications. A growing body of literature demonstrates the benefits of increasing patients' knowledge, specific skills, and self-efficacy in managing their disease [4,5]. It has been shown that to be effective, care of patients with chronic disease requires self-management education with formulation of a mutually understood care plan and careful and continuous communication with a case manager [6–8].

As for all chronic diseases, self-management strategies are highly important for patients who have COPD. Patients and families must learn to engage in self-management activities that promote health and prevent complications and ensure patients' involvement in daily management decisions. As the disease progresses to different stages and complications, education based on self-management principles in the continuum of care helps patients and families adapt to COPD-related changes and maintain healthy behaviors.

At the end of this article, the reader will be able to understand the newest scientific concepts and advances in the field of self-management in COPD, recognize the importance of self-management education and what might be needed to enhance behavior modification, and translate these advances into strategies and specific interventions in clinical practice.

Chronic illness management: theoretical foundations and models

Self-management is a component of a health care management process that is commonly called disease management. Although disease management has no universally accepted definition, the Disease Management Association of America has defined disease management as a "system of coordinated health care interventions and communications for populations with conditions in which patient self-care is significant" (www.dmaa.org/definition.html). Disease management is further characterized as supporting the physician-patient relationship using evidence-based practices and

* Corresponding author. COPD Clinic and Pulmonary Rehabilitation Program, Montreal Chest Institute, Mcgill University Health Center, 3650 St., Urbain, Room K1.30, Montreal, Quebec H2X 2P4, Canada.
 E-mail address: jean.bourbeau@mcgill.ca
(J. Bourbeau).

0272-5231/07/$ - see front matter © 2007 Elsevier Inc. All rights reserved.
doi:10.1016/j.ccm.2007.06.002

patient empowerment and evaluating outcomes on an ongoing basis for improvement of patient health.

A key element in effective disease management is patient self-management education. Self-management applies to any formalized patient education program aimed at teaching skills needed to carry out medical regimens specific to the chronic disease and guide health behavior change for patients to control their disease and improve their well-being. Self-management does require an approach as part of a continuum of care that incorporates not only teaching various disease related topics but also implementing strategies to change specific behavior in patients [9,10]. Behavior modification implies the implementation of healthy and new lifestyle behaviors that are better adapted to a patient's need. It also implies the appropriate use of many skills (eg, proper use of medication and inhalation devices, breathing techniques, such as pursed-lip breathing). Providing patients who have COPD with the self-management skills they need to properly manage their chronic disease should be considered as important as writing the correct medication prescription.

Chronic illness management is based on models that have high relevance for the implementation of practice better adapted to patients who have COPD. These models are not competing but serve different purposes and are complementary. The "chronic care model" has been proposed as a solution to improve management and prevent complications and outcomes in patients with chronic disease. The chronic care model has essential elements that encourage

high-quality chronic disease care [11–13]. Self-management strategy and support are important components of the chronic care model, but to be successful it does require an approach that incorporates not only teaching various disease contents but also implementing strategies to change behavior in patients. Changes in behavior are caused by enhancement of self-efficacy, which is the confidence an individual has in response to specific actions and the ability to perform these actions [10]. This is based on the "self-management model (self-efficacy)." Finally, the "precede-proceed model" [14] has been proposed to help in the development of self-management education programs. Each of these models is considered in further detail in this article.

Chronic care model of disease management

Critical components of effective chronic disease care are (1) self-management approach, (2) delivery system design, (3) decision support, and (4) clinical information systems (Fig. 1) [11–13]. Patient interactions with an integrated team that includes a skilled health professional case manager are key components of effective chronic disease management. The chronic care disease management model requires more than a case manager, however. The care delivery system must be designed to provide planned chronic care. Regular patient follow-up and communication with health care providers are essential for effective management of chronic disease throughout its trajectory of changes. Health care providers also should be trained to support the physician and the patient. Therapies given should be based on evidence-based practice guidelines.

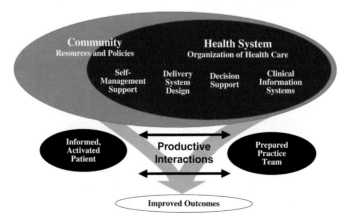

Fig. 1. Chronic care model components. (*From* Wagner EH. Chronic disease management: what will it take to improve care for chronic illness? Effect Clin Pract 1998;1:3; with permission.)

Shared care between family physicians and specialists produces the best outcomes and increases the likelihood that patients receive guideline-directed care [15]. The final component in the chronic care model, which is often lacking, involves integrating a computerized clinical information system into clinical practice. This system can be used to improve chronic care by keeping registries for planning individual and population-based care, implementing automated reminders for the primary care team to comply with clinical guidelines, and providing individual feedback to physicians and clinical practices regarding their performance in specific chronic illness care measures.

Self-management model (self-efficacy)

Self-management strategy and support are crucial components of the chronic care model. The needs of patients suffering from a chronic disease to adjust or change roles as a result of their illness and successfully manage their day-to-day lives are high priorities in self-management. The self-management model assists patients in acquiring skills necessary to adjust their behavior to manage their own illness and, more importantly, to gain the confidence to apply these skills on a daily basis, which means increasing their self-efficacy [10]. This is a rather important causal chain that is presented as a simple illustration in Fig. 2. Health care providers must consider and work on many factors if we want to change patient behavior and expect to have an impact on patient health. According to Lorig and Holman [16] problem solving, decision making, resource use, formation of patient-provider

partnership, action planning, and self-tailoring are the most important general self-management skills that individuals should acquire to manage chronic disease.

Self-efficacy, which is the individual's belief in his or her ability to execute necessary actions in response to specific situations, is considered in the social cognitive theory as a predictor of behavioral change [17,18]. Self-efficacy influences actions that individuals choose to perform and maintain and the effort they invest. Individuals choose an action only if they believe that they are capable of doing it and will benefit from it. As part of patient education, several strategies can be used to enhance self-efficacy, including (1) focusing on past performance accomplishments and building on successful experiences, (2) using peer observation and role models (group education), (3) enlisting verbal persuasion from health professionals, and (4) performing self-evaluation of physical/emotional state and impact of symptom recognition. Compared with traditional care plans, self-management education programs require fewer lectures, promote more active participation of patients, and must focus more on practice and acquisition of new skills, including decision making and problem solving to have an impact on self-efficacy leading to behavioral changes.

Precede/proceed model

The precede-proceed model for health program planning from Green and Kreuter [14] is helpful in the development of self-management education programs for patients who suffer from chronic diseases, such as COPD. This model has been

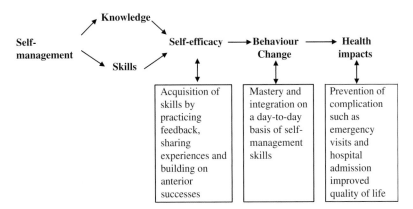

Fig. 2. Effective chronic illness care model: self-management. (*Data from* Bourbeau J, Nault D, Dang-Tan T. Self-management and behaviour modification in COPD. Patient Educ Couns 2004;52(3):271–7.)

the basis for the development of the self-management program "Living Well with COPD." This model helps to (1) define the goals, objectives, and organizational structure that can support a patient's self-management of the disease, (2) identify the potential participant's learning needs based on factors that can influence behavior change, (3) plan the educational interventions in relation to the identified needs, (4) describe the specific self-management skills leading to behavior changes, and (5) define patient outcomes in terms of expected behavior changes.

According to the precede-proceed model, three types of factors can influence the adoption and the maintenance of healthy behaviors:

- *The predisposing factors* refer to the existing knowledge, beliefs, attitudes, and values of the person toward his or her health condition and the behavior changes expected. An important predisposing factor to behavior change is the person's level of self-efficacy.
- *The facilitating factors or barriers* are based on the person's past life experiences, knowledge, and skills already acquired and the accessibility of services and financial resources.
- *The reinforcing factors* depend on the person's social support network and successful past life experiences.

Consideration and review of these factors is important in formulating individualized patient-centered self-management plans tailored to meet individual patient's needs. In the planning of self-management education programs, health professionals should ensure that (1) interactions and collaboration between the learners and the educators will occur, (2) the education is based on a patient's learning needs and is provided on an individual or group basis through methods that enhance self-efficacy, motivation for change, and maintenance of behavior changes, (3) emphasis is put on the mastery of self-management skills through practice, constructive feedback, and reinforcement, and (4) evaluation of behavior changes and patient outcomes is done.

Measuring the benefits of self-management in chronic obstructive pulmonary disease

Self-management strategies for disease management have been studied in chronic respiratory diseases, such as COPD and asthma. A recent Cochrane review on self-management in asthma showed a decrease in hospitalizations (RR 0.64, 95% CI 0.50–0.82), emergency room visits (0.82, 95% CI 0.73–0.94), and unscheduled clinic visits (0.68, 95% CI 0.56–0.81) [19]. The review showed that the most successful self-management education programs combine the use of a written action plan, self-monitoring, and regular medical reviews. Although the success of self-management in asthma provides encouragement that similar strategies might work with COPD, differences between the two diseases do not allow direct extrapolation from one disease to the other [20].

Seeking "truth": totality of available evidence

The results of an early Cochrane systematic review on educating patients who have COPD on self-management were inconclusive [21]. The authors concluded that more research was needed. Other randomized clinical trials have been published since this 2002 Cochrane review [22–24]. Taylor and colleagues [25] published the most recent systematic review of randomized controlled trials on innovations in chronic disease management for COPD. These trials included education on medication and smoking cessation, breathing techniques, and fitness [9]. Only two studies mentioned providing a supply of drugs or a prescription to be filled by patients in the event of an exacerbation. Trials using brief interventions after a hospital admission—both approximately 1 month in duration—found no evidence to support their implementation [2]. Meta-analysis of the three studies that reported quality-of-life outcomes (measured by the St. George's respiratory questionnaire score) found no significant beneficial effect (except one study with a benefit at 4 months but not at 12 months) [22]. Two of the five long-term studies (approximately 1 year in duration) reported a reduction in hospital admission and emergency room visits. The author conclusions were that data were too sparse to exclude any clinically relevant benefit.

Although randomized trials should represent the benchmark or gold standard for determining "truth," many published trials on self-management in COPD have major methodologic limitations. Often, studies that claim to assess self-management education in COPD do not provide complete information allowing readers to evaluate if the intervention met the criteria for true self-management education. In many studies, the focus is primarily on the intervention elements and not on the educational process (teaching self-management, emphasizing day-to-day controls and health behavior, and enhancing self-efficacy). Few studies emphasize continual communication, which is key in the successful self-management program. None of the studies conducted to date assesses if the intervention resulted in intended changes in patient behavior. The question remains in negative studies as to whether the intervention failed to show a benefit or whether it was a failure to intervene.

In addition to problems associated with the intervention, studies with no beneficial effect of self-management may have been underpowered. Surprisingly, this limitation of the studies is rarely brought to the attention of the reader or is brought as a potential explanation for negative results. Finally, no single consistent set of outcomes is reported, and nonvalidated measurements often are used to assess outcomes. It is important to reach consensus on a list of desired outcomes (psychosocial, intended changes in patient behavior, biomedical and service outcomes) and standardize the way these outcomes are measured. With a lack of consistency in the intervention, poor reporting of the self-management process (with potential of enhancing behavior modification), and use of nonstandardized measure outcomes, it is difficult to compare the outcomes of one trial to another. Consequently, review of the sum of available trials, such as is reported in meta-analyses, is not likely to be the best approach in seeking "truth" or helping us define key components of successful self-management in COPD. Standardized methods and properly designed studies should be adopted to ensure comparability of clinical trial results and enable the field of COPD self-management to become a discipline with a "high level" evidence base.

Seeking "truth": knowledge gained from specific trials

New studies that involve self-management, an integrated team with a skilled health professional case manager, and a delivery care system designed to provide planned chronic care are providing emerging evidence of benefits in patients who have COPD, including reduced admissions and hospital bed days [22,26]. Much of the evidence on self-management education comes from a Canadian multifaceted self-management program, "Living Well with COPD," which was one of the first studies to produce conclusive results [9,22].

Patients included in the study had moderate to severe COPD and at least one previous exacerbation that required hospital admission. The foundations of the intervention were based on (1) the chronic care model with self-management program and a delivery system that included communication with a well trained case-manager, (2) self-management strategies with emphasis on self-efficacy leading to behavioral changes, and (3) the precede/proceed model in planning the self-management education program development and delivery of "Living Well with COPD." The program "Living Well with COPD" included self-management education with patient workbooks and a written action plan provided by a trained health professional case manager, seven to eight individual education sessions with specific skill acquisitions for day-to-day management of their disease, and monthly telephone self-use of health-promoting contacts to follow-up to ensure continuous communication and reinforce self-health behaviors.

Patients were encouraged to follow a home exercise program without direct supervision three times per week. The exercise program was not mandatory; nor was it done under the supervision of a health care provider. The action plan was customized for each patient and included a contact list and symptom monitoring list for different situations (eg, stress, environment change, and respiratory tract infection), each of which were linked to appropriate therapeutic actions. It included a self-initiated prescription of antibiotic and prednisone to be used in the event of an acute exacerbation (defined as at least two of the following three symptom changes: increase in dyspnea, sputum, or sputum purulence). It also included safeguards to call the case manager if symptoms became worse despite the use of antibiotics or prednisone. Patients were received follow-up for 1 year.

In the Canadian randomized clinical trial [22], the active intervention, when compared with usual care, reduced hospital admissions by 40% ($P = .01$) and admissions for other health problems by 57% ($P = .01$). In the intervention group, 23.7% of the exacerbations resulted in a hospital admission compared with 32.5% in the usual care group. Emergency department visits were reduced by 41% ($P = .02$) and unscheduled physician visits by 59% ($P = .003$). In the intervention group, 31.7% of exacerbations resulted in an emergency room visit compared with 44.4% in the usual care group. Health status assessed with the St. George's respiratory questionnaire showed a statistically significant difference for the impact subscale and total score at 4 months and difference for the impact score that almost reached statistical significance at 12 months ($P = .05$). Importantly, these differences at 4 and 12 months reached the minimal clinical important difference of -4 (improvement of health). The study also demonstrated that reduction in hospital admission and emergency room visits could be maintained after a 2-year period (Fig. 3) [27]. This is the first study showing the sustainability of self-management benefits.

More recently, an economic analysis showed results that also hold promise for economic benefits of self-management [28]. Fig. 4 demonstrates the cost comparisons of self-management versus usual care based on several hypothetical scenarios for a care manager's patient caseload. Assuming realistic caseloads per case manager of 30, 50, and 70 patients, the mean difference between the two groups reached statistical significance at a caseload of 50 and 70 patients per case manager. From the third-party payer perspective, this could represent cost savings of more than $2000 per patient per year. The cost saving was mainly driven by the number of hospitalizations prevented, which reflects the capacity of a self-management program to meet the changing needs of patients who have moderate to severe COPD.

Key components of successful self-management

The literature suggests the need for multicomponent, interconnected changes to current practice to improve the process and outcomes of

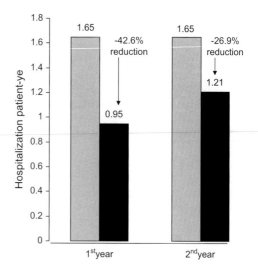

Fig. 3. Difference in all-cause hospitalizations between patients who have COPD in the self-management and usual care groups according to the first- and second-year follow-up. (*Data from* Gadoury MA, Schwartzman K, Rouleau M, et al. Self-management reduces both short- and long-term hospitalisation in COPD. Eur Respir J 2005;26(5):853–7.)

chronic diseases [29]. Diabetes and depression have been the subjects of the largest volume of research in effective management of chronic illness. A recent Cochrane collaboration review showed that the only interventions to achieve improvements in patient outcomes, such as glycemic control, were those with a strong patient-oriented component [30]. Similarly, research

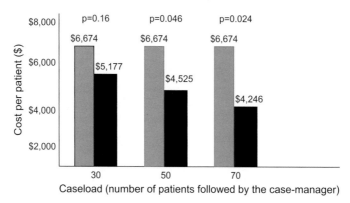

Fig. 4. Cost comparison between self-management and usual care groups according to several scenarios of COPD patient caseloads. The base-case scenario of 14 patients reflects the organization of the trial. Scenarios of 30 and 50 patients' and 70 patients' home and outpatient settings were based on tabulation of the average time spent for patient visits, travel, and telephone contacts. (*Data from* Bourbeau J, Collet JP, Schwartzman K, et al. Economic benefits of self-management education in COPD. Chest 2006;130:1704–11.)

on improving care for depression showed that a trained care team is essential to ensure patient support for self-management [31,32].

A review of 29 randomized trials involving 5039 patients who had chronic heart failure showed that strategies incorporating multidisciplinary team follow-up decreased hospitalizations that resulted from heart failure (RR 0.74, 95% CI 0.63–0.87), all-cause hospitalizations (RR 0.81, 95% CI 0.71–0.92), and mortality (risk ratio 0.75, 95% CI 0.59–0.96) [11]. Programs that focused on enhancing patient self-care activities decreased hospitalizations that resulted from heart failure (RR 0.66, 95% CI 0.52–0.83) and all-cause hospitalizations (RR 0.73, 95% CI 0.57–0.93) but had no effect on mortality (RR 1.14 95% CI 0.67–1.94). Finally, strategies that used telephone contact and advised patients to see their primary care physician in the event of deterioration decreased hospitalizations that resulted from heart failure (RR 0.75, 95% CI 0.57–0.99) but had no effect on all-cause hospitalizations (RR 0.98, 95% CI 0.80–1.20) or mortality (RR 0.91, 95% CI 0.67–1.29).

To be effective, the chronic care approach requires self-management within a delivery system designed to provide planned chronic care. Self-management education includes a mutually understood care plan and careful and continuous communication with a case manager [6–8]. This finding is consistent with the growing body of literature, which demonstrates the benefit of efforts to increase patients' knowledge, specific skills, and self-efficacy in managing their disease. Success of self-management education depends on (1) the educational process (self-management model) and (2) educational topics (intervention elements). It is imperative to realize that improving knowledge, although necessary, is an insufficient sole outcome of a self-management program. Less time should be spent by care providers teaching pathophysiology of the disease, and more time should be spent teaching the appropriate use of specific disease-related skills in the context of daily life.

Success of self-management: the educational process

Patient education on self-management involves not only lecture-based teaching but also promotion of learning by helping the patient and family improve knowledge, increase self-confidence, and take charge of the disease by pursuing actions that allow the prevention and management of disease symptoms and integration of self-care behaviors. Teaching and learning are parts of an interactive process that involves the patient and family, the health care professional educator, the disease itself, and the environment [33]. The style of teaching must change from the traditional, didactic format to that of self-management (Table 1). Health educators in self-management should ensure that patients acquire the confidence and the specific skills to manage their disease on a daily basis.

Ideally this goal should be supported by a case manager whose role is to optimize disease control and follow-up with empowerment. Patients need reassurance and re-enforcement of appropriate behavior. The keys to self-management are strong collaboration and good communication between the patient, the health professional case manager, and the medical team. A meta-analysis done on a wide variety of chronic illnesses showed that combining education of patients and reminders (prompts to remind patients to perform specific tasks) was associated with improved disease control [8]. Providing patients who have COPD with the tools and skills they need and making sure they can use these specific skills to properly manage their disease on a daily basis is as important as writing the correct prescription and ensuring that the patient takes his or her medication.

Success of self-management: the educational topics

Proven effective interventions should be the main focus of our self-management educational approach. These educational topics include (1)

Table 1
Style of teaching: traditional versus self-management education

Style of teaching	Specific feature
Traditional	• Provision of information related to the patient's condition and therapy in didactic sessions
Self-management	• Teaches self-management skills • Emphasizes day-to-day illness symptom control and health behavior (eg, medication use plus exercise) • Increases self-efficacy

smoking cessation, (2) proper prescription and use of medication, (3) breathing techniques and positioning, (4) regular exercise and physical activities, and (5) early recognition of exacerbation and prompt treatment. Self-management education programs represent a window of opportunity that health professionals should try to exploit for smoking cessation interventions.

Self-management also may help to enhance patient compliance to medications. Improving patient self-efficacy in breathing strategies, such as pursed lips breathing, forward leaning position, and energy conservation [34–36], can help a patient manage dyspnea and remain able to perform desired daily activities. Self-management also has potential use in interventions such as exercise training or rehabilitation programs, in which long-term adherence to behaviors learned depends on self-efficacy and other behavioral variables, as demonstrated in studies of elderly and chronically ill populations. Exercise self-efficacy has been found to be the most consistent predictor of adherence to physical activity [37–39]. Outcome expectancies, defined as the estimate of expected benefits from regular exercise, are also associated with adherence [37].

With the recognition of the impact of COPD exacerbations on patient symptoms, functional status, and health-related quality of life comes the knowledge that prevention of exacerbations and early treatment is an important goal of COPD therapy. To date, treatment has focused mainly on drug therapy to decrease admission rates, decrease length of stay, and hasten recovery. Little attention has been paid to early treatment of exacerbations. The East London cohort has just shown that delay/failure to visit a professional to initiate antibiotic and corticosteroid treatment has serious consequences, including increased emergency visits or hospitalizations [40]. The study suggested that the sooner treatment is initiated after onset of symptoms, the shorter the duration of the illness. The use of action plans to help patients recognize symptom changes, implement self-care, and self-initiate a customized prescription (antibiotics and corticosteroids) in the event of an exacerbation has been suggested as a promising strategy.

For example, the results of a recent Cochrane review showed that action plans used in COPD help patients recognize and react appropriately to an exacerbation by promptly self-initiating antibiotics and oral steroids [41]. We have yet to prove, however, that these changes to patient behavior significantly reduce morbidity and use of costly health services, such as emergency department visits and hospital admissions. New study results suggest that an action plan as part of a strategy that promotes self-management education may play a key role in reducing emergency visits and hospitalization risk, as demonstrated in a subanalysis of a previously successful randomized controlled trial [22]. There were fewer exacerbations in the intervention group compared with the control group, for which antibiotics and prednisone were used, which resulted in fewer hospitalizations (16.5% versus 35.1%, $P = .001$) and emergency visits (33.1% versus 72.3%, $P < .001$) because of early treatment [42].

Helpful action plan strategies also should include adoption of healthy behaviors, such as eating a proper diet, maintaining good sleep habits, and engaging in regular home exercise. In a recent study that compared enhanced follow-up to conventional follow-up (only visits to their physician), Brooks and colleagues [43] documented adherence to home exercises in patients who have COPD after completion of a pulmonary rehabilitation program. The most consistently reported reasons for nonadherence were chest infections and disease exacerbations. As part of the action plans, these episodes of worsening symptoms must be recognized, and patients need reassurance and reinforcement of appropriate behavior. Patients who experienced failure may need to be reassessed more carefully so as to understand causes of this failure and provide the necessary treatment.

Application of the chronic care model with self-management education for patients who have chronic obstructive pulmonary disease

Chronic care model applied to chronic obstructive pulmonary disease management

To improve outcomes in chronic disease management, active collaboration between the patient and the practice team is necessary. This goal cannot be achieved without a health care system organization that supports patient self-management and provides a delivery system design in which partners' roles are well defined and long-term follow-up is assured through integrated services [5].

Self-management support within an integrated delivery system

For patients to become managers of their illness, the support of a practice team—in which the roles of the team members are well defined—seems important for the achievement of COPD self-management. The treating physician is in charge of evaluating patient health condition, prescribing the overall optimal disease treatment, and referring patients to the appropriate resources when needed. Patients must play an active role in the care decisions process. The case manager is the contact and resource person for patients and can be located in hospital or in a community center. In the self-management model, case managers are used to empower patients with sufficient knowledge and confidence to take over the responsibility of managing the illness [44]. The other health professionals involved in the care of patients either in hospital or in the community, including the physician, act as consultants who provide education on specific skills related to their domain of expertise if needed and provide support and give reinforcement throughout follow-up.

Regular follow-up and coordination of care are the responsibilities of the treating physician and case manager. To ensure an efficient follow-up, they must (1) assess a patient's general health condition and needs on a regular basis, (2) help the patient/family integrate the skills and healthy behaviors learned into daily life, (3) provide a written action plan with a prescription to be self-administered in case of a COPD exacerbation and support the use of this action plan until the patient demonstrates complete mastery of skills, and (4) make proper referrals to other care providers within hospital and in the community, if needed.

Decision support

Care decisions should be based on best practice guidelines and quality control process. COPD self-management education programs for patients and families should include interventions that already have scientific validity. "Living Well with COPD" (www.livingwellwithcopd.com) (password: copd) is a good example of a self-management education program that has demonstrated significant results in a randomized controlled trial [22,27]. The patient education process established in this program guides health professionals in assessing patient readiness and motivation to learn, set mutual realistic learning goals and objectives with patient and family, use efficient educational methods, implement individualized or group educational interventions, and evaluate patient outcomes.

The essential steps in self-management education using the example of the program "Living Well with COPD"

The first critical step in helping patients and families to engage in the learning experience is to ask them to identify what they know about the illness, what concerns or problems they have in relation to the disease itself and its impact, and what strategies they are already using to cope and live with the disease [45]. Another essential step toward the achievement of patient and family learning goals and objectives is choosing educational methods that (1) take a patient's style of coding, storing, and retrieving information and his or her learning style into account, (2) enhance self-efficacy, and (3) best support the integration of knowledge and skills required for self-management. Use of a combination of educational methods is likely more effective for ensuring learning retention [33,46]. Table 2 demonstrates methods used in disease management education for patients who have COPD to manage their disease. These different educational methods are efficient ways to facilitate the self-management learning process in patients who have COPD [47].

The most important step leading to the learners' acquisition of knowledge and mastery of skills required for the integration of expected self-care behaviors is the implementation of educational interventions. Interventions useful for

Table 2
Efficient educational methods to be used either in individual or group sessions for patients who have chronic obstructive pulmonary disease for self-management

Method	Individual	Group
Interactive lecturing	▲	▲
Motivational interviewing techniques	▲	▲
Case scenarios	▲	▲
Demonstrations and practice	▲	▲
Constructive feedback and reinforcement	▲	▲
Group exchanges or discussion	—	▲
Peer observation (use of an expert patient)	—	▲
Learning contracts (homework, goals achievement)	▲	▲
Written material given to patients adapted to their level of literacy	▲	▲

patients who have COPD and their families include smoking cessation, breathing control, conservation of energy, management of anxiety and stress, prevention and management of exacerbations, and adoption of healthy life habits. Presenting material from the program "Living Well with COPD," Table 3 lists the specific skills to master and healthy behaviors to adopt and maintain in COPD self-management.

Evaluating patient comprehension, attitudes, and self-efficacy, the skills mastered and healthy behaviors adopted should be done throughout the

Table 3
Self-management skills and healthy behaviors for self-management of chronic obstructive pulmonary disease

Healthy behavior	Self-management skill (strategy)
Live in a smoke-free environment	Quit smoking and remain nonsmoker and avoid second-hand smoke
Comply with your medication	Take medication as prescribed on a regular basis and use proper inhalation techniques
Manage your breathing	Use according to directives: • the pursed-lip breathing technique • the forward body positions • the coughing techniques
Conserve your energy	Prioritize your activities, plan your schedule, and pace yourself
Manage your stress and anxiety	Use your relaxation and breathing techniques Try to solve one problem at a time Talk about your problems and do not hesitate to ask for help Maintain a positive attitude
Prevent and manage aggravations of your symptoms (exacerbations)	Get your flu shot every year and your vaccine for pneumonia Identify and avoid factors that can make your symptoms worse Use your plan of action according to the directives (recognition of symptoms deterioration and actions to perform) Contact your resource person when needed
Maintain an active life	Maintain physical activities (eg, activities of daily living, walking, climbing stairs) Exercise regularly (according to a prescribed home exercise program)
Keep a healthy diet	Maintain a healthy weight Eat food high in protein Eat smaller meals more often (5–6 meals/d)
Have good sleep habits	Maintain a routine Avoid heavy meals and stimulants before bedtime Relax before bedtime
Maintain a satisfying sex life	Use positions that require less energy Share your feelings with your partner Do not limit yourself to intercourse, create a romantic atmosphere Use your breathing, relaxation and coughing techniques
Get involved in leisure activities	Choose leisure activities that you enjoy Choose environments in which your symptoms are not aggravated Pace yourself through the activities while using your breathing techniques Respect your strengths and limitations
Plan your trips	Get a list from your doctor of current medical diagnoses, allergies, and medications Have enough medication for the duration of the trip and make the proper arrangements if you are on home oxygen Bring your plan of action, including a supply of antibiotics and prednisone Make sure you have adequate health insurance

learning process to determine if the pre-established goals and objectives are met. Methods such as direct questioning, problem solving, simulations, direct observation, summarizing in own words, and repetition of key instructions can be used to supplement information, correct misunderstandings and mistakes in a constructive way, and reinforce newly acquired skills and behaviors. For goals and objectives that are unmet, the educational plan should be revised and education repeated through other efficient interventions and methods. More information is provided as part of the reference guides for the health professional on the Web site specific to the self-management program "Living Well with COPD" www.livingwellwithcopd.com (password: copd).

Summary

Self-management education is an important new adjunct to the management of COPD, and it is applicable to a broad cross-section of patients. We have provided evidence that self-management can positively impact a patient' life, reduce hospital admissions, and potentially save costs. To be effective, however, self-management must be part of a continuum of care with access to a case manager. This approach of care through a continuum of self-management is interesting because it does not require specialized resources and could be implemented within normal practice. We have illustrated that self-management strategies and support do not require a new breed of health professionals but rather some revamping of currently existing health care delivery systems and current health professionals' education and training.

Understanding which interventions (self-management processes and topics) are most effective is important for guiding future development in self-management programs. Some conclusions still can be drawn while we are awaiting further research. Successful programs are based on organization and practice that (1) include self-management COPD care strategies, (2) ensure that patients have confidence self-efficacy and specific skills to be used on a day-to-day basis, and (3) are supported by a practice team case manager to optimize disease control and follow-up.

References

[1] Celli BR, MacNee W. Standrads for the diagnosis and treatment of patients with COPD: a summary of the ATS/ERS position paper. Eur Respir J 2004;23:932–46.

[2] Pauwels RA, Buist AS, Calverley PM, et al. Global strategy for the diagnosis, management, and prevention of chronic obstructive pulmonary disease. NHLBI/WHO Global Initiative for Chronic Obstructive Lung Disease (GOLD) workshop summary. Am J Respir Crit Care Med 2001;163(5): 1256–76.

[3] Nici L, Donner C, Wouters E, et al. American Thoracic Society/European Respiratory Society statement on pulmonary rehabilitation. Am J Respir Crit Care Med 2006;173(12):1390–413.

[4] Von Korff M, Gruman J, Schaefer J, et al. Collaborative management of chronic illness. Ann Intern Med 1997;127(12):1097–102.

[5] Wagner EH, Glasgow RE, Davis C, et al. Quality improvement in chronic illness care: a collaborative approach. Jt Comm J Qual Improv 2001;27(2):63–80.

[6] Piette JD, Weinberger M, Kraemer FB, et al. Impact of automated calls with nurse follow-up on diabetes treatment outcomes in a Department of Veterans Affairs health care system: a randomized controlled trial. Diabetes Care 2001;24(2):202–8.

[7] Simon GE, VonKorff M, Rutter C, et al. Randomised trial of monitoring, feedback, and management of care by telephone to improve treatment of depression in primary care. BMJ 2000;320(7234): 550–4.

[8] Weingarten SR, Henning JM, Badamgarav E, et al. Interventions used in disease management programmes for patients with chronic illness: which ones work? Meta-analysis of published reports. BMJ 2002;325(7370):925–8.

[9] Bourbeau J, Nault D, Dang-Tan T. Self-management and behaviour modification in COPD. Patient Educ Couns 2004;52(3):271–7.

[10] Lorig K. Chronic disease self-management: a model for tertiary prevention. Am Behav Sci 1996;39(6): 676–83.

[11] McAlister FA, Lawson FM, Teo KK, et al. A systematic review of randomized trials of disease management programs in heart failure. Am J Med 2001;110(5):378–84.

[12] Norris SL, Nichols PJ, Caspersen CJ, et al. The effectiveness of disease and case management for people with diabetes: a systematic review. Am J Prev Med 2002;22(4 Suppl):15–38.

[13] Wagner EH. More than a case manager. Ann Intern Med 1998;129(8):654–6.

[14] Green LW, Kreuter MW. Health promotion planning: an educational and environmental approach. 3rd edition. London: Mayfield Publishing Company; 1999.

[15] Willison DJ, Soumerai SB, McLaughlin TJ, et al. Consultation between cardiologists and generalists in the management of acute myocardial infarction: implications for quality of care. Arch Intern Med 1998;158(16):1778–83.

[16] Lorig KR, Holman H. Self-management education: history, definition, outcomes, and mechanisms. Ann Behav Med 2003;26(1):1–7.

[17] Bandura A. Social learning theory. Englewood Cliffs (NJ): Prentice Hall; 1977.

[18] Bandura A. The assessment and predictive generality of self-percepts of efficacy. J Behav Ther Exp Psychiatry 1982;13(3):195–9.

[19] Gibson PG, Powell H, Coughlan J, et al. Self-management education and regular practitioner review for adults with asthma. Cochrane Database Syst Rev 2003;1:CD001117.

[20] Gallefoss F, Bakke PS, Rsgaard PK. Quality of life assessment after patient education in a randomized controlled study on asthma and chronic obstructive pulmonary disease. Am J Respir Crit Care Med 1999;159(3):812–7.

[21] Monninkhof EM, van der Valk PD, van der PJ, et al. Self-management education for chronic obstructive pulmonary disease. Cochrane Database Syst Rev 2003;1:CD002990.

[22] Bourbeau J, Julien M, Maltais F, et al. Reduction of hospital utilization in patients with chronic obstructive pulmonary disease: a disease-specific self-management intervention. Arch Intern Med 2003; 163(5):585–91.

[23] Hermiz O, Comino E, Marks G, et al. Randomised controlled trial of home based care of patients with chronic obstructive pulmonary disease. BMJ 2002; 325:938–42.

[24] Monninkhof E, van der Valk P, van der Palen J, et al. Effects of a comprehensive self-management programme in patients with chronic obstructive pulmonary disease. Eur Respir J 2003;22(5):815–20.

[25] Taylor SJ, Candy B, Bryar RM, et al. Effectiveness of innovations in nurse led chronic disease management for patients with chronic obstructive pulmonary disease: systematic review of evidence. BMJ 2005;331(7515):485–8.

[26] Rea H, McAuley S, Stewart A, et al. A chronic disease management programme can reduce days in hospital for patients with chronic obstructive pulmonary disease. Intern Med J 2004;34(11):608–14.

[27] Gadoury MA, Schwartzman K, Rouleau M, et al. Self-management reduces both short- and long-term hospitalisation in COPD. Eur Respir J 2005; 26(5):853–7.

[28] Bourbeau J, Collet JP, Schwartzman K, et al. Economic benefits of self-management education in COPD. Chest 2006;130:1704–11.

[29] Rothman AA, Wagner EH. Chronic illness management: what is the role of primary care? Ann Intern Med 2003;138(3):256–61.

[30] Renders CM, Valk GD, Griffin SJ, et al. Interventions to improve the management of diabetes in primary care, outpatient, and community settings: a systematic review. Diabetes Care 2001;24(10): 1821–33.

[31] Callahan CM. Quality improvement research on late life depression in primary care. Med Care 2001; 39(8):772–84.

[32] Von Korff M, Unutzer J, Katon W, et al. Improving care for depression in organized health care systems. J Fam Pract 2001;50:530–1.

[33] Kumm S, Hicks V, Shupe S, et al. You can help your clients change. Dimens Crit Care Nurs 2002;21(2): 72–7.

[34] Gosselink R. Breathing techniques in patients with chronic obstructive pulmonary disease (COPD). Chron Respir Dis 2004;1:163–72.

[35] Gosselink R, Troosters T, Decramer M. Exercise training in COPD patients: the basic questions. Eur Respir J 1997;10(12):2884–91.

[36] Grandevia B. The spirogram of gross expiratory tracheobronchial collapse in emphysema. Q J Med 1963;32:23–31.

[37] Brassington GS, Atienza AA, Perczek RE, et al. Intervention-related cognitive versus social mediators of exercise adherence in the elderly. Am J Prev Med 2002;23(2 Suppl):80–6.

[38] Jette AM, Rooks D, Lachman M, et al. Home-based resistance training: predictors of participation and adherence. Gerontologist 1998;38(4):412–21.

[39] McAuley E, Lox C, Duncan TE. Long-term maintenance of exercise, self-efficacy, and physiological change in older adults. J Gerontol 1993;48(4):218–24.

[40] Wilkinson TM, Donaldson GC, Hurst JR, et al. Early therapy improves outcomes of exacerbations of chronic obstructive pulmonary disease. Am J Respir Crit Care Med 2004;169(12):1298–303.

[41] Turnock AC, Walters EH, Walters JA, et al. Action plans for chronic obstructive pulmonary disease. Cochrane Database Syst Rev 2005;CD005047.

[42] Sedeno MF, Nault D, Hamd D, et al. A written action plan for early treatment of COPD exacerbations: an important component to the reduction of hospitalizations [abstract]American Thoracic Society 2006;3:A603.

[43] Brooks D, Krip B, Mangovski-Alzamora S, et al. The effect of postrehabilitation programmes among individuals with chronic obstructive pulmonary disease. Eur Respir J 2002;20(1):20–9.

[44] Zwarenstein M, Stephenson B, Johnson L. Case management: effects on professional practice and health care outcomes. Cochrane Database Syst Rev 2000;4:CD000050.

[45] Weston-Eborn R, Sitzman K. Creating teaching plans for the adult learner. Home Healthc Nurse 2005;23(3):192–4.

[46] Nault D, Dagenais J, Perreault V, et al. Comprehensive management of COPD. In: Decker BC, editor. Comprehensive management of COPD. Hamilton (Ontario): BC Decker, Inc; 2002. p. 301–18.

[47] Lange N, Tigges BB. Influence positive change with motivational interviewing. Nurse Pract 2005;30(3): 44–53.

ELSEVIER
SAUNDERS

Clin Chest Med 28 (2007) 629–638

CLINICS
IN CHEST
MEDICINE

New Approaches in Pulmonary Rehabilitation

Nicolino Ambrosino, MD*, Gerardo Palmiero, MD,
Soo-Kyung Strambi, PT

Pulmonary Unit, Cardio-Thoracic Department, University Hospital, Pisa, Via Paradisa 2-Cisanello, 56124 Pisa, Italy

Chronic obstructive pulmonary disease (COPD) affects 6% of the general population and is a leading cause of morbidity and mortality worldwide. It is a heterogeneous disorder resulting from dysfunction of the small and large airways and destruction of the lung parenchyma and vasculature in highly variable combinations [1,2]. Breathlessness and reduction in exercise capacity are the main complaints of patients who have COPD. Over time, these symptoms progress relentlessly, reducing patients' ability to face activities of daily living [3].

Patients who have mild to severe COPD may obtain improvement in dyspnea, exercise capacity, and health-related quality of life (HRQOL) as a result of exercise training within pulmonary rehabilitation, a comprehensive treatment that has grown tremendously in scientific interest over the past several years [4].

Mechanisms of dyspnea during exercise in chronic obstructive pulmonary disease

Dyspnea is "a term used to characterize a subjective experience of breathing discomfort that consists of qualitatively distinct sensations that vary in intensity. The experience derives from interactions among multiple physiological, psychological, social and environmental factors, and may induce secondary physiological and behavioral responses" [5]. Different pathophysiologic factors may contribute to dyspnea during exercise in patients who have COPD: increased intrinsic mechanical loading on inspiratory muscles resulting from

the intrinsic positive end-expiratory pressure (PEEPi), airflow limitation, inspiratory muscle weakness, increased ventilatory demand relative to capacity, gas exchange abnormalities, and cardiovascular factors [6]. In COPD, dyspnea during exercise correlates with lung hyperinflation (as assessed by inspiratory capacity) which, in turn, results in severe "neuromechanical dissociation" [7].

Peripheral (skeletal) muscle function and pulmonary rehabilitation

Peripheral muscle function is another important determinant of exercise capacity in COPD [8]. Many patients who have COPD have significant skeletal muscle dysfunction, characterized by structural and functional disturbances [8]. Peripheral muscle wasting and reduced body weight also are common findings in advanced COPD and have a negative impact on patients' survival, as in several other chronic diseases [8–10]. Gains in muscle mass and strength and in body weight are associated with better exercise tolerance and survival [11]. The potential role of pharmacologic approaches to address this problem (eg, anabolic steroid, growth hormone, and testosterone supplementation) still is uncertain [11,12]. In contrast, the role of multidisciplinary pulmonary rehabilitation, including exercise training in improving skeletal muscle dysfunction, is well defined [4].

The improvements in exercise tolerance of patients who have COPD induced by training have been found to be based on physiologic changes, such as improved muscle function [13,14] and altered breathing pattern, with a higher tidal volume (V_T) and lower breathing frequency leading to a reduced dead space–to–V_T ratio and, thus, to a lower ventilatory requirement for

---

* Corresponding author.
E-mail address: n.ambrosino@ao-pisa.toscana.it
(N. Ambrosino).

0272-5231/07/$ - see front matter © 2007 Elsevier Inc. All rights reserved.
doi:10.1016/j.ccm.2007.06.001

chestmed.theclinics.com

exercise [15]. Intensive training increases the levels of aerobic enzymes and the capillary density of exercised muscle [16] and counteracts the increased exercise-associated oxidative stress of patients who have COPD [17]. The intensity of exercise training is of key importance in determining specific outcomes [13]. Although low-intensity training leads to improved exercise endurance, usually in the absence of physiologic gains in aerobic fitness, high-intensity training improves performance of maximal and submaximal exercise tests and induces cardiorespiratory and peripheral muscle adaptations [13–16]. Some patients, however, may not be able to exercise at an intensity sufficient to achieve these benefits. Given the demonstrated value of exercise training [4], extensive recent research has focused on new approaches to improve the effectiveness of exercise training and muscle function [18]. For example, a review of the literature from 1966 to 2006 (PubMed) shows 1345 articles under the terms, COPD and pulmonary rehabilitation (Fig. 1). For the purpose of this article, those articles have been reviewed according the following terms: COPD and exercise and (1) mechanical ventilation (76 studies, including two meta-analyses); (2) electrical stimulation (eight studies); (3) interval training (24 articles, including three meta-analyses); (4) oxygen (726 studies, including three meta-analyses); and (5) biofeedback (five studies). Each of these interventions has emerged as a potentially important adjunct to conventional pulmonary rehabilitation, to improve the exercise tolerance of patients who have COPD.

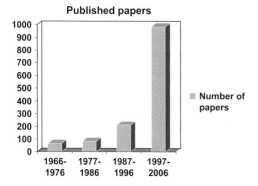

Published papers

Fig. 1. Number of articles dealing with COPD and pulmonary rehabilitation, per decade, published from 1966 to January 1, 2007. (*Data from* National Library of Medicine and National Institutes of Health. Available at: http://www.pubmed.gov. Accessed January 1, 2007.)

Ventilatory assistance during exercise

In recent years, there has been increasing interest in the use of noninvasive positive pressure ventilation (NPPV) to increase exercise capacity [18]. Assisted ventilation, by unloading respiratory muscles, might allow patients to train at higher levels of exercise intensity. Using proportional assist ventilation (PAV), a recently proposed modality of assisted ventilation [19], it is shown that work of breathing (WOB) needed to sustain heavy-intensity exercise of healthy trained cyclists correlated to a reduction in leg blood flow and had a significant influence on exercise performance [20,21]. In other words, during leg exercise, there may be a competition for blood flow between respiratory and limb muscles that may be minimized by use of assisted ventilation during exercise. In another study, PAV prevented exercise-induced diaphragmatic fatigue [22]. Because intrinsic mechanical loading and functional inspiratory muscle weakness in COPD contribute to dyspnea, assisted ventilation should provide a symptomatic benefit by unloading and assisting the overburdened ventilatory muscles. Unloading of the respiratory muscles by assisted ventilation in turn may reduce the blood requirement of inspiratory muscles and may allow a switch of blood flow from respiratory to limb muscles. Several laboratory studies have examined the acute effects of different modalities of ventilatory assistance on dyspnea and exercise tolerance in advanced COPD [18,23,24].

Continuous positive airway pressure

Theoretically, continuous positive airway pressure (CPAP) should reduce the inspiratory threshold load on the inspiratory muscles of patients who have COPD and hyperinflation and enhance neuromuscular coupling, thus improving dyspnea and exercise tolerance [25–28]. CPAP, however, counterbalances, at least in part, PEEPi (ie, the inspiratory threshold load) [29]. CPAP also is shown to reduce the WOB and increase exercise tolerance in patients who have cystic fibrosis [30]. For maximal benefit, CPAP should be titrated on an individual basis to optimize comfort. Nevertheless, theoretically this implies the measurement of PEEPi, which is difficult to perform on a routine basis [29].

Pressure support ventilation

Inspiratory pressure support (IPS) is a form of mechanical ventilation that can assist ventilation effectively when applied noninvasively to patients in acute and chronic respiratory failure. Pressure support is a pressure-targeted mode in which each breath is patient triggered and supported [31]. IPS can improve dyspnea and exercise capacity by reducing the excessive load placed on inspiratory muscles when patients who have COPD exercise [32–38]. Patients who have severe COPD can sustain exercise-induced lactatemia longer if assisted with IPS [39].

Proportional assist ventilation

PAV is a mode of partial ventilatory assistance endowed with characteristics of proportionality and adaptability to the intensity and timing of spontaneous ventilatory pattern by providing inspiratory flow and pressure in proportion to patient effort [19]. Several laboratory studies show that PAV can increase exercise capacity of patients who have COPD [40–43].

Controlled mechanical ventilation

Assist-control ventilation is a combination mode of ventilation in which the ventilator delivers a positive pressure breath at a preset V_T in response to a patient's inspiratory effort. The ventilator also delivers breaths at a preset rate if no patient effort occurs within the preselected time period [44]. This modality of assisted ventilation was delivered through nasal masks during exercise in patients who had pulmonary tuberculosis sequelae and kyphoscoliosis, resulting in a significant improvement in breathlessness and increase in exercise endurance [45,46]. Its use is not yet studied in patients who have COPD.

Ventilatory assistance and pulmonary rehabilitation

The message of the physiologic studies (discussed previously) can be summarized as follows: acute NPPV, either CPAP, IPS, or PAV, during exercise reduces dyspnea and WOB and enhances exercise tolerance in patients who have COPD. Nevertheless, the role of NPPV as a routine component of pulmonary rehabilitation, if any, is still to be defined. This is an important issue, because most patients who have moderate to severe COPD are candidates for pulmonary rehabilitation, and a majority of patients facing lung transplantation or lung volume reduction surgery are required to attend rehabilitation programs [47,48]. Given the established usefulness of NPPV in increasing exercise tolerance and reducing

dyspnea in an acute (laboratory) setting [18], the next step is to evaluate whether or not assisted ventilation can be used as an aid during exercise training sessions. This is a different issue, as conflicting results are reported to date. One randomized controlled study [49] finds no additional benefit from providing assisted ventilation (in PAV modality) on exercise tolerance, dyspnea, or health status when compared with training alone. In contrast, a similar study [50] finds that after PAV-assisted training, mean training intensity, and peak work rate were higher than after nonassisted training. Isoworkload lactatemia after training was reduced to a greater extent in the assisted than in unassisted patients. Moreover, a significant inverse relationship was found between reduction in isoworkload lactatemia after training during the constant work rate test and peak work rate achieved during the last week of training. This was considered a marker of true physiologic training effect. Other investigators have confirmed benefits of addition of NPPV to pulmonary rehabilitation [51–53].

Despite promising, although conflicting, results, the use of ventilatory assistance during exercise training programs is unlikely to have a role in routine pulmonary rehabilitation settings. Some potential problems with the use of NIPPV in pulmonary rehabilitation are

1. NPPV interfaces. During high-intensity exercise, patients may breathe through their mouth rather than their nose, thus requiring a full-face mask or mouthpiece. Use of full-face masks during exercise may be less comfortable than nasal mask interfaces, hence reducing patient compliance.

2. Comorbidities. Many patients who have COPD have significant comorbidities, including a high proportion of ischemic cardiac disease [54]. It is of concern that reduction of dyspnea with this kind of "mechanical doping" [55] might allow patients to exercise at a higher intensity and, as such, expose unaware and ischemic patients who have COPD to a load greater than their coronary ischemic threshold.

3. Practicalities. In a study by Bianchi and colleagues [49], a high rate of drop-outs resulting from lack of compliance in the ventilated group and a mean 17-minute time spent to set the ventilator and supervise the training session during NPPV were practical drawbacks to the addition of mask ventilation during a high-intensity training

program. It might not be practical or worth-while to submit patients to unpleasant equip-ment (eg, mask and related troubles), given the need for constant supervision of an indi-vidual operator to check for leaks and to reset the ventilator when needed and given a substantial risk for lack of patient compli-ance. Furthermore, to deliver NPPV during exercise training, a one-to-one patient-therapist ratio is needed, which in turn adds to the cost of the rehabilitation program. This is a particularly important concern, es-pecially in light of the recognized benefits of well-conducted standard exercise training programs that do not require complex and sophisticated machinery or a personalized physiotherapist [4,55].

Nighttime noninvasive positive pressure ventilation and daytime exercise

It is possible to use NPPV in another way to improve results of pulmonary rehabilitation. Pa-tients who have severe stable COPD and are undergoing home nocturnal NPPV and daytime exercise training showed a significant improve-ment in exercise capacity and HRQOL compared with patients undergoing exercise training alone [56]. The hypothesis that the observed increased exercise performance with nocturnal NPPV may be associated with increased quadriceps strength was not confirmed [57,58].

Electrical stimulation of peripheral muscles

Low-volt neuromuscular electrical stimulation (NMES) is used by physical therapists to improve muscle performance by stimulating motor nerves to cause a muscle contraction. NMES is used to increase performance of healthy muscles and is associated with increased mass, strength, and endurance of normally and abnormally inner-vated muscles in a wide range of pathologic conditions. NMES retards muscle wasting during denervation immobilization and optimizes recov-ery of muscle strength during rehabilitation [18]. It is used to assist respiratory function in patients who have spinal cord injury and in patients who have skeletal muscle dysfunction and exercise in-tolerance resulting from congestive heart failure [59].

Pulmonary rehabilitation in active patients who have COPD may normalize the electrical activity of skeletal muscles during incremental dynamic exercise. The electromyographic signal confirms neuromuscular changes after endurance training [60]. Passive training of specific locomo-tor muscle groups by means of NMES might be tolerated better than whole body exercise in patients who have severe COPD. Small controlled studies of this technique in patients who have severe COPD are reported with encouraging results [61–64].

The major advantage of NMES over conven-tional exercise training is considered the lack of ventilatory or cardiac stress during passive mus-cular activity, reflecting the reduced muscle mass involved. Thus, NMES may be a particularly beneficial mode of exercise training for those patients who have COPD who are unable to perform conventional exercise because of severe ventilatory limitation and dyspnea. Furthermore, NMES may be used even during periods of COPD exacerbations, which are associated with loss of muscle strength and mass [63]. There are negative studies in non-COPD patient populations, how-ever, in which no significant change in neurophys-iologic status, aerobic performance, or clinical status occurred after electrostimulation [65,66]. Thus, these studies must be considered prelimi-nary, and at present NMES still should be consid-ered an experimental tool in pulmonary rehabilitation. In particular, further randomized trials using larger patient samples and longer fol-low-up periods are needed. Also, the optimal pro-tocols for stimulation settings are yet to be determined [18].

Timing and intensity of exercise in pulmonary rehabilitation

The optimal duration of pulmonary rehabili-tation programs has yet to be established. Short-ened supervised programs seem equivalent to longer supervised programs at comparable time points [67,68].

Interval training is characterized by repeated bouts of high-intensity exercise interspersed with recovery periods (light exercise or rest). In healthy subjects, interval training with rest during a re-covery period has been studied widely and, in some studies, shows better results than continuous training [69]. In patients who have COPD, inter-val training is shown capable of inducing physio-logic training effects [8]. The most common interval training protocol studied in these patients is moderate- to high-intensity exercise alternated with low-intensity exercise. High-intensity interval exercise training is equally effective as moderately intense, constant-load exercise training in inducing peripheral muscle adaptations; however, interval training is associated with fewer disturbing symptoms during training [70]. As such, an "intermittent" training modality may be tolerated better and allows a greater amount of work to be performed in most patients who have severe COPD [71]. This, in turn, may allow some patients who are incapable of performing high-intensity, constant-load exercise still to achieve physiologic gains in aerobic fitness.

Strength training enhances muscle growth and strength and may be associated with less dyspnea than aerobic exercise in patients who have COPD. The combination of strength and aerobic training seems an appropriate physiologically complete approach [8].

Whole body exercises (cycling, walking, and stair climbing) result in higher cardiopulmonary stress than arm cranking and resistance training. Dyspnea is higher during cycling than resistance training. The lower cardiopulmonary stress during resistance training results in fewer disturbing symptoms [72]. Studies demonstrate the effectiveness of one-legged exercise at the same muscle-specific intensity in extending the duration of exercise among patients who have COPD [73].

The use of a rollator walker improves the biomechanical efficiency of walking and breathing by repositioning the body forward, anchoring the upper extremities, and assuming a small amount of the user's weight. Rollators may improve performance on exercise tests, especially among more impaired individuals. These improvements are accompanied by patient preference for assisted walking in addition to reducing dyspnea and adding a greater sense of safety. Despite several reports on the short-term beneficial effects of rollators [74,75], further evaluations of rollator effectiveness, including objective monitoring of usage, are required to establish longer-term benefits.

Oxygen supplementation

Supplemental oxygen has the potential to increase exercise tolerance of patients who have hypoxemic COPD by several different mechanisms: hypoxic stimulation of the carotid bodies is reduced, pulmonary circulation vasodilates, and arterial oxygen content increases. The latter two mechanisms potentially may reduce carotid body stimulation at heavy levels of exercise by increasing oxygen delivery to the exercising muscles and reducing carotid body stimulation by lactic acidemia. The main mechanism for oxygen's effect on exercise tolerance recently has been clarified [76].

Ambulatory oxygen therapy has been shown widely to increase exercise performance and to relieve exercise breathlessness in patients who have COPD [77–79]. A systematic review [80] of the short-term efficacy of ambulatory oxygen from single-assessment studies in COPD has been published recently. Thirty-one studies (33 data sets; 534 participants) met the inclusion criteria of the review. Oxygen improved the primary outcomes relating to endurance and maximal exercise capacity. Oxygen also improved breathlessness, oxygen saturation, and minute ventilation at isotime with endurance exercise testing.

Studies indicate that reduction in lung hyperinflation plays an important role in the oxygen-related relief of dyspnea [78,79]. Supplemental oxygen generally increases exercise tolerance even in patients who have only mild to moderate hypoxemia (ie, levels of hypoxemia not severe enough to meet guidelines for long-term oxygen therapy) [81–83]. Short-term oxygen supplementation also prevents exercise-induced oxidative stress in patients who have COPD and who are normoxemic and muscle wasted [84].

Despite the positive results of these physiologic studies, there is evidence [85] that mild hypoxemia accelerates peripheral muscle adaptation, suggesting that supplemental oxygen during training of patients who are mildly hypoxemic may not be advantageous. This seems confirmed by previous studies of patients who had COPD trained while using supplemental oxygen, which failed to demonstrate benefits [86–90]. In contrast with those studies, a more recent study [91] showed that patients who had COPD and were nonhypoxemic trained with oxygen supplementation were able to reach a greater training intensity and endurance more rapidly than patients trained without it. Combining the benefits of bronchodilators (reduced hyperinflation) and oxygen (reduced ventilatory drive) also shows additive effects on exercise endurance in patients who have COPD and are normoxic [92].

Air-heliox mixtures

Heliox breathing can improve dyspnea and increase high-intensity exercise endurance capacity in moderate to severe COPD by reducing airflow limitation and dynamic hyperinflation [93–95]. Combining heliox and hyperoxia delays dynamic hyperinflation and improves respiratory mechanics, which translates into added improvements in exercise tolerance in the laboratory setting [96]. The role of heliox breathing, if any, in routine exercise of patients who have COPD during pulmonary rehabilitation has yet to be defined.

Biofeedback

Biofeedback refers to techniques to teach self-control over physiologic functions. People might be taught to increase or decrease the activity of internal bodily functions. The most common application of biofeedback is stress management, by teaching relaxation of major muscle groups. More recently, patients have tried to modify such autonomic functions as vasomotor activity, heart rate, blood pressure, and bronchomotor tone using biofeedback. Several biofeedback techniques have been applied to patients who have pulmonary disorders in the context of pulmonary rehabilitation programs. In respiratory biofeedback, a signal relating to some respiratory function is monitored and displayed to a patient, who tries to modify that function. Biofeedback is used in patients who have asthma, emphysema, and pulmonary fibrosis and to improve gas exchange and reduce the WOB. Techniques vary from relaxation and stress management to patient self-control. Electromyography, incentive spirometry, airway resistance signals, and pulse oximetry are used [97]. Training patients in pursed-lips breathing guided by oximetry and decreasing the time of weaning from mechanical ventilation are examples of biofeedback application in respiratory patients [98,99]. Application of biofeedback to exercise in patients who have COPD is less studied and results are not promising to date [100]. This issue requires further investigation.

Summary

The new positive conclusion of this review is an old one: multidisciplinary pulmonary rehabilitation in its consolidated "old" modalities, as evaluated by evidence-based medicine, is a valuable adjunct to pharmacologic or surgical treatment of COPD [4]. Exercise training is a key cornerstone component of pulmonary rehabilitation. The value of studies supporting the use of the new strategies discussed in this review in the clinical management of patients who have COPD varies substantially among the different techniques. Clinical trials designed to establish that a given intervention yields superior results compared with standard interventions generally are difficult to perform because of the wide variability of responses to exercise interventions among patients. At present, the modalities discussed should be considered for use as adjuncts to a well-designed comprehensive respiratory rehabilitation program, including other interventions, such as conventional exercise training, education, nutrition, and psychologic counseling [4,18].

References

[1] Global initiative for chronic obstructive lung disease. Workshop report, global strategy for diagnosis, management, and prevention of COPD. Update Sept 2005. Bethesda (MD): National Institutes of Health, National Heart, Lung and Blood Institute; 2005 Available at: www.goldcopd.com. Accessed January 1, 2007.

[2] Celli BR, MacNee W, Agusti A, et al. Standards for the diagnosis and treatment of patients with COPD: a summary of the ATS/ERS position paper. Eur Respir J 2004;23:932–46.

[3] Pitta F, Troosters T, Spruit MA, et al. Characteristics of physical activities in daily life in chronic obstructive pulmonary disease. Am J Respir Crit Care Med 2005;171:972–7.

[4] Nici L, Donner C, Wouters E, et alon behalf of the ATS/ERS pulmonary rehabilitation writing committee. American thoracic society/European respiratory society statement on pulmonary rehabilitation. Am J Respir Crit Care Med 2006; 173:1390–413.

[5] American Thoracic Society. Dyspnea. Mechanisms, assessment and management: a consensus statement. Am J Respir Crit Care Med 1999;159: 321–40.

[6] Ambrosino N, Serradori M. Dyspnea, linguistic and biological descriptors. Chron Respir Dis 2006;3:117–22.

[7] O'Donnell DE, Webb KA. Exertional breathlessness in patients with chronic airflow limitation: the role of hyperinflation. Am Rev Respir Dis 1993;148:1351–7.

[8] Saey D, Maltais F. Role of peripheral muscle function in rehabilitation. In: Donner CF, Ambrosino N, Goldstein RS, editors. Pulmonary rehabilitation. London: Arnold Pub; 2005. p. 80–90.

[9] Vestbo J, Prescott E, Almdal T, et al. Body mass, fat-free body mass, and prognosis in patients with chronic obstructive pulmonary disease from

a random population sample. Findings from the Copenhagen city heart study. Am J Respir Crit Care Med 2006;173:79–83.

[10] Jee SH, Sull JW, Park J, et al. Body-mass index and mortality in Korean men and women. N Engl J Med 2006;355:779–87.

[11] Schols AMWJ, Wouters EFM. Nutrition and metabolic therapy. In: Donner CF, Ambrosino N, Goldstein RS, editors. Pulmonary rehabilitation. London: Hodder Arnold; 2005. p. 229–35.

[12] Casaburi R, Bhasin S, Cosentino L, et al. Effects of testosterone and resistance training in men with chronic obstructive pulmonary disease. Am J Respir Crit Care Med 2004;170:870–8.

[13] Casaburi R, Patessio A, Ioli F, et al. Reduction in exercise lactic acidosis and ventilation as a result of exercise training in patients with obstructive lung disease. Am Rev Respir Dis 1991;143:9–18.

[14] Casaburi R, Porszasz J, Burns MR, et al. Physiologic benefits of exercise training in rehabilitation of severe COPD patients. Am J Respir Crit Care Med 1997;155:1541–51.

[15] Gigliotti F, Coli C, Bianchi R, et al. Exercise training improves exertional dyspnea in patients with COPD: evidence of the role of mechanical factors. Chest 2003;123:1794–802.

[16] Maltais F, LeBlanc P, Simard C, et al. Skeletal muscle adaptation to endurance training in patients with chronic obstructive pulmonary disease. Am J Respir Crit Care Med 1996;154:442–7.

[17] Mercken EM, Hageman GJ, Schols AM, et al. Rehabilitation decreases exercise-induced oxidative stress in chronic obstructive pulmonary disease. Am J Respir Crit Care Med 2005;172:994–1001.

[18] Ambrosino N, Strambi S. New strategies to improve exercise tolerance in chronic obstructive pulmonary disease. Eur Respir J 2004;24:313–22.

[19] Younes M. Proportional assist ventilation. In: Tobin MJ, editor. Principles and practice of mechanical ventilation. 2nd edition. New York: McGraw-Hill inc; 2006. p. 335–64.

[20] Harms CA, Babcock MA, McClaran SR, et al. Respiratory muscle work compromises leg blood flow during maximal exercise. J Appl Physiol 1997;82:1573–83.

[21] Harms CA, Wetter TJ, St Croix CM, et al. Effects of respiratory muscle work on exercise performance. J Appl Physiol 2000;89:131–8.

[22] Babcock MA, Pegelow DF, Harms CA, et al. Effects of respiratory muscle unloading on exercise-induced diaphragm fatigue. J Appl Physiol 2002;93:201–6.

[23] Ambrosino N. Exercise and noninvasive ventilatory support. Monaldi Arch Chest Dis 2000;55:242–6.

[24] van't Hul A, Kwakkel G, Gosselink R. The acute effects of noninvasive ventilatory support during exercise on exercise endurance and dyspnea in patients with chronic obstructive pulmonary disease:

a systematic review. J Cardiopulm Rehabil 2002;22:290–7.

[25] Lougheed MD, Webb KA, O'Donnell DE. Breathlessness during induced hyperinflation in asthma: role of the inspiratory threshold load. Am J Respir Crit Care Med 1995;152:911–20.

[26] O'Donnell DE, Sanii R, Younes M. Improvement in exercise endurance in patients with chronic airflow limitation using continuous positive airway pressure. Am Rev Respir Dis 1988;138:1510–4.

[27] O'Donnell DE, Sanii R, Giesbrecht G, et al. Effect of continuous positive airway pressure on respiratory sensation in patients with chronic obstructive pulmonary disease during submaximal exercise. Am Rev Respir Dis 1988;138:1185–91.

[28] Petrof BJ, Calderini E, Gottfried SB. Effect of CPAP on respiratory effort and dyspnoea during exercise in severe COPD. J Appl Physiol 1990;69:179–88.

[29] Rossi A, Polese G, Brandi G, et al. Intrinsic positive end-expiratory pressure (PEEPi). Intensive Care Med 1995;21:522–36.

[30] Henke KG, Regnis JA, Bye PTP. Benefits of continuous positive airway pressure during exercise in cystic fibrosis and relationship to disease severity. Am Rev Respir Dis 1993;148:1272–6.

[31] Brochard L. Pressure support ventilation. In: Tobin MJ, editor. Principles and practice of mechanical ventilation. 2nd edition. New York: McGraw-Hill inc; 2006. p. 221–50.

[32] Wysocki M, Meshaka P, Richard JC, et al. Proportional-assist ventilation compared with pressure-support ventilation during exercise in volunteers with external thoracic restriction. Crit Care Med 2004;32:409–14.

[33] Kyroussis D, Polkey MI, Keilty SE, et al. Exhaustive exercise slows inspiratory muscle relaxation rate in chronic obstructive pulmonary disease. Am J Respir Crit Care Med 1996;153:787–93.

[34] Polkey MI, Kyroussis D, Mills GH, et al. Inspiratory pressure support reduces slowing of inspiratory muscle relaxation rate during exhaustive treadmill walking in severe COPD. Am J Respir Crit Care Med 1996;154:1146–50.

[35] Keilty SE, Ponte J, Fleming TA, et al. Effect of inspiratory pressure support on exercise tolerance and breathlessness in patients with severe stable chronic obstructive pulmonary disease. Thorax 1994;49:990–6.

[36] Maltais F, Reissmann H, Gottfried SB. Pressure support reduces inspiratory effort and dyspnea during exercise in chronic airflow obstruction. Am J Respir Crit Care Med 1995;151:1027–33.

[37] Kyroussis D, Polkey MI, Hamnegard CH, et al. Respiratory muscle activity in patients with COPD walking to exhaustion with and without pressure support. Eur Respir J 2000;15:649–55.

[38] van't Hul A, Gosselink R, Hollander P, et al. Acute effects of inspiratory pressure support during

exercise in patients with COPD. Eur Respir J 2004; 23:34–40.

[39] Polkey MI, Hawkins P, Kyroussis D, et al. Inspiratory pressure support prolongs exercise induced lactataemia in severe COPD. Thorax 2000;55: 547–9.

[40] Dolmage TE, Goldstein RS. Proportional assist ventilation and exercise tolerance in subjects with COPD. Chest 1997;111:948–54.

[41] Bianchi L, Foglio K, Pagani M, et al. Effects of proportional assist ventilation on exercise tolerance in COPD patients with chronic hypercapnia. Eur Respir J 1998;11:422–7.

[42] Hernandez P, Maltais F, Gursahaney A, et al. Proportional assist ventilation may improve exercise performance in severe chronic obstructive pulmonary disease. J Cardiopulm Rehabil 2001;21: 135–42.

[43] Poggi R, Appendini L, Polese G, et al. Noninvasive proportional assist ventilation and pressure support ventilation during arm elevation in patients with chronic respiratory failure. A preliminary, physiologic study. Respir Med 2006;100:972–9.

[44] Mancebo J. Assist-control ventilation. In: Tobin MJ, editor. Principles and practice of mechanical ventilation. 2nd edition. New York: McGraw-Hill inc; 2006. p. 183–200.

[45] Tsuboi T, Ohi M, Cjin K, et al. Ventilatory support during exercise in patients with pulmonary tuberculosis sequelae. Chest 1997;112:1000–7.

[46] Highcock MP, Smith IE, Shneerson JM. The effect of noninvasive intermittent positive-pressure ventilation during exercise in severe scoliosis. Chest 2002;121:1555–60.

[47] Make B. Pulmonary rehabilitation and lung volume reduction surgery. In: Donner CF, Ambrosino N, Goldstein RS, editors. Pulmonary rehabilitation. London: Arnold Pub; 2005. p. 297–303.

[48] Gay SE, Martinez FJ. Pulmonary rehabilitation and transplantation. In: Donner CF, Ambrosino N, Goldstein RS, editors. Pulmonary rehabilitation. London: Arnold Pub; 2005. p. 304–11.

[49] Bianchi L, Foglio K, Porta R, et al. Lack of additional effect of adjunct of assisted ventilation to pulmonary rehabilitation in mild COPD patients. Respir Med 2002;96:359–67.

[50] Hawkins P, Johnson LC, Nikoletou D, et al. Proportional assist ventilation as an aid to exercise training in severe chronic obstructive pulmonary disease. Thorax 2002;57:853–9.

[51] van 't Hul A, Gosselink R, Hollander P, et al. Training with inspiratory pressure support in patients with severe COPD. Eur Respir J 2006;27: 65–72.

[52] Johnson JE, Gavin DJ, Usar M, et al. Effects of training with heliox and noninvasive positive pressure ventilation on exercise ability in patients with severe COPD. Chest 2002;122:464–72.

[53] Costes F, Agresti A, Court-Fortune I, et al. Noninvasive ventilation during exercise training improves exercise tolerance in patients with chronic obstructive pulmonary disease. J Cardiopulm Rehabil 2003;23:307–13.

[54] Le Jemtel TH, Padeletti M, Jelic S. Diagnostic and therapeutic challenges in patients with coexistent chronic obstructive pulmonary disease and chronic heart failure. J Am Coll Cardiol 2007;49:171–80.

[55] Ambrosino N. Assisted ventilation as an aid to exercise training: a mechanical doping? Eur Respir J 2006;27:3–5.

[56] Garrod R, Mikelsons C, Paul EA, et al. Randomized controlled trial of domiciliary noninvasive positive pressure ventilation and physical training in severe chronic obstructive pulmonary disease. Am J Respir Crit Care Med 2000;162:1335–41.

[57] Schonhofer B, Zimmermann C, Abramek P, et al. Non-invasive mechanical ventilation improves walking distance but not quadriceps strength in chronic respiratory failure. Respir Med 2003;97: 818–24.

[58] Langbein WE, Maloney C, Kandare F, et al. Pulmonary function testing in spinal cord injury: effects of abdominal muscle stimulation. J Rehabil Res Dev 2001;38:591–7.

[59] Quittan M, Wiesinger GF, Sturm B, et al. Improvement of thigh muscles by neuromuscular electrical stimulation in patients with refractory heart failure: a single-blind, randomized, controlled trial. Am J Phys Med Rehabil 2001;80:206–14.

[60] Gosselin N, Lambert K, Poulain M, et al. Endurance training improves skeletal muscle electrical activity in active COPD patients. Muscle Nerve 2003;28:744–53.

[61] Neder JA, Sword D, Ward SA, et al. Home based neuromuscular electrical stimulation as a new rehabilitative strategy for severely disabled patients with chronic obstructive pulmonary disease (COPD). Thorax 2002;57:333–7.

[62] Bourjeily-Habr G, Rochester CL, Palermo F, et al. Randomised controlled trial of transcutaneous electrical muscle stimulation of the lower extremities in patients with chronic obstructive pulmonary disease. Thorax 2002;57:1045–9.

[63] Zanotti E, Felicetti G, Maini M, et al. Peripheral muscle strength training in bed-bound patients with COPD receiving mechanical ventilation. Effect of electrical stimulation. Chest 2003;124:292–6.

[64] Vivodtzev I, Pepin JL, Vottero G, et al. Improvement in quadriceps strength and dyspnea in daily tasks after 1 month of electrical stimulation in severely deconditioned and malnourished COPD. Chest 2006;129:1540–8.

[65] Vengust R, Strojnik V, Pavlovic V, et al. The effect of electrostimulation and high load exercises in patients with patellofemoral joint dysfunction. A preliminary report. Pflugers Arch 2001;442(Suppl 1): 153–4.

[66] Perez M, Lucia A, Rivero JL, et al. Effects of trans-cutaneous short-term electrical stimulation on M. vastus lateralis characteristics of healthy young men. Pflugers Arch 2002;443:866–74.

[67] Clini E, Foglio K, Bianchi L, et al. In-hospital short-term training program in patients with chronic airway obstruction (CAO). Chest 2001; 120:1500–5.

[68] Sewell L, Singh SJ, Williams JEA, et al. How long should outpatient pulmonary rehabilitation be? A randomised controlled trial of 4 weeks versus 7 weeks. Thorax 2006;61:767–72.

[69] Coppoolse R, Schols AMWJ, Baarends EM, et al. Interval versus continuous training in patients with severe COPD: a randomized clinical trial. Eur Respir J 1999;14:258–63.

[70] Vogiatzis I, Terzis G, Nanas S, et al. Skeletal muscle adaptations to interval training in patients with advanced COPD. Chest 2005;128:3838–45.

[71] Sabapathy S, Kingsley RA, Schneider DA, et al. Continuous and intermittent exercise responses in individuals with chronic obstructive pulmonary disease. Thorax 2004;59:1026–31.

[72] Probst VS, Troosters T, Pitta F, et al. Cardiopulmonary stress during exercise training in patients with COPD. Eur Respir J 2006;27:1110–8.

[73] Dolmage TE, Goldstein RS. Response to one-legged cycling in patients with COPD. Chest 2006;129:325–32.

[74] Gupta RB, Brooks D, Lacasse Y, et al. Effect of rollator use on health-related quality of life in individuals with COPD. Chest 2006;130:1089–95.

[75] Gupta R, Goldstein R, Brooks D. The acute effects of a rollator in individuals with COPD. J Cardiopulm Rehabil 2006;26:107–11.

[76] Somfay A, Porszasz J, Lee SM, et al. Effect of hyperoxia on gas exchange and lactate kinetics following exercise onset in non-hypoxemic COPD patients. Chest 2002;121:393–400.

[77] Ambrosino N, Giannini D, D'Amico I. How good is the evidence for ambulatory oxygen in chronic obstructive pulmonary disease. Chron Respir Dis 2004;3:125–6.

[78] Somfay A, Porszasz J, Lee SM, et al. Effect of oxygen on hyperinflation and exercise endurance in non-hypoxemic COPD patients. Eur Respir J 2001;18:77–84.

[79] O'Donnell DE, Bain DJ, Webb KA. Factors contributing to relief of exertional breathlessness during hyperoxia in chronic airflow limitation. Am J Respir Crit Care Med 1997;155:530–5.

[80] Bradley JM, Lasserson T, Elborn S, et al. A systematic review of randomized controlled trials examining the short-term benefit of ambulatory oxygen in COPD. Chest 2007;131:278–85.

[81] O'Donnell DE, D'Arsigny C, Webb KA. Effects of hyperoxia on ventilatory limitation during exercise in advanced chronic obstructive pulmonary disease. Am J Respir Crit Care Med 2001;163:892–8.

[82] Stevenson NJ, Calverley PMA. Effect of oxygen on recovery from maximal exercise in patients with chronic obstructive pulmonary disease. Thorax 2004;59:668–72.

[83] Fujimoto K, Matsuzawa Y, Yamaguchi S, et al. Benefits of oxygen on exercise performance and pulmonary hemodynamics in patients with COPD with mild hypoxemia. Chest 2002;122: 457–63.

[84] van Helvoort HAC, Heijdra YF, Heunks LMA, et al. Supplemental oxygen prevents exercise-induced oxidative stress in muscle-wasted patients with chronic obstructive pulmonary disease. Am J Respir Crit Care Med 2006;173:1122–9.

[85] Terrados N, Jansson E, Sylven C, et al. Is hypoxia a stimulus for synthesis of oxidative enzymes and myoglobin? J Appl Physiol 1990;68:2369–72.

[86] Garrod R, Paul EA, Wedzicha JA. Supplemental oxygen during pulmonary rehabilitation in patients with COPD with exercise hypoxaemia. Thorax 2000;55:539–43.

[87] Fichter J, Fleckenstein J, Stahl C, et al. Effect of oxygen (FI02: 0.35) on the aerobic capacity in patients with COPD. Pneumologie 1999;53:121–6.

[88] McDonald CF, Blyth CM, Lazarus MD, et al. Exertional oxygen of limited benefit in patients with chronic obstructive pulmonary disease and mild hypoxemia. Am J Respir Crit Care Med 1995;152:1616–9.

[89] Rooyackers JM, Dekhuijzen PN, Van Herwaarden CL, et al. Training with supplemental oxygen in patients with COPD and hypoxaemia at peak exercise. Eur Respir J 1997;10:1278–84.

[90] Wadell K, Henriksson-Larsen K, Lundgren R. Physical training with and without oxygen in patients with chronic obstructive pulmonary disease and exercise-induced hypoxaemia. J Rehabil Med 2001;33:200–5.

[91] Emtner M, Porszasz J, Burns M, et al. Benefits of supplemental oxygen in exercise training in non-hypoxemic COPD patients. Am J Respir Crit Care Med 2003;68:1034–42.

[92] Peters MM, Webb KA, O'Donnell DE. Combined physiological effects of bronchodilators and hyperoxia on exertional dyspnoea in normoxic COPD. Thorax 2006;61:559–67.

[93] Palange P, Crimi E, Pellegrino R, et al. Supplemental oxygen and heliox: 'new' tools for exercise training in chronic obstructive pulmonary disease. Curr Opin Pulm Med 2005;11:145–8.

[94] Palange P, Valli G, Onorati P, et al. Effect of heliox on lung dynamic hyperinflation, dyspnea, and exercise endurance capacity in COPD patients. J Appl Physiol 2004;97:1637–42.

[95] Laude EA, Duffy NC, Baveystock C, et al. The effect of helium and oxygen on exercise performance in chronic obstructive pulmonary disease. A randomized crossover trial. Am J Respir Crit Care Med 2006;173:865–70.

[96] Eves ND, Petersen SR, Haykowsky MJ, et al. He-
     lium-hyperoxia, exercise, and respiratory mechan-
     ics in chronic obstructive pulmonary disease. Am
     J Respir Crit Care Med 2006;174:763–71.

[97] Esteve F, Blanc-Gras N, Gallego J, et al. The effects
     of breathing pattern training on ventilatory func-
     tion in patients with COPD. Biofeedback Self
     Regul 1996;21:311–21.

[98] Tiep BL, Burns M, Kao D, et al. Pursed lips breath-
     ing training using ear oximetry. Chest 1986;90:218–23.

[99] Holliday JE, Hyers TM. The reduction of weaning
     time from mechanical ventilation using tidal vol-
     ume and relaxation biofeedback. Am Rev Respir
     Dis 1990;141:1214–20.

[100] Collins E, Fehr l, Bannert C, et al. Effect of ventila-
      tion-feedback training on endurance and perceived
      breathlessness during constant work-rate leg-cycle
      exercise in patients with COPD. J Rehabil Res
      Dev 2003;40:35–44.

ELSEVIER
SAUNDERS

Clin Chest Med 28 (2007) 639–653

CLINICS
IN CHEST
MEDICINE

Update in Surgical Therapy for Chronic Obstructive Pulmonary Disease

David J. Lederer, MD, MS[a,b], Selim M. Arcasoy, MD, FCCP, FACP[a,b],*

[a]Division of Pulmonary, Allergy, and Critical Care Medicine, Columbia University College of Physicians
and Surgeons, Lung Transplantation Program, PH-14 East, Room 104, New York, NY 10032, USA
[b]New York Presbyterian Hospital of Columbia and Cornell University,
622 West 168th Street, New York, NY 10032, USA

Chronic obstructive pulmonary disease (COPD) is characterized by progressive and irreversible airflow limitation. It is caused primarily by exposure to tobacco smoke, and less commonly to other noxious stimuli or by alpha$_1$-antitrypsin deficiency. COPD is one of the leading causes of death and disability worldwide, with incapacitating symptoms in severe cases [1]. Smoking cessation and oxygen supplementation when needed are the only treatments known to impact outcomes, whereas other medical therapies and pulmonary rehabilitation are aimed mainly at limiting symptoms and exacerbations of disease. Therefore, numerous surgical therapies have been attempted over the last century in an effort to improve lung function and symptomatic debility, but only three have stood the test of time. This article reviews bullectomy for giant bullae, lung volume reduction surgery (LVRS) and lung transplantation for the treatment of advanced COPD, focusing on patient selection and clinical outcomes for the practicing pulmonologist.

This work was supported in part by Grant No. RR024157 from the National Institutes of Health.

Dr. Lederer is a coinvestigator of a clinical trial for bronchoscopic lung volume reduction sponsored by Broncus Technologies.

* Corresponding author. Division of Pulmonary, Allergy, and Critical Care Medicine, Columbia University College of Physicians and Surgeons, Lung Transplantation Program, PH-14 East, Room 104, New York, NY 10032.

E-mail address: sa2059@columbia.edu
(S.M. Arcasoy).

Bullectomy

Giant bullae (bullae occupying greater than one third of the hemithorax) may compress adjacent lung and lead to dyspnea and reduced exercise capacity by impairing lung mechanics and gas exchange [2]. In uncontrolled studies, giant bullectomy improves forced expiratory volume in 1 second (FEV$_1$), total lung capacity (TLC), 6-minute walk distance (6MWD), dyspnea, and quality of life [2–4]. Less than half of patients, however, derive a long-term benefit from bullectomy [3,5]. Bullectomy should be reserved for patients who are symptomatic despite optimal medical therapy, who have a single well-defined giant bulla with adjacent vascular crowding and relatively normal parenchyma in other lung zones along with only a modest decline in spirometry, and increased trapped gas volume with near-normal gas exchange [1]. Older patients who have significant comorbid illnesses, pulmonary hypertension, chronic bronchitis and respiratory tract infections, severe reduction in FEV$_1$ with obstructive physiology, significantly impaired diffusing capacity for carbon monoxide (DLCO) and gas exchange, and multiple smaller bullae are not considered appropriate candidates [1].

Lung volume reduction surgery

Historical aspects

In the 1950s, Brantigan described 33 emphysema patients who underwent bilateral LVRS and autonomic denervation in an attempt to increase radial traction on the airways and thereby improve expiratory airflow [6,7]. LVRS was not performed widely in the initial years following these publications in light of the high surgical mortality and sparse physiological data reported.

Subsequent experience with LVRS was largely unimpressive until 1995, when Cooper and colleagues [8] reported a 76% relative improvement in mean FEV_1 and no mortality in 20 patients undergoing bilateral LVRS by means of median sternotomy. This study marked the beginning of an era of enthusiastic single-center reports of patients undergoing LVRS using variable surgical techniques and with low reported morbidity and mortality rates [9]. These studies, however, were limited by the lack of control arms and failure to account for loss to follow-up. Widespread application of LVRS for advanced pulmonary emphysema in the mid-1990s prompted an analysis of Medicare claims data, revealing a 23% mortality rate at 1 year, a proportion much higher than that suggested by literature [10,11]. Driven by the questionable effectiveness of LVRS and its high potential cost, the Centers for Medicare and Medicaid Services (CMS) stopped payments for LVRS in December 1995 and joined the National Heart, Lung, and Blood Institute and the Agency for Healthcare Research and Quality in funding the National Emphysema Treatment Trial (NETT), the largest randomized trial of LVRS performed to date.

Surgical procedure

The currently accepted surgical approach is to perform stapled wedge resection of 25% to 30% of the most diseased areas of the lungs based on the distribution of emphysema evident on preoperative perfusion scan and CT [12]. Buttressing the staple line with bovine pericardium reduces the duration of air leaks [13]. Postoperative management focuses on early extubation and ambulation, pain control, and airway clearance. Common early postoperative complications include prolonged air leak (50% last 7 days or more), arrhythmia (24%), and pneumonia (18%) [14,15].

Bilateral LVRS is preferred over unilateral LVRS, as it offers greater improvements in FEV_1 and dyspnea with similar complication rates, and in one study, a lower mortality rate [16]. Median sternotomy and bilateral video-assisted thoracoscopic surgical (VATS) approaches lead to similar outcomes [17]. VATS, however, has been associated with a lower incidence of respiratory failure [18] and a shorter length of stay [17].

Clinical outcomes and patient selection

The NETT was the largest and most informative of the seven published randomized trials of LVRS versus medical therapy for pulmonary emphysema (Table 1) [12,19–26]. The NETT randomized 1218 patients who have moderate-to-severe emphysema to receive bilateral LVRS or medical treatment alone at 17 centers in the United States. All patients received optimal medical therapy and underwent pulmonary rehabilitation before randomization.

The NETT results were published in 2003 after a median follow-up time of 2.4 years and again in 2006 after a median follow-up time of 4.3 years [12,23]. Although overall mortality did not differ between treatment arms in the initial report, patients randomized to LVRS had a 6.6% lower absolute mortality rate during the extended follow-up period than those in the medical arm ($P = .02$; Table 2) [23,27]. The 90-day mortality rate, however, was sixfold higher in the surgical arm (7.9% versus 1.3%, $P<.001$), a finding not unexpected when comparing a surgical intervention with medical therapy alone. Improvements in exercise capacity (defined as an increase of more than 10 W during cycle ergometry) and health-related quality of life were more frequent in the surgical arm (see Table 2). Consistent with prior observational studies of LVRS [9], those in the surgical arm were also more likely to have improvements in FEV_1, 6MWD, and dyspnea.

One of the goals of the NETT was to identify subgroups of patients who derived greater benefit or harm from LVRS [11]. In post hoc analyses, the investigators found that outcomes varied by upper lobe predominance of radiographic emphysema and maximal exercise capacity. The findings within each subgroup are described, followed by a discussion of the strengths and limitations of these analyses.

Emphysema patients who should not undergo lung volume reduction surgery

After the first 1033 patients were randomized in the NETT, the data and safety monitoring board identified a subgroup at high risk of early mortality in the surgical arm of the study [28]. Study subjects with an FEV_1 of 20% predicted or less, who also had either a DLCO of 20% predicted or less, a homogeneous pattern of emphysema on CT had a fourfold increased risk of death at 1 year (43 versus 10 deaths per 100 patient-years in the LVRS and medical arms,

Table 1
Randomized trials of lung volume reduction surgery

Lead author	Total number randomized	FEV$_1$ criteria	Emphysema pattern	Surgical approach	Follow-up time	Mortality at follow-up[a]	Improved outcomes in LVRS arm
Criner [19]	37	<30%	Diffuse bullous	MS	3 months	LVRS: 3 deaths (9%) Medical: 0 deaths (0%)	FEV$_1$, QOL
Geddes [20]	48	>500 mL	No restriction	MS or VATS	12 months	LVRS: 5 deaths (21%) Medical: 3 deaths (12%)	FEV$_1$, QOL
Pompeo [21,22]	60	≤40%	Heterogeneous	VATS	6 months	LVRS: 2 deaths (7%) Medical: 1 death (3%)	FEV$_1$, dyspnea, WD, PaO$_2$, QOL
NETT [12,23][b]	1218	≤45%	Bilateral	MS or VATS	4.3 yrs	LVRS: 283 deaths (47%) Medical: 324 deaths (53%)	Exercise capacity
Goldstein [24]	55	<40%	Heterogeneous	MS or VATS	12 months	LVRS: 4 deaths (14%) Medical: 1 death (4%)	FEV$_1$, dyspnea, WD, QOL
Hillderdal [25]	106	≤35%	Heterogeneous	MS or VATS	12 months	LVRS: 7 deaths (13%) Medical: 2 deaths (4%)	FEV$_1$, WD, QOL
Miller [26]	62	≤40%	No restriction	MS	24 months	LVRS: 5 deaths (16%) Medical: 4 deaths (13%)	FEV$_1$, WD, QOL

All studies included pulmonary rehabilitation in both arms except Pompeo (LVRS without rehabilitation versus rehabilitation alone).

Abbreviations: FEV$_1$, forced expiratory volume in 1 sec; LVRS, lung volume reduction surgery; MS, median sternotomy; NETT, National Emphysema Treatment Trial; PaO$_2$, arterial partial pressure of oxygen; QOL, quality-of-life; VATS, video-assisted thoracoscopic surgery; WD, walking distance.

[a] Except for the NETT, none of the mortality differences were statistically significant ($P > .05$).

[b] Only extended follow-up of NETT data is included in the table [23].

respectively, $P < .001$). Eleven of the 70 high-risk patients in the surgical arm died within 30 days of surgery compared with 0 of the 70 high-risk patients in the medical arm (16% versus 0%, $P < .001$). Similar outcomes were reported after extended follow-up of these patients (Fig. 1 and see Table 2) [23,27].

In addition, patients who have nonupper lobe-predominant emphysema and a high exercise capacity (>25 W for women and >40 W for men) do not appear to benefit from LVRS. Such patients who were randomized to the surgical arm of the NETT had a higher mortality rate than those in the medical arm at 1 year (see Fig. 1 and Table 2; 16% versus 3%, respectively, $P = .001$) [12]. Furthermore, no improvement in exercise capacity was seen in the surgical arm in this subgroup. Hence, these patients should not be considered for LVRS.

Patients who should be considered for lung volume reduction surgery

Nonhigh-risk patients who meet the accepted selection criteria for LVRS (Table 3) and who have

a low baseline maximal exercise capacity (≤25 W for women and ≤40 W for men) and upper lobe-predominant emphysema on CT should be considered for LVRS. Those in the surgical arm of this subgroup had an improvement in survival (see Fig. 1 and Table 2; 12% versus 24% mortality at 2 years in the LVRS and medical arms, respectively, $P = .01$) and were more likely to have improvements in exercise capacity (30% versus 2% at 2 years, respectively, $P < .001$) and quality of life (44% versus 10% at 2 years, respectively, $P < .001$) than those in the medical arm [23].

Patients who have questionable benefit from lung volume reduction surgery

Randomization to the surgical arm did not provide a survival benefit to those with high baseline exercise capacity and upper lobe-predominant emphysema (see Fig. 1 and Table 2), but was associated with an increased likelihood of improvement in exercise capacity (16% versus 4%, $P < .001$) and quality of life (41% versus 10%, $P < .001$) at 2 years compared with the medical arm [23]. Careful clinical judgment by

Table 2
Outcomes of the National Emphysema Treatment Trial

	All patients		High risk		Upper lobe low exercise		Upper lobe high exercise		Nonupper lobe low exercise		Nonupper lobe high exercise	
	LVRS	Medical	LVRS	Medical	LVRS	Medical	LVRS	Medical	LVRS	Medical	LVRS	Medical
No.	608	610	70	70	139	151	206	213	84	65	109	111
90-day mortality	8%	1%	28%[a]	0%	3%	3%	3%	1%	8%[a]	0%	10%[a]	1%
1-y mortality	13%[a]	8%	37%[a]	9%	9%	13%	7%	3%	14%	15%	16%[a]	3%
2-y mortality	18%	17%	49%[a]	23%	12%[a]	24%	12%	10%	23%	32%	17%	8%
Overall mortality[b]	47%[a]	53%	73%	77%	45%[a]	60%	46%	42%	57%	66%[b]	44%	41%
Improved exercise capacity at 2 y	15%[a]	3%	7%	3%	30%[a]	2%	16%[a]	4%	14%	7%	3%	4%
Improved QOL at 2 y	32%[a]	8%	11%[a]	1%	44%[a]	10%	41%[a]	10%	27%[a]	6%	19%	9%

Abbreviations: HE, high exercise capacity; LE, low exercise capacity; LVRS, lung volume reduction surgery; NETT, National Emphysema Treatment Trial; NUL, nonupper lobe emphysema; QOL, quality-of-life; UL, upper lobe emphysema. See text for definitions of NETT subgroups.

[a] $P < 0.05$ compared with medical therapy.

[b] Median follow-up time of 4.3 years.

Data from Naunheim KS, Wood DE, Mohsenifar Z, et al. Long-term follow-up of patients receiving lung volume-reduction surgery versus medical therapy for severe emphysema by the National Emphysema Treatment Trial Research Group. Ann Thorac Surg 2006;82(2):431–43; and Lenfant C. Will lung volume reduction surgery be widely applied? Ann Thorac Surg 2006;82(2):385–7.

an experienced multidisciplinary team should be exercised when considering LVRS for patients in this subgroup.

Patients with predominantly nonupper lobe emphysema and low exercise capacity in the surgical arm did not have a survival (see Fig. 1 and Table 2) or exercise capacity benefit, but they were more likely to have improved quality of life at 2 years (27% versus 6%, $P = .002$) compared with the medical arm [23]. This benefit should be interpreted cautiously. Patients in the NETT were not blinded to treatment arm assignment, leaving open the possibility of over-reporting of subjective benefit in the surgical arm. Without clear evidence of clinical benefit, LVRS only should be performed in highly selected cases in this subgroup.

Strengths and criticisms of the National Emphysema Treatment Trial

In articles accompanying NETT publications, criticisms were raised regarding multiple comparisons and post hoc subgroup analyses [27,29,30]. Although there remain concerns about a high type I error rate (ie, that the benefit and harm observed in the subgroups were caused by chance) and confounding (ie, that the benefit and harm in subgroups were caused by unmeasured factors that varied by subgroup and themselves directly

influenced outcomes), two arguments suggest that the NETT results are, in fact, valid.

First, the NETT was a large, well-designed, multicenter, randomized trial, providing the highest level of evidence of safety and efficacy of an intervention. The NETT represents the most rigorous study of a surgical intervention conducted to date.

Second, the investigators performed conservative tests to assess the differences in effect sizes across subgroups (tests for interaction). The p value for the test for interaction across the four nonhigh-risk subgroups in the NETT was .004, close to multiple comparison-corrected p value of .003 [30], suggesting that the differences in outcomes between subgroups were unlikely to have been caused by chance alone.

Other studies of lung volume reduction surgery

Several smaller randomized trials of LVRS have been published (see Table 1) [19–22,24–26]. These trials have been limited by small sample size, variability in patient selection criteria, short follow-up time, and failure to account for loss to follow-up and drop-outs in the evaluation of outcomes.

Not unexpectedly, none of these trials showed an effect of LVRS on mortality. In the largest trial, which had a 12-month follow-up, seven deaths occurred in the LVRS arm, and two

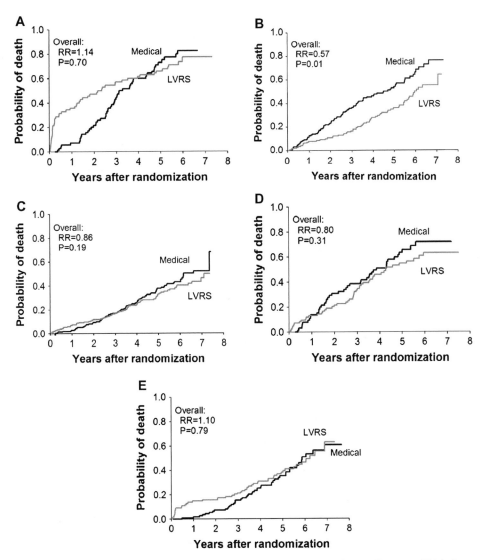

Fig. 1. Kaplan-Meier survival estimates for the five subgroups of the National Emphysema Treatment Trial after a median follow-up time of 4.3 years. (*A*) High-risk group. (*B*) Upper lobe predominant/low exercise capacity group. (*C*) Upper lobe predominant/high exercise capacity group. (*D*) Nonupper lobe predominant/low exercise capacity group. (*E*) Nonupper lobe predominant/high exercise capacity group. See text for definitions of subgroups. p-values are for the comparison between survival rates at last follow-up. (*Adapted from* Naunheim KS, Wood DE, Mohsenifar Z, et al. Long-term follow-up of patients receiving lung-volume-reduction surgery versus medical therapy for severe emphysema by the National Emphysema Treatment Trial Research Group. Ann Thorac Surg 2006;82(2):431–43; with permission from the Society of Thoracic Surgeons.)

deaths occurred in the medical arm ($P = .49$) [25]. In no study were deaths more frequent in the medical arm. Despite the inherent shortcomings of these trials, they typically have shown improvements in FEV_1, quality-of-life, walking distance, and dyspnea following LVRS (see Table 1) [19–21,24–26].

A recent meta-analysis of these randomized trials and the NETT confirmed the overall increase in early mortality after LVRS [31]. The number needed to harm at 90 days was 16, indicating that for every 16 patients undergoing LVRS, one extra death would occur within 90 days. The number needed to harm was four for

Table 3
Selection criteria for lung volume reduction surgery

	Inclusion criteria	Exclusion criteria
General	Consistent with emphysema	Prior lung transplant
	BMI $\leq$ 31.1 kg/m^2 (men)	Prior LVRS
	BMI $\leq$ 32.3 kg/m^2 (women)	Prior median sternotomy
	Prednisone dose $\leq$ 20 mg daily	Prior lobectomy
	Appropriate surgical candidate	Bronchiectasis
	Nonsmoking $\geq$ 4 months	Recurrent pulmonary infections with
	Plasma cotinine $\leq$ 13.7 ng/mL	sputum production
		Significant cardiac disease[a]
Radiographic	HRCT evidence of bilateral emphysema	Diffuse emphysema unsuitable for LVRS
Physiologic	FEV$_1$ $\leq$ 45% predicted ($\geq$ 15% if	FEV$_1$ $\leq$ 20% + DLCO $\leq$ 20%
	$\geq$ 70 years)	FEV$_1$ $\leq$ 20% + homogeneous
	TLC $\geq$ 100% predicted	emphysema on CT
	RV $\geq$ 150% predicted	Nonupper lobe predominant emphysema
	PaCO$_2$ $\leq$ 60 mm Hg	with high exercise capacity
	PaO$_2$ $\geq$ 45 mm Hg	Systolic PAP $\geq$ 45 mm Hg
	6MWD $\geq$ 140 m after pulmonary	Mean PAP $\geq$ 35 mm Hg
	rehabilitation	

Abbreviations: 6MWD, 6-minute walk distance; BMI, body mass index; DLCO, diffusing capacity for carbon monoxide; FEV$_1$, forced expiratory volume in 1 second; LVRS, lung volume reduction surgery; PaCO$_2$, arterial partial pressure of carbon dioxide; PaO$_2$, arterial partial pressure of oxygen; PAP, pulmonary artery pressure; RV, residual volume; TLC, total lung capacity.

[a] Significant cardiac conditions: left ventricular ejection fraction <45%, coronary artery disease, arrhythmia, uncontrolled hypertension.

Data from Fishman A, Martinez F, Naunheim K, et al. A randomized trial comparing lung volume reduction surgery with medical therapy for severe emphysema. N Engl J Med 2003;348(21):2059–73.

the high-risk group and 27 for the nonhigh-risk group of the NETT [31]. This meta-analysis did not examine long-term survival after LVRS and did not include the extended follow-up of NETT subjects [23]. The authors warn about the questionable validity of the multiple subgroup analyses of the NETT, but conclude that the "benefit of surgery in surviving patients was significant in terms of quality of life, exercise capacity, and lung function" [31].

Long-term follow-up after LVRS has been reported by the Washington University group [32]. In patients who had complete 5-year follow-up, FEV$_1$, 6MWD, and DLCO improved after surgery and returned close to preoperative values by 5 years [32]. These findings suggest that LVRS may provide lasting benefit in selected patients who have severe emphysema.

LVRS has been performed successfully in patients with early stage nonsmall cell lung cancer, both as a technique to resect the cancer, and as a concomitant procedure in cancer-free lung zones to improve lung function [33]. In this regard, LVRS may permit lung cancer resection

in selected patients whose lung function otherwise would prohibit such definitive therapy [34–37].

Physiological benefit and mechanisms of improvement

Numerous studies have demonstrated improvements in lung physiology and mechanics following LVRS for emphysema. Increases in FEV$_1$ and forced vital capacity (FVC) and decreases in TLC and residual volume hyperinflation typically are observed after LVRS [9,32,38]. The NETT reported a 6% absolute increase in FEV$_1$% (21% relative increase) in nonhigh-risk survivors 12 months after LVRS [12].

Although it is not surprising that a surgical reduction in lung volume leads to a lower TLC, it is not immediately obvious why removing emphysematous lung would improve expiratory airflow, increase FVC, and reduce residual volume hyperinflation. Multiple mechanisms appear to be involved (Box 1), but the most important factor may be the increase in lung elastic recoil observed after LVRS (Fig. 2) [39–42]. Sciurba and

<table>
<tr><td>

Box 1. Physiological effects of lung volume reduction surgery

Lung mechanics
Improved lung elastic recoil
Improved airway diameter
Improved lung homogeneity
Decreased intrinsic positive
    end-expiratory pressure

Chest wall mechanics
Decreased inward recoil at
    end-expiratory lung volume
Respiratory muscle function
Increased inspiratory muscle length
Improved geometry and mechanical
    effectiveness of inspiratory muscles
Expiratory derecruitment of abdominal
    muscles

Gas exchange
Improved alveolar ventilation
Increased mixed venous arterial oxygen
    tension

Pulmonary circulation
Improved right ventricular function

─────────

Adapted from Marchand E, Gayan-Ramirez
G, De Leyn P, et al. Physiological basis of im-
provement after lung volume reduction surgery
for severe emphysema: where are we? Eur
Respir J 1999;13(3):686–96; with permission.

</td></tr>
</table>

Lung volume reduction surgery

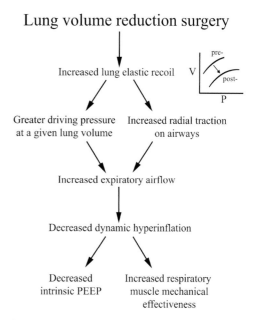

Fig. 2. A simplified model of the physiological effects of lung volume reduction.

6 months after surgery. Similarly, Ciccone and colleagues [32] found that continuous oxygen use dropped from 45% preoperatively to 11% at 6 months, and oxygen use during exercise dropped from 92% preoperatively to 50% at 6 months.

Cost-effectiveness

The cost-effectiveness of LVRS was called into question in an article published alongside the initial NETT results [47]. The overall health care-related costs and the number of hospital days, outpatient care days, and nursing home admissions in the LVRS arm of the NETT exceeded those of the medical arm in the first postrandomization year [47]. In the second year, however, LVRS was associated with reduced overall health care-related costs and fewer hospital days and emergency room visits.

Interventions typically are considered cost-effective when the cost per quality-adjusted life-year (QALY) is under $50,000 to $100,000. The high upfront costs of LVRS and the questionable overall benefit contribute to the high cost-effectiveness ratio of LVRS: $190,000 per QALY gained at 3 years and still only $140,000 per QALY gained at 5 years [47,48]. For the low-exercise/upper lobe-predominant subgroup, the cost-effectiveness ratio was $98,000 per QALY at 3 years and $77,000 per

colleagues [42] showed that lung elastic recoil increased in 16 of 20 patients after LVRS. Those with an increase in lung elastic recoil experienced greater improvements in residual volume hyperinflation and 6MWD than others in whom lung elastic recoil did not increase.

Other factors, such as dynamic hyperinflation and diaphragmatic function, also improve after LVRS [41,43,44]. These and other changes outlined in Fig. 2 likely contribute to improvements in exercise capacity and exertional dyspnea after LVRS by increasing maximal minute ventilation during exercise, permitting greater maximal oxygen consumption [12,32,41,42,45,46].

Some patients are able to discontinue supplemental oxygen use following LVRS. Mineo and colleagues [22] showed that while 63% of patients undergoing LVRS used supplemental oxygen preoperatively, only 7% were still using oxygen

QALY at 5 years [47,48]. Estimates for the less favorable subgroups ranged from $240,000 to $330,000 per QALY at 5 years [48].

Nevertheless, CMS approved reimbursement for LVRS procedures performed on or after Jan. 1, 2004, at NETT-designated centers and Medicare-approved lung transplant centers [49]. CMS has restricted LVRS to severe emphysema patients who:

Meet the inclusion and exclusion criteria of the NETT

Do not fall into the high-risk group

Have upper-lobe predominant emphysema *or* nonupper lobe-predominant emphysema with low maximal exercise capacity (see Table 3) [50]

Bronchoscopic lung volume reduction

Given the peri- and postoperative mortality risk of LVRS, nonsurgical approaches to lung volume reduction are an attractive alternative. Bronchoscopic techniques, including endobronchial valve placement, the use of endobronchial polymers, and bronchial fenestration, are being studied [51]. Early experience with endobronchial valves suggests improvement in lung volume, gas exchange, and exercise capacity [52,53]. A recent multicenter study, however, found no improvement in these factors [54]. Concerns regarding pneumothorax and postobstructive pneumonia and the lack of clinical endpoints in these early reports should be addressed by adequately designed clinical trials.

Lung transplantation

Although the history of human lung transplantation dates back to 1963, successful results could not be achieved until after 1981 when the first successful combined heart–lung transplantation was performed for pulmonary hypertension [55]. Early experience in transplantation for COPD in the late 1980s started with bilateral lung transplantation (BLT), with the first report of successful single lung transplantation (SLT) by Mal and colleagues in 1989 [56,57]. Since then, COPD has become the major indication for lung transplantation, accounting for 46% of all lung transplants performed worldwide between January 1995 and June 2005 [58].

Timing and patient selection

Lung transplantation, an incredibly complicated and risky treatment modality for advanced pulmonary diseases, targets two main objectives: to prolong survival and to enhance quality of life. To reach and maintain these objectives, lung transplant recipients have to pay a very high price that includes an intricate post-transplant lifestyle with the need for lifelong medical monitoring and the never-ending potential for multiple complications resulting in unsatisfactory long-term outcomes [59,60].

In COPD, lung transplantation is indicated for end-stage disease failing medical and other surgical therapies, or not amenable to previously discussed surgical options, at a time when the benefits of transplantation are predicted to outweigh its risks. Such timing has proven to be extremely difficult to access because of two important facts. First, despite incapacitating symptoms and severe disability, patients on the transplant waiting list who have COPD have a significantly better survival than patients with other pulmonary disorders. Second, it has been difficult to demonstrate a clear-cut survival benefit from transplantation in this disorder [61]. Nonetheless, selection criteria for transplantation and lung allocation systems are directly responsible for the prognosis of patients both on the waiting list and after transplantation, with demonstration of a survival benefit from lung transplantation in several studies from Europe [62,63].

Patient selection criteria for lung transplantation were revised recently by the Pulmonary Scientific Council of the International Society for Heart and Lung Transplantation (ISHLT) [64]. The current general guidelines for patient selection and contraindications are summarized in Box 2. Within each diagnostic category, separate criteria for patient referral and transplantation were proposed in the revised document. For COPD, a recently described composite multidimensional prognostic score, the BODE index, was emphasized in patient selection (Table 4). The components of the BODE index are body mass index (BMI), the degree of airflow obstruction ($FEV_1\%$), severity of dyspnea (modified Medical Research Council dyspnea scale), and exercise capacity (6MWD) [65]. This index was shown in a prospective study by Celli and colleagues [65] to accurately predict prognosis in COPD. For instance, patients who had the highest

<hr>

Box 2. General guidelines for the selection of lung transplant candidates

Indications and general prerequisites
Chronic advanced lung disease without effective medical therapy
Perceived survival benefit from lung transplantation
Well informed candidate with demonstrated compliance, motivation, and health behavior

Contraindications
Absolute
  Malignancy in the last 2 years with the exception of skin basal cell and squamous cell
    tumors. A 5-year disease-free interval is recommended.
  Untreatable advanced nonpulmonary organ dysfunction (eg, heart, liver, kidney)
  Incurable chronic extrapulmonary infection (active hepatitis B, hepatitis C, HIV infection)
  Severe chest wall and spinal deformity
  Documented noncompliance with therapy and/or medical follow-up
  Substance (eg, tobacco, alcohol, illicit drugs) addiction within the last 6 months
  Severe psychiatric illness
  Lack of a reliable social support system
  Relative
  Age older than 65 years
  Unstable or critical illness (eg, shock, sepsis)
  Invasive mechanical ventilation
  Severe obesity with body mass index (BMI) greater than 30 kg/m^2
  Severe limitation in functional status with poor rehabilitation potential
  Infection with highly resistant or virulent microorganisms
  Severe and symptomatic osteoporosis
  Chronic medical illnesses with end-organ damage

<hr>

Data from Orens JB, Estenne M, Arcasoy S, et al. International guidelines for the selection of lung transplant candidates: 2006 update—a consensus report from the Pulmonary Scientific Council of the International Society for Heart and Lung Transplantation. J Heart Lung Transplant 2006;25(7):745–55.

quartile of BODE index (scores of 7 to 10) had 80% mortality at 52 months. However, the prognostic value and practical utility of BODE index have not been confirmed in patients who have advanced COPD nearing transplantation, and similar to other prognostic criteria, it may not be able to discriminate patients who have a very poor short-term outlook from those who have a better prognosis in this subset of patients.

Another important update to the patient selection criteria originated from the early findings of the NETT. As discussed earlier, a group of patients was identified to be at high risk for mortality following LVRS, but also had a median survival of approximately 3 years with medical therapy, suggesting that these patients are likely to benefit from lung transplantation [28]. Because of the short median survival of this group of patients on medical therapy and unacceptably high mortality following LVRS, the criteria that define

high risk for LVRS also were included as an indication for transplantation in the revised transplant guidelines. The current guidelines for patient referral and transplantation in COPD are summarized in Box 3.

Until recently, donor lung allocation in the United States was based solely on the waiting time with no consideration of disease severity except in idiopathic pulmonary fibrosis, for which a 90-day credit was granted. In May 2005, a revised allocation scoring system was put into place to give priority to patients who are most likely to die on the waiting list and at the same time have an acceptable post-transplant survival. Not unexpectedly, this system resulted in significantly lower lung allocation scores in COPD compared with idiopathic pulmonary fibrosis and cystic fibrosis, diseases that traditionally have been associated with high waitlist mortality, and in turn led to decreased percentage of transplants for COPD.

Table 4
Components of the BODE index

Variable	Points on BODE index			
	0	1	2	3
FEV$_1$, % predicted	≥ 65	50–64	36–49	≤ 35
6-min walk distance, meters	≥ 350	250–349	150–249	≤ 149
MMRC dyspnea scale	0–1	2	3	4
Body mass index	> 21	≤ 21		

A score from 0 to 3 is assigned for each of the 4 BODE components. These scores are summed to generate the BODE index, which ranges from 0 to 10.

Abbreviations: FEV$_1$, forced expiratory volume in 1 second; MMRC, modified Medical Research Council.

Adapted from Celli BR, Cote CG, Marin JM, et al. The body-mass index, airflow obstruction, dyspnea, and exercise capacity index in chronic obstructive pulmonary disease. N Engl J Med 2004;350(10):1005–12; with permission. Copyright © 2004 Massachusetts Medical Society.

Future studies of the revised patient selection guidelines and the new lung allocation system will be important to determine the impact of these changes on the overall survival of patients who have COPD.

Survival after lung transplantation

In the 2006 ISHLT Registry Report, the median survival following lung transplantation for COPD was 4.8 years, with 1-, 5-, and 10-year survival rates of 82%, 49%, and 19%, respectively [58]. Although the 1-year survival rate is superior to most other pulmonary diseases, and the 5-year survival rate is fairly similar among all diseases, the 10-year survival of COPD patients is among the worst. The poor long-term survival likely reflects the more advanced age of recipients who have COPD, along with the presence of significant medical comorbidities. As one would expect, the median survival after lung transplantation for emphysema caused by alpha-1 antitrypsin deficiency is 5.3 years, with a somewhat better 10-year survival rate of 32%, which may relate to the younger age of these recipients [58]. It is important to note that large single-center studies have reported significantly better outcomes in COPD, particularly following BLT, with 10-year survival of 43%, very close to the 5-year survival figure of 49% in the ISHLT Registry [66]. Pretransplant ventilator use, hospitalization, chronic steroid therapy, and older recipient age have been

---

Box 3. Guidelines for patient referral and lung transplantation in chronic obstructive pulmonary disease

Guidelines for referral
BODE index greater than 5

Guidelines for transplantation
BODE index of 7 to 10 or at least one of the following criteria:
Hospitalization for exacerbation associated with acute hypercapnia (PaCO$_2$>50 mm Hg)
Pulmonary hypertension or cor pulmonale despite oxygen therapy
FEV$_1$ of less than 20% predicted and either DLCO of less than 20% or homogeneous disease distribution on CT

Abbreviations: BODE, body mass index, airflow obstruction, dyspnea, and exercise capacity index; DLCO, diffusing capacity for carbon monoxide; FEV$_1$, forced expiratory volume in 1 second; PaCO$_2$, arterial partial pressure of carbon dioxide.

Data from Orens JB, Estenne M, Arcasoy S, et al. International guidelines for the selection of lung transplant candidates: 2006 update—a consensus report from the Pulmonary Scientific Council of the International Society for Heart and Lung Transplantation. J Heart Lung Transplant 2006;25(7):745–55.

---

identified as recipient-related risk factors for 1-year post-transplant mortality in the registry [58]. Long-term post-transplant mortality in COPD, similar to other diagnoses, is influenced mainly by the development of chronic graft dysfunction and infections.

An area of controversy that relates to survival is the optimal transplant procedure in COPD: SLT versus BLT. ISHLT Registry data and several studies have shown improved survival following BLT [58,67]. Although the results from the ISHLT Registry may have been affected by preferential use of BLT in younger patients, combined data from the ISHLT registry and United Network for Organ Sharing, and other single-center and multicenter studies have revealed a survival advantage of BLT, even when patients were stratified by age [58,67–69]. The survival advantage is realized mainly during long-term follow-up beyond the first 2 years and perhaps applies only to younger patients; however, data in older age group (> 60 years) are scant and not conclusive [69]. The physiologic basis for a survival advantage after BLT potentially includes the achievement of superior lung function, avoidance of native lung complications, and possibly lower incidence of chronic allograft dysfunction. The ultimate decision on the optimal transplant procedure for patients who have COPD will have to weigh the potential survival advantage of BLT against the ability to offer SLT to two candidates in need, particularly in the context of the current donor organ shortage.

Functional outcomes after lung transplantation

Patients experience a significant improvement in pulmonary function (more after BLT compared with SLT), exercise capacity, and health-related quality of life following lung transplantation [68,70,71]. $FEV_1\%$ reaches a near-normal level of approximately 80% after BLT and peaks around 50% to 60% after SLT [68,70–72]. Interestingly, the rate of bronchiolitis obliterans syndrome (BOS) has been reported to be significantly lower in recipients of BLT, although the mechanisms underlying this important difference between groups are unclear [67,68]. Gas exchange improves to a larger extent with BLT relative to SLT [71]. 6MWD increases significantly after both BLT and SLT, with a higher mean distance by 100 to 400 feet following BLT, which is of questionable clinical significance [70,71]. Maximal exercise testing reveals resolution of ventilatory limitation to exercise, but abnormally low maximal oxygen consumption between 40% and 60% that has been attributed to peripheral muscle dysfunction [72,73]. Several studies have shown an improvement in health-related quality of life following lung transplantation, but this important outcome warrants further research to determine the longitudinal impact of transplantation [74,75]. Furthermore, ISHLT Registry data reveal that most patients live without any activity limitations, and approximately 40% go back to part-time or full-time work, which is remarkable considering the universal presence of severe pretransplant disability [58]. It is important to note, however, that most of these outcome variables, along with health status, decline over time with the development of BOS [74,76].

Complications of lung transplantation

Lung transplantation is associated with high short- and long-term mortality related to numerous potential complications. In the first post-transplant year, noncytomegalovirus (CMV) infection and graft failure are the two most common causes of death [58]. Thereafter, obliterative bronchiolitis and non-CMV infection are the leading causes of death, together accounting for over half of the deaths [58]. It is important to recognize, however, that approximately 35% of deaths that occur after the first 5 years following lung transplantation are caused by malignancy, cardiovascular, and other medical complications [58]. Although transplant-specific complications affect patients who have COPD in a similar frequency as patients who have other diseases, the lower 10-year post-transplant survival in patients who have COPD suggests that other medical comorbidities, such as malignancy or cardiac disease, may be more common, possibly related to more advanced age of this patient population, highlighting the importance of comprehensive and multidisciplinary medical management postoperatively to optimize long-term outcomes [59,77]. For further information, the reader is referred to recent comprehensive reviews on complications of lung transplantation [59,60,77].

Lung volume reduction surgery before or after lung transplantation

Many patients are considered simultaneously for LVRS and lung transplantation, and some meet criteria for both procedures (Fig. 3). For patients who have less severe disease and are deemed appropriate candidates for LVRS, this procedure should be offered first. In addition, some patients who are older, have significant medical comorbidities, and lack of adequate social support may be considered more appropriate for LVRS than lung transplantation, provided that they meet physiologic and anatomic criteria. In instances where both procedures are considered feasible, initial performance of LVRS may result in sufficient improvement in symptoms and physiologic derangements such that lung transplantation may be avoided or deferred for several years. Although lung transplantation results in significantly better lung function, gas exchange, and 6MWD compared with LVRS, a delay in exposure to the risks and limited long-term survival of lung transplantation by first pursuing LVRS certainly can be considered a desirable outcome [78].

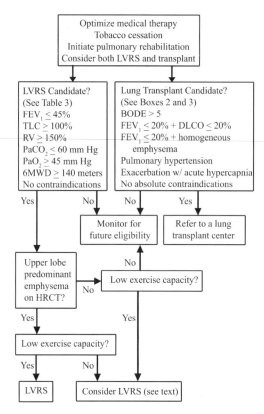

Fig. 3. Clinical approach to the surgical management of advanced chronic obstructive pulmonary disease.

Patients who do not respond to LVRS or who deteriorate after an initially successful LVRS may be bridged to lung transplantation [79].

Numerous investigators have reported their experience performing LVRS in those who are candidates for both procedures. The largest series included 99 transplant candidates who underwent bilateral LVRS [79]. No control arm was included. Three- and 5-year survival rates after LVRS were 91% and 75%, respectively. Although 15 subsequently underwent transplantation, none required transplantation within 2 years of LVRS. Based on these results and those of additional smaller series [80], LVRS appears to be a reasonable alternative to lung transplantation in patients with emphysema who are candidates for both procedures.

The outcomes of lung transplantation after LVRS also have been studied, because of concerns regarding surgical difficulty in lung explantation because of adhesions. The largest study to address this issue was an analysis of the United Network for Organ Sharing database [81]. Of 791 patients

who had emphysema undergoing lung transplantation, 50 patients had previously undergone LVRS. There were no differences in early graft dysfunction, prolonged air leak rate, length of stay, or overall survival between groups. This report suggests that lung transplantation may be performed safely after LVRS.

In rare instances, unilateral LVRS may be performed after transplantation in an SLT recipient whose native emphysematous lung is acutely or chronically hyperinflated with compression of the allograft and reduction in pulmonary function. In the acute setting early after SLT, surgery tends to be risky, and conservative medical and ventilatory management is advised. In chronic native lung hyperinflation, the differentiation of primary allograft dysfunction caused by BOS from extrinsic graft compression is challenging, but anecdotal reports of benefit from LVRS of the native lung (without such distinction in the pathophysiology of lung dysfunction) exist [82,83].

Summary

A small subset of patients who have advanced COPD may be eligible for surgical therapy. Bullectomy for giant bullae, LVRS, and lung transplantation are the three possible interventions that may benefit stringently selected and motivated patients. Appropriate patient and procedural selection, diligent postoperative management, and continued advancement in these therapeutic modalities through basic and clinical research are keys to the future success of surgical therapy of COPD.

References

[1] Celli BR, MacNee W. Standards for the diagnosis and treatment of patients with COPD: a summary of the ATS/ERS position paper. Eur Respir J 2004; 23(6):932–46.

[2] Snider GL. Reduction pneumoplasty for giant bullous emphysema. Implications for surgical treatment of nonbullous emphysema. Chest 1996;109(2): 540–8.

[3] Palla A, Desideri M, Rossi G, et al. Elective surgery for giant bullous emphysema: a 5-year clinical and functional follow-up. Chest 2005; 128(4):2043–50.

[4] Schipper PH, Meyers BF, Battafarano RJ, et al. Outcomes after resection of giant emphysematous bullae. Ann Thorac Surg 2004;78(3):976–82.

[5] Pearson MG, Ogilvie C. Surgical treatment of emphysematous bullae: late outcome. Thorax 1983; 38(2):134–7.

[6] Brantigan OC, Mueller E. Surgical treatment of pulmonary emphysema. Am Surg 1957;23:789–804.

[7] Brantigan OC, Mueller E, Kress MB. A surgical approach to pulmonary emphysema. Am Rev Respir Dis 1959;80(1 Part 2):194–206.

[8] Cooper JD, Trulock EP, Triantafillou AN, et al. Bilateral pneumectomy (volume reduction) for chronic obstructive pulmonary disease. J Thorac Cardiovasc Surg 1995;109(1):106–16.

[9] Flaherty KR, Martinez FJ. Lung volume reduction surgery for emphysema. Clin Chest Med 2000; 21(4):819–48.

[10] Huizenga HF, Ramsey SD, Albert RK, et al. Estimated growth of lung volume reduction surgery among Medicare enrollees: 1994 to 1996. Chest 1998;114(6):1583–7.

[11] National Emphysema Treatment Trial Research Group. Rationale and design of The National Emphysema Treatment Trial: a prospective randomized trial of lung volume reduction surgery. Chest 1999; 116(6):1750–61.

[12] Fishman A, Martinez F, Naunheim K, et al. A randomized trial comparing lung volume reduction surgery with medical therapy for severe emphysema. N Engl J Med 2003;348(21):2059–73.

[13] Stammberger U, Klepetko W, Stamatis G, et al. Buttressing the staple line in lung volume reduction surgery: a randomized three-center study. Ann Thorac Surg 2000;70(6):1820–5.

[14] DeCamp MM, Blackstone EH, Naunheim KS, et al. Patient and surgical factors influencing air leak after lung volume reduction surgery. Ann Thorac Surg 2006;82(1):197–206.

[15] Naunheim KS, Wood DE, Krasna MJ, et al. Predictors of operative mortality and cardiopulmonary morbidity in the National Emphysema Treatment Trial. J Thorac Cardiovasc Surg 2006;131(1):43–53.

[16] McKenna RJ Jr, Brenner M, Fischel RJ, et al. Should lung volume reduction for emphysema be unilateral or bilateral? J Thorac Cardiovasc Surg 1996;112(5):1331–8.

[17] McKenna RJ Jr, Benditt JO, DeCamp M, et al. Safety and efficacy of median sternotomy versus video-assisted thoracic surgery for lung volume reduction surgery. J Thorac Cardiovasc Surg 2004; 127(5):1350–60.

[18] Kotloff RM, Tino G, Bavaria JE, et al. Bilateral lung volume reduction surgery for advanced emphysema. A comparison of median sternotomy and thoracoscopic approaches. Chest 1996;110(6):1399–406.

[19] Criner GJ, Cordova FC, Furukawa S, et al. Prospective randomized trial comparing bilateral lung volume reduction surgery to pulmonary rehabilitation in severe chronic obstructive pulmonary disease. Am J Respir Crit Care Med 1999;160(6): 2018–27.

[20] Geddes D, Davies M, Koyama H, et al. Effect of lung volume reduction surgery in patients with severe emphysema. N Engl J Med 2000;343(4): 239–45.

[21] Pompeo E, Marino M, Nofroni I, et al. Reduction pneumoplasty versus respiratory rehabilitation in severe emphysema: a randomized study. Ann Thorac Surg 2000;70(3):948–53.

[22] Mineo TC, Ambrogi V, Pompeo E, et al. Impact of lung volume reduction surgery versus rehabilitation on quality of life. Eur Respir J 2004;23(2):275–80.

[23] Naunheim KS, Wood DE, Mohsenifar Z, et al. Long-term follow-up of patients receiving lung volume reduction surgery versus medical therapy for severe emphysema by the National Emphysema Treatment Trial Research Group. Ann Thorac Surg 2006;82(2):431–43.

[24] Goldstein RS, Todd TR, Guyatt G, et al. Influence of lung volume reduction surgery (LVRS) on health-related quality of life in patients with chronic obstructive pulmonary disease. Thorax 2003;58(5): 405–10.

[25] Hillerdal G, Lofdahl CG, Strom K, et al. Comparison of lung volume reduction surgery and physical training on health status and physiologic outcomes: a randomized controlled clinical trial. Chest 2005; 128(5):3489–99.

[26] Miller JD, Malthaner RA, Goldsmith CH, et al. A randomized clinical trial of lung volume reduction surgery versus best medical care for patients with advanced emphysema: a two-year study from Canada. Ann Thorac Surg 2006;81(1):314–20.

[27] Lenfant C. Will lung volume reduction surgery be widely applied? Ann Thorac Surg 2006;82(2): 385–7.

[28] National Emphysema Treatment Trial Group. Patients at high risk of death after lung-volume-reduction surgery. N Engl J Med 2001;345(15):1075–83.

[29] Drazen JM, Epstein AM. Guidance concerning surgery for emphysema. N Engl J Med 2003;348(21): 2134–6.

[30] Ware JH. The National Emphysema Treatment Trial—how strong is the evidence? N Engl J Med 2003;348(21):2055–6.

[31] Tiong LU, Davies R, Gibson PG, et al. Lung volume reduction surgery for diffuse emphysema. Cochrane Database Syst Rev 2006;(4):CD001001.

[32] Ciccone AM, Meyers BF, Guthrie TJ, et al. Long-term outcome of bilateral lung volume reduction in 250 consecutive patients with emphysema. J Thorac Cardiovasc Surg 2003;125(3): 513–25.

[33] Mentzer SJ, Swanson SJ, Mentzer SJ, et al. Treatment of patients with lung cancer and severe emphysema. Chest 1999;116(6 Suppl):477S–9S.

[34] Choong CK, Meyers BF, Battafarano RJ, et al. Lung cancer resection combined with lung volume reduction in patients with severe emphysema. J Thorac Cardiovasc Surg 2004;127(5):1323–31.

[35] DeRose JJ Jr, Argenziano M, El-Amir N, et al. Lung reduction operation and resection of pulmonary nodules in patients with severe emphysema. Ann Thorac Surg 1998;65(2):314–8.

[36] Edwards JG, Duthie DJ, Waller DA, et al. Lobar volume reduction surgery: a method of increasing the lung cancer resection rate in patients with emphysema. Thorax 2001;56(10):791–5.

[37] McKenna RJ Jr, Fischel RJ, Brenner M, et al. Combined operations for lung volume reduction surgery and lung cancer. Chest 1996;110(4):885–8.

[38] Lederer DJ, Thomashow BM, Ginsburg ME, et al. Lung volume reduction surgery for pulmonary emphysema: Improvement of the BODE index after one year. J Thorac Cardiovasc Surg 2007;133(6): 1434–8.

[39] Gelb AF, Zamel N, McKenna RJ Jr, et al. Mechanism of short-term improvement in lung function after emphysema resection. Am J Respir Crit Care Med 1996;154(4 Pt 1):945–51.

[40] Marchand E, Gayan-Ramirez G, De Leyn P, et al. Physiological basis of improvement after lung volume reduction surgery for severe emphysema: where are we? Eur Respir J 1999;13(3):686–96.

[41] Martinez FJ, de Oca MM, Whyte RI, et al. Lung volume reduction improves dyspnea, dynamic hyperinflation, and respiratory muscle function. Am J Respir Crit Care Med 1997;155(6):1984–90.

[42] Sciurba FC, Rogers RM, Keenan RJ, et al. Improvement in pulmonary function and elastic recoil after lung reduction surgery for diffuse emphysema. N Engl J Med 1996;334(17):1095–9.

[43] Cassart M, Hamacher J, Verbandt Y, et al. Effects of lung volume reduction surgery for emphysema on diaphragm dimensions and configuration. Am J Respir Crit Care Med 2001;163(5):1171–5.

[44] Tschernko EM, Wisser W, Wanke T, et al. Changes in ventilatory mechanics and diaphragmatic function after lung volume reduction surgery in patients with COPD. Thorax 1997;52(6):545–50.

[45] Benditt JO, Lewis S, Wood DE, et al. Lung volume reduction surgery improves maximal O_2 consumption, maximal minute ventilation, O_2 pulse, and dead space-to-tidal volume ratio during leg cycle ergometry. Am J Respir Crit Care Med 1997; 156(2 Pt 1):561–6.

[46] Tschernko EM, Gruber EM, Jaksch P, et al. Ventilatory mechanics and gas exchange during exercise before and after lung volume reduction surgery. Am J Respir Crit Care Med 1998;158(5 Pt 1): 1424–31.

[47] Ramsey SD, Berry K, Etzioni R, et al. Cost effectiveness of lung volume reduction surgery for patients with severe emphysema. N Engl J Med 2003; 348(21):2092–102.

[48] Ramsey SD, Shroyer AL, Sullivan SD, et al. Updated evaluation of the cost-effectiveness of lung volume reduction surgery. Chest 2007;131(3): 823–32.

[49] Ramsey SD, Sullivan SD. Evidence, economics, and emphysema: Medicare's long journey with lung volume reduction surgery. Health Aff (Millwood) 2005;24(1):55–66.

[50] Centers for Medicare and Medicaid Services. Administrative file: CAG-00115R, lung volume reduction surgery (LVRS): coverage decision for lung volume reduction surgery, August 20, 2003. Available at: http://www.cms.hhs.gov/determinationprocess/ downloads/id96.pdf. Accessed March 23, 2007.

[51] Maxfield RA. New and emerging minimally invasive techniques for lung volume reduction. Chest 2004; 125(2):777–83.

[52] Hopkinson NS, Toma TP, Hansell DM, et al. Effect of bronchoscopic lung volume reduction on dynamic hyperinflation and exercise in emphysema. Am J Respir Crit Care Med 2005;171(5):453–60.

[53] Wan IY, Toma TP, Geddes DM, et al. Bronchoscopic lung volume reduction for end-stage emphysema: report on the first 98 patients. Chest 2006; 129(3):518–26.

[54] Wood DE, McKenna RJ Jr, Yusen RD, et al. A multicenter trial of an intrabronchial valve for treatment of severe emphysema. J Thorac Cardiovasc Surg 2007;133(1):65–73.

[55] Reitz BA, Wallwork JL, Hunt SA, et al. Heart-lung transplantation: successful therapy for patients with pulmonary vascular disease. N Engl J Med 1982; 306(10):557–64.

[56] Mal H, Andreassian B, Pamela F, et al. Unilateral lung transplantation in end-stage pulmonary emphysema. Am Rev Respir Dis 1989;140(3):797–802.

[57] Patterson GA, Cooper JD, Dark JH, et al. Experimental and clinical double lung transplantation. J Thorac Cardiovasc Surg 1988;95(1):70–4.

[58] Trulock EP, Edwards LB, Taylor DO, et al. Registry of the International Society for Heart and Lung Transplantation: twenty-third official adult lung and heart-lung transplantation report–2006. J Heart Lung Transplant 2006;25(8):880–92.

[59] Arcasoy SM, Wilt J. Medical complications after lung transplantation. Semin Respir Crit Care Med 2006;27(5):508–20.

[60] Knoop C, Estenne M. Acute and chronic rejection after lung transplantation. Semin Respir Crit Care Med 2006;27(5):521–33.

[61] Hosenpud JD, Bennett LE, Keck BM, et al. Effect of diagnosis on survival benefit of lung transplantation for end-stage lung disease. Lancet 1998;351(9095): 24–7.

[62] Charman SC, Sharples LD, McNeil KD, et al. Assessment of survival benefit after lung transplantation by patient diagnosis. J Heart Lung Transplant 2002;21(2):226–32.

[63] De Meester J, Smits JM, Persijn GG, et al. Listing for lung transplantation: life expectancy and transplant effect, stratified by type of end-stage lung disease: the Eurotransplant experience. J Heart Lung Transplant 2001;20(5):518–24.

[64] Orens JB, Estenne M, Arcasoy S, et al. International guidelines for the selection of lung transplant candidates: 2006 update—a consensus report from the Pulmonary Scientific Council of the International Society for Heart and Lung Transplantation. J Heart Lung Transplant 2006;25(7):745–55.

[65] Celli BR, Cote CG, Marin JM, et al. The body-mass index, airflow obstruction, dyspnea, and exercise capacity index in chronic obstructive pulmonary disease. N Engl J Med 2004;350(10):1005–12.

[66] de Perrot M, Chaparro C, McRae K, et al. Twenty-year experience of lung transplantation at a single center: influence of recipient diagnosis on long-term survival. J Thorac Cardiovasc Surg 2004; 127(5):1493–501.

[67] Hadjiliadis D, Chaparro C, Gutierrez C, et al. Impact of lung transplant operation on bronchiolitis obliterans syndrome in patients with chronic obstructive pulmonary disease. Am J Transplant 2006;6(1):183–9.

[68] Cassivi SD, Meyers BF, Battafarano RJ, et al. Thirteen-year experience in lung transplantation for emphysema. Ann Thorac Surg 2002;74(5): 1663–9.

[69] Meyer DM, Bennett LE, Novick RJ, et al. Single vs bilateral, sequential lung transplantation for end-stage emphysema: influence of recipient age on survival and secondary endpoints. J Heart Lung Transplant 2001;20(9):935–41.

[70] Pochettino A, Kotloff RM, Rosengard BR, et al. Bilateral versus single lung transplantation for chronic obstructive pulmonary disease: intermediate-term results. Ann Thorac Surg 2000;70(6):1813–8.

[71] Sundaresan RS, Shiraishi Y, Trulock EP, et al. Single or bilateral lung transplantation for emphysema? J Thorac Cardiovasc Surg 1996;112(6):1485–94.

[72] Levine SM, Anzueto A, Peters JI, et al. Medium-term functional results of single lung transplantation for end-stage obstructive lung disease. Am J Respir Crit Care Med 1994;150(2):398–402.

[73] Schwaiblmair M, Reichenspurner H, Muller C, et al. Cardiopulmonary exercise testing before and after lung and heart–lung transplantation. Am J Respir Crit Care Med 1999;159(4 Pt 1):1277–83.

[74] Gross CR, Savik K, Bolman RM 3rd, et al. Long-term health status and quality of life outcomes of lung transplant recipients. Chest 1995;108(6):1587–93.

[75] TenVergert EM, Essink-Bot ML, Geertsma A, et al. The effect of lung transplantation on health-related quality of life: a longitudinal study. Chest 1998; 113(2):358–64.

[76] van den Berg JW, van Enckevort PJ, TenVergert EM, et al. Bronchiolitis obliterans syndrome and additional costs of lung transplantation. Chest 2000;118(6):1648–52.

[77] Arcasoy SM. Medical complications and management of lung transplant recipients. Respir Care Clin N Am 2004;10(4):505–29.

[78] Gaissert HA, Trulock EP, Cooper JD, et al. Comparison of early functional results after volume reduction or lung transplantation for chronic obstructive pulmonary disease. J Thorac Cardiovasc Surg 1996;111(2):296–306.

[79] Meyers BF, Yusen RD, Guthrie TJ, et al. Outcome of bilateral lung volume reduction in patients with emphysema potentially eligible for lung transplantation. J Thorac Cardiovasc Surg 2001;122(1):10–7.

[80] Tutic M, Lardinois D, Imfeld S, et al. Lung volume reduction surgery as an alternative or bridging procedure to lung transplantation. Ann Thorac Surg 2006;82(1):208–13.

[81] Nathan SD, Edwards LB, Barnett SD, et al. Outcomes of COPD lung transplant recipients after lung volume reduction surgery. Chest 2004;126(5): 1569–74.

[82] Anderson MB, Kriett JM, Kapelanski DP, et al. Volume reduction surgery in the native lung after single lung transplantation for emphysema. J Heart Lung Transplant 1997;16(7):752–7.

[83] Moy ML, Loring SH, Ingenito EP, et al. Causes of allograft dysfunction after single lung transplantation for emphysema: extrinsic restriction versus intrinsic obstruction. J Heart Lung Transplant 1999;18(10):986–93.

ELSEVIER
SAUNDERS

Clin Chest Med 28 (2007) 655–662

CLINICS
IN CHEST
MEDICINE

Index

Note: Page numbers of article titles are in **boldface** type.

0272-5231/07/$ - see front matter © 2007 Elsevier Inc. All rights reserved.
doi:10.1016/S0272-5231(07)00079-2

chestmed.theclinics.com